Prediction, Prevention and Genetic Counseling in IDDM

Prediction, Prevention and Genetic Counseling in IDDM

Edited by

JERRY P. PALMER

University of Washington, Seattle, USA

John Wiley & Sons

Chichester · New York · Brisbane · Toronto · Singapore

Other Wiley Editorial Offices

John Wiley & Sons, Inc., 605 Third Avenue,
New York, NY 10158-0012, USA

Jacaranda Wiley Ltd, 33 Park Road, Milton,
Queensland 4064, Australia

John Wiley & Sons (Canada) Ltd, 22 Worcester Road,
Rexdale, Ontario M9W 1L1, Canada

John Wiley & Sons (Asia) Pte Ltd, 2 Clementi Loop #02–01,
Jin Xing Distripark, Singapore 0512

Library of Congress Cataloging-in-Publication Data

Prediction, prevention, and genetic counseling in IDDM / edited by
    Jerry P. Palmer.
        p.   cm. – (Practical diabetes)
    Includes bibliographical references and index.
    ISBN 0 471 95525 6 (alk. paper)
    1. Diabetes – Genetic aspects.   2. Diabetes – Prevention.
  3. Genetic counseling.   I. Palmer, Jerry P.   II. Series: Practical
  diabetes (Chichester, England)
      [DNLM: 1. Diabetes Mellitus, Insulin-Dependent – diagnosis.
  2. Diabetes Mellitus, Insulin-Dependent – etiology.   3. Diabetes
  Mellitus, Insulin-Dependent – prevention & control.   4. Genetic
  Counseling.   5. Disease Progression.   WK 810 D5397 1996]
  RC660.D546 1996
  616.4'62–dc20
  DNLM/DLC
  for Library of Congress   95-38949
                                                                  CIP

British Library Cataloguing in Publication Data

A catalogue record for this book is available from the British Library

ISBN 0-471-95525-6

Typeset in 10/12pt Palatino by Vision Typesetting, Manchester.
Printed and bound in Great Britain by Biddles Ltd, Guildford.
This book is printed on acid-free paper responsibly manufactured from sustainable forestation,
for which at least two trees are planted for each one used for paper production.

Contents

List of Contributors

MARK A. ATKINSON *Department of Pathology, University of Florida College of Medicine, PO Box 100275, Gainesville, FL 32610-0275, USA*

POLLY BINGLEY *Dept of Diabetes and Metabolism, St Bartholomew's Hospital, 3rd Floor Dominion House, 59 Bartholomew Close, West Smithfield, London EC1A 7BE*

EZIO BONIFACIO *Department of Internal Medicine, Istituto Scientifico San Raffaele, Via Olgettina 60, 20132 Milan, Italy*

MARK A. BOWMAN *Department of Pathology, University of Florida College of Medicine, PO Box 100275, Gainesville, FL 32610-0275, USA*

BRETT CHARLTON *Stanford University School of Medicine, Division of Immunology and Rheumatology, Stanford, CA 94305-5111, USA*

MICHAEL R. CHRISTIE *Department of Medicine, King's College Hospital, Bessemer Rd, London SE5 9PJ*

ELEANOR COLLE *2300 Tupper St, Dept of Metabolism Rm E316, The Montreal Children's Hospital, Montreal, PQ Canada H3H 1P5*

H.-MICHAEL DOSCH *Research Institute, The Hospital for Sick Children, University of Toronto, 555 University Avenue, Toronto, Ontario, Canada M5G LX8*

JOHN DUPRE *University Hospital, University of Western Ontario, 339 Windermere Rd, PO Box 5339, Station A, London, Ontario, Canada N6A 5A5*

ROBERT B. ELLIOTT *Department of Pediatrics, University of Auckland, School of Medicine, Auckland, New Zealand*

C. GARRISON FATHMAN — *Stanford University School of Medicine, Division of Immunology and Rheumatology, Stanford, CA 94305-5111, USA*

EDWIN GALE — *Dept of Diabetes and Metabolism, St Bartholomew's Hospital, 3rd Floor Dominion House, 59 Bartholomew Close, West Smithfield, London EC1A 7BE*

CARRIE GARBER — *Division of Medical Genetics, Cedars-Sinai Medical Center, 8700 Boulevard, Los Angeles, CA 90048-1865, USA*

CARLA GREENBAUM — *Seattle Veterans Administration, Endocrinology Dept (111), 1660 South Columbian Way, Seattle, WA 98108, USA*

RICHARD JACKSON — *Joslin Diabetes Center, 1 Joslin Place, Boston, MA 02215, USA*

HOWARD JACOB — *Cardiovascular Research Center, MGH-East, Harvard Medical School, Boston, MA 02129, USA*

WOLFRAM J. P. KARGES — *Research Institute, The Hospital for Sick Children, University of Toronto, 555 University Avenue, Toronto, Ontario, Canada M5G LX8*

EDWARD H. LEITER — *Senior Staff Scientist, The Jackson Laboratory, Bar Harbor, ME 04609, USA*

ÅKE LERNMARK — *Robert H. Williams Laboratory, Department of Medicine, University of Washington, Seattle, WA 98195, USA*

DAVID K. McCULLOCH — *Diabetes Clinical Research Unit, Virginia Mason Research Center, 1100 Ninth Avenue, PO Box 900, Seattle, WA 98111, USA*

ROBERT McEVOY — *Division of Diabetes and Endocrinology, Department of Pediatrics, Mount Sinai School of Medicine, New York, NY 10029, USA*

JEFFREY MAHON — *University Hospital, University of Western Ontario, 339 Windermere Rd, PO Box 5339, Station A, London, Ontario, Canada N6A 5A5*

THOMAS MANDRUP-POULSEN — *Steno Diabetes Center, Niels Steensensvej 2, SO21 DK 2820, Gentofte, Denmark*

JENNIFER B. MARKS   *Behavioral Medical Research Center (D-110), 1500 NW 12th Avenue, Jackson Medical Towers, 14th Floor, Miami, FL 33136, USA*

ERROL MARLISS   *McGill Nutrition and Food Science Center, Royal Victoria Hospital, 687 Pine Avenue W, Montreal, Canada H3A 1A1*

VIVEK MEHTA   *Division of Endocrinology, Metabolism and Nutrition, Department of Veterans Affairs Medical Center, 1660 South Columbian Way, Seattle, WA 98106, USA*

GERRY NEPOM   *Director Immunology and Diabetes, Virginia Mason Research Center, 1000 Seneca St, Seattle, WA 98101, USA*

JØRN NERUP   *Steno Diabetes Center, Niels Steensensvej 2, SO21 DK 2820, Gentofte, Denmark*

JANICE NESS   *Children's Hospital and Medical Center, Dept of Pediatrics, 4800 Sand Point Way NE, Seattle, WA 98105, USA*

TIHAMER ORBAN   *Joslin Diabetes Center, 1 Joslin Place, Boston, MA 02215, USA*

JERRY P. PALMER   *Division of Endocrinology, Metabolism and Nutrition, Department of Veterans Affairs Medical Center, 1660 South Columbian Way, Seattle, WA 98106, USA*

ANNA PETTERSSON   *Karolinska Institute, Department of Molecular Medicine, Karolinska Hospital – L1:02, S-171 76 Stockholm, Sweden*

FLEMMING POCIOT   *Steno Diabetes Center, Niels Steensensvej 2, SO21 DK 2820, Gentofte, Denmark*

LESLIE J. RAFFEL   *Division of Medical Genetics, Cedars-Sinai Medical Center, 8700 Boulevard Los Angeles-CA 90048-1865, USA*

JEROME I. ROTTER   *Division of Medical Genetics, Cedars-Sinai Medical Center, 8700 Boulevard Los Angeles-CA 90048-1865, USA*

ALICIA SCHIFFRIN   *2300 Tupper St, Dept of Metabolism Rm E316, The Montreal Children's Hospital, Montreal, PQ Canada H3H 1P5*

FRASER SCOTT   *Nutrition Research Division, Health Protection Branch,*
                       Banting Research Center, 3 West Tunney's Pasture,
                       Ottawa K1A 0L2, Canada

AKIRA SHIMADA   *Stanford University School of Medicine, Division of*
                       Immunology and Rheumatology, Stanford, CA
                       94305-5111, USA

JAY S. SKYLER   *Behavioral Medical Research Center (D-110), 1500 NW*
                       12th Avenue, Jackson Medical Towers, 14th Floor,
                       Miami, FL 33136, USA

NANCY M. THOMAS   *Division of Diabetes and Endocrinology, Department of*
                       Pediatrics, Mount Sinai School of Medicine, New York,
                       NY 10029, USA

HOWARD L. WEINER   *Center for Neurologic Diseases, LMRC – Room 102A,*
                       Brigham and Women's Hospital, 221 Longwood Avenue,
                       Boston, MA 02115 USA

JEAN-FRANCOIS   *McGill Nutrition and Food Science Center, Royal*
   YALE   *Victoria Hospital, 687 Pine Avenue W, Montreal,*
                       Canada H3A 1A1

JI-WON YOON   *Laboratory of Viral and Immunopathogenesis of Julia*
                       MacFarlane Diabetes Research Center, University of
                       Calgary, 3330 Hospital Drive NW, Calgary, Canada,
                       T3N 4N1

Preface

Since the recognition around 1960 that insulin dependent diabetes (IDDM) and non-insulin dependent diabetes (NIDDM) were distinct disease processes both causing hyperglycemia, enormous strides have been made in our understanding of the IDDM or type I diabetes disease process. In approximately 35 years this area has evolved and advanced to the point where we can now identify, amongst nondiabetic people, those at highest risk of subsequent IDDM and our knowledge of the pathogenesis of IDDM, even though incomplete, is being used in clinical trials to try to prevent the development of clinical IDDM. It is truly remarkable to contemplate that within my investigative career, we may have progressed from recognizing IDDM as a distinct cause of hyperglycemia to being able to intervene and prevent at least some cases of this disease.

In this book we have tried to provide the reader, in a single volume, with an up-to-date summary of the world's data on the prediction, prevention, and genetic counseling of IDDM. Each of the chapters has been written by the most authoritative international investigators in each respective area. We have tried to balance each chapter such that it is useful to both physicians caring for patients with IDDM and their families and to scientists investigating IDDM.

I would like to dedicate this book to all those who have contributed to making it possible. IDDM investigators world-wide and the thousands of patients and their families who have in the past and continue to volunteer for research studies deserve recognition. All of the authors were responsive to my editorial requests, and I thank my staff at the University of Washington Diabetes Endocrinology Research Center and the Seattle Veterans Affairs Medical Center and the staff at John Wiley and Sons Ltd for their help. And finally, I would like to thank my wife, Christine, for her understanding and support in my bringing this book to completion.

Part 1

INTRODUCTION

1

The Natural History of the IDDM Disease Process

VIVEK MEHTA and JERRY P. PALMER
Division of Endocrinology, Metabolism and Nutrition, Seattle Veterans Affairs
Medical Center, Seattle, USA

Insulin-dependent diabetes mellitus (IDDM) affects about 0.2% of the population of the United States, with a peak age on onset of 11–12 years. These patients have a deficiency of insulin resulting from damage and destruction of the insulin producing β cells of the islets of Langerhans in the pancreas, and continuous hormone replacement therapy is needed.

The steps in the pathogenesis of IDDM have only partially been defined and many of the genes that determine IDDM susceptibility are unidentified. Even though any scheme is partially speculative and incomplete, we will provide a model of the disease process as an overview based upon data from studies of the natural history of this disease. In our model, the genetically susceptible patient was exposed to an initiating event or unexposed to some protective event which allowed autoimmunity to develop and to continue until a significant portion of the β cells were damaged and/or destroyed. The IDDM disease process does not come with guarantees, no outcome is assured. Some individuals will remain at one of the stages for long periods of time before progressing. Some individuals stay so long at one of the stages that in practical terms they never progress to clinical IDDM (Figure 1.1).

GENETICS

From the earliest studies of patients with autoimmune disorders, it was observed that some of these diseases run in families. Approximately 5% of

Prediction, Prevention and Genetic Counseling in IDDM. Edited by Jerry P. Palmer.
© 1996 John Wiley & Sons Ltd.

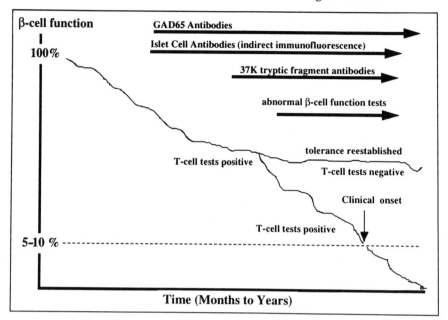

Figure 1.1. Hypothetical natural history of autoimmune diabetes. The complex nature and timing of many necessary events can perhaps explain why the time course for disease is variable for IDDM patients. Some individuals take longer than others to reach clinical IDDM. Interestingly, some individuals only proceed part way, and never completely progress to clinical IDDM

first degree relatives of individuals with Type 1 diabetes also have the disease. Nearly 50% of identical twins are concordant for the disease. While a strong familial influence is evident, it should be emphasized that most individuals who develop IDDM do not have a first degree relative with IDDM.

The genetic component of various autoimmune diseases was more firmly established by human leukocyte antigen (HLA) typing which showed that some HLA alleles occur in higher frequencies in patients with these diseases than in the general population. Analysis of Type 1 diabetes demonstrates both positive and negative associations with HLA genes. HLA-DR3 and/or HLA-DR4 is observed in 90–95% of Caucasians with this disease but in only 40% of normals. Nearly half of the IDDM patients are HLA-DR3/DR4 heterozygotes in contrast to 5% of normals. In addition, affected siblings tend to share at least one and frequently both HLA haplotypes[1,2]. HLA-DQ alleles are even more strongly associated with IDDM than DR. Since diabetic patients with a family history of diabetes and those without show the same genetic markers, susceptibility at the gene level is probably similar for both groups. Not only are class II genes associated with diabetes susceptibility, some class II haplotypes confer protection from IDDM. For example, haplotypes bearing DR2 alleles usually protect from diabetes independently of whether the other HLA haplotype contains a high-risk allele[3].

The genes primarily responsible for diabetes susceptibility are in the major histocompatibility complex (MHC). The MHC genes determine the rapidity with which skin grafts or other transplanted tissue is rejected. This region of the genome probably contains at least 100 genes but only a few have been identified. The MHC region contains genes for heat shock proteins, tumor necrosis factor, transporters, accessory molecules and the MHC[4]. The classic histocompatibility genes are extremely polymorphic and include HLA-A, B, and C molecules (class I histocompatibility antigens) and the "immune response genes" DP, DQ, and DR (class II histocompatibility antigens). Differences in the nucleotide sequences among individuals determine amino acid polymorphisms of histocompatibility molecules such that essentially no two unrelated individuals are identical for histocompatibility molecules. Crystallographic studies have shown that the histocompatibility molecule has a complicated three-dimensional structure with a peptide binding groove. The polymorphic amino acids of the histocompatibility molecule determine binding affinities for peptide.

Animal studies have provided additional data which support the hypothesis that genes in the MHC are involved in IDDM. Investigators working with the non-obese diabetic (NOD) mouse, an animal model of IDDM, suggest that the generation and progression of the autoimmune response is predominantly associated with the MHC linked gene, although other genes may be involved[5]. Recently it was shown that the NOD mouse and a closely related non-obese mouse differ in terms of one amino acid residue in the DQβ chain. Some have suggested that the presence of an aspartate in that position confers resistance whereas its absence seems to relate to an increased susceptibility to diabetes[6]. Other investigators have demonstrated that specific amino acids in the α chain[7] may also be important. Slight modifications in the amino acid sequence of the MHC molecule can significantly alter which antigen is presented to a T cell. This may explain the strength of the associations to IDDM.

Several mechanisms have been postulated to account for the association of autoimmune diseases with MHC sequences. During thymic education, T cells are exposed to various peptides attached to the antigen-binding clefts of MHC molecules and this recognition determines the selection of developing T lymphocytes. If the MHC molecules in the thymus of an individual fails to bind a self-protein with high affinity, T cells reactive with this self-antigen may escape clonal deletion. On the other hand, the observed protective effect, apparently conveyed by HLA-DQβ, may be the result of a functional MHC molecule capable of binding and presenting the self-antigens responsible for insulitis during thymic education. This would result in the deletion or inactivation of T cells specific for this self-antigen. It has also been hypothesized that microbial antigens which resemble self-molecules are presented on the

MHC molecules of "susceptible" individuals creating T-cell responses against the microbe resulting in cross-reactions and an autoimmune response. Another hypothesis is that one role of class II MHC molecules might be to influence the activation of T-cell suppressor cells, whose function is to regulate autoimmune reactions. Lastly, it has been proposed that the protection afforded by some HLA alleles may be the result of high affinity binding of the diabetogenic antigens intracellularly. This would prevent their surface expression and subsequent presentation to the immune system[8].

Our understanding of exactly how genetics relates to IDDM is still in the formative stages. It is too simplistic to suggest that individuals either inherit "protection" or "susceptibility". With further research, we might be able to explain on a genetic level why some individuals are more likely to: (1) have their immune tolerance broken and thus, initiate autoimmunity; (2) have immune recognition of multiple islet-specific target antigens; and (3) lack the normal mechanisms to suppress anti-islet autoimmunity. The genetics of IDDM are complicated because it is possible that one may inherit a predisposition for autoimmunity or may inherit a failure to protect against autoimmunity. It should also be noted that disease-associated HLA sequences are found in healthy individuals and, conversely, that alleles commonly present in normal individuals are also found in some patients with autoimmune diseases. Therefore, the expression of a particular HLA gene is not by itself the cause of any autoimmune disease but is likely to be one of several factors that contribute to autoimmunity.

AUTOIMMUNITY

The concept of an autoimmune pathogenesis for IDDM is supported by the observation that patients who die shortly after the onset of the disease often exhibit an infiltrate of mononuclear cells in and around the islets of Langerhans.

The presence of circulating antibodies against components of β cells of the islets in the large majority of all newly diagnosed IDDM patients suggests an autoimmune origin. During the pre-clinical period prior to diagnosis, a number of immune markers can also be detected. These include antibodies to GAD (glumatic acid decarboxylase), cytoplasmic islet cells, insulin, islet cell surface and carboxypeptidase H (Table 1.1).

Most patients develop these antibodies years before the appearance of clinical symptoms, either prior to or concomitant with a decreasing production of insulin by the β cells. A number of human studies have shown that the pattern of autoantibodies expressed can be predictive of progression to diabetes. Individuals with high titer ICA as well as either IAA and/or a decrease in first-phase insulin response have been reported to be at very high risk for Type 1 diabetes[9-11]. Because GAD antibodies have been detected in

Table 1.1. Islet cell autoantigens of insulin-dependent diabetes (from reference 40, with permission)

Autoantigen	Characteristics
Sialoglycolipid	Target of ICA in humans, GM2-1, non-beta-cell specific.
Glutamate decarboxylase	Target of 64 kD antigen/GAD antibody in humans and animal models of IDD, two forms (GAD-65 and GAD-67), cellular immune antigen, synaptic like microvesicle protein, disease-modifying antigen.
Insulin	Target of IAA in humans and non-obese diabetic (NOD) mice, cellular immune antigen, disease-modifying antigen.
Insulin receptor	Target of autoantibodies in humans determined by bioassay.
38 kDa	Target of 38 kDa antigen in humans, induced by cytomegalovirus, localized in insulin secretory granules, cellular immune antigen, multiple antigens of this molecular mass?
Bovine serum albumin	Target of BSA antibody, antigen in humans and animal models of IDD, contains ABBOS peptide, has molecular mimic to beta cell p69 protein (PM-1), disease-modifying antigen.
Glucose transporter	Target of autoantibodies in humans, inhibits glucose stimulation, GLUT-2 directed?
hsp 65	Target of autoantibodies and cellular immunity in NOD mice, disease-modifying antigen, contains p277 peptide.
Carboxypeptidase H	Target of autoantibodies in humans, identified by immunoscreening of islet cDNA, insulin secretory granule protein.
52 kDa	Target of autoantibodies in humans and NOD mice, molecular mimic with rubella virus.
ICA12/ICA512	Target of autoantibodies in humans, identified by immunoscreening of islet cDNA, homology to CD45.
150 kDa	Target of autoantibodies in humans, beta cell specific, membrane associated.
RIN polar	Target of autoantibodies in humans and NOD mice, present on insulinoma cells

individuals up to eight years prior to onset, correlate with progressively impaired β-cell function, and have a prolonged persistence after disease onset, some argue that GAD may be a more specific marker for the autoimmune process[12,13]. These antibodies were also detected in the sera from diabetic BB rats and non-obese diabetic (NOD) mice as early as the time of weaning. Today, these antibodies are generally regarded as a response to the β-cell antigens released during the destruction of β cells, rather than the cause of β-cell destruction.

In addition to the obvious humoral component, considerable evidence now implicates cell-mediated immune mechanisms in the pathogenesis of IDDM. Attempts have been made to replace β cells by transplanting pancreatic tissue from non-diabetic monozygotic twins to the diabetic sibling. However, an inflammatory infiltrate develops in the islets of Langerhans of the transplanted pancreas and the β cells are destroyed by the immune response of the diabetic recipient. Recently, another study reported that blood donated from a diabetic to a non-diabetic caused the onset of IDDM[14]. In animal studies, non-diseased mice were converted to the diseased state after receiving injections of T-cell subsets[15]. These observations strongly suggest that sensitized cytotoxic T lymphocytes are the effector cells in IDDM.

The immune response consists of two functional pathways: humoral and cellular. At the molecular level, the pathways have been characterized in terms of functional subsets of CD4+T cells. Th1 cells that produce interleukin-2 and interferon-γ mediate delayed type hypersensitivity reactions; Th2 cells that produce interleukins 4, 5, 6 and 10 mediate humoral immunity and allergy (Table 1.2)[16]. Factors such as the mouse strain, MHC haplotype, the nature and dose of antigen, route of immunization, and the type of antigen-presenting cell and the cytokines released are important in determining the nature of the immune response (Th1 compared with Th2)[17].

Table 1.2. Cytokines produced by Th1- and Th2-cell subsets of T cells

Cytokine produced	Th1-cell subset		Th2-cell subset	
	Mouse	Human	Mouse	Human
IL-2	+	++	−	−
IFN-γ	++	++	−	−
TNF-β	++	++	−	−
TNF-α	++	++	+	+
GM-CSF	++	+	+	++
IL-3	++	+	++	++
IL-4	−	−	++	++
IL-5	−	−	++	++
IL-10	−	+	++	++

Values for mouse Th1 and Th2-cell subsets are proportions of mouse CD4+T-cell clones producing a given cytokine. Values for human Th1- and Th2-cell subsets are proportions of human T-cell clones producing a given cytokine. ++, Large proportion; +, small proportion; −, none (from reference 41, with permission).

GAD may be a key molecule at a critical juncture in the autoimmune process of IDDM. Although somewhat controversial, a study by Harrison provided evidence that increased T-cell immune response to GAD (Th1) predicts a progression to clinical IDDM whereas antibodies to GAD do not[18]. This finding is consistent with a Th1 directed immune response eliciting IDDM whereas a Th2 response, even to the same islet antigens, fails to confer β-cell damage (Figure 1.2).

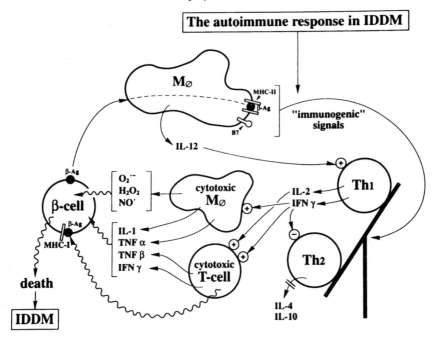

Figure 1.2. An illustration of the immune system cells that may be involved in the autoimmune destruction of the pancreatic β cells. The T cells, predominantly the Th1 cells, are activated by the antigen–MHC II complex, accessory molecules on the antigen presenting cell, and other immunogenic signals. The antigen activated Th1 cells release IL-2 and IFN-γ which inhibits the Th2 cell production of IL-4 and IL-10. In addition, the Th1 released cytokines activate macrophages and cytotoxic T cells. These effector cells destroy islet β cells by a variety of mechanisms including oxygen free radicals, NO*, and cytokines (from reference 41, with permission)

ENVIRONMENTAL FACTORS

While it is possible that some individuals are genetically predetermined to develop an aberrant immunologic response and others are genetically protected from this response, it is very likely that environmental factors are involved in the disease onset and/or progression. Whether environmental factors in general act to increase or decrease one's overall risk is controversial.

Environmental insult or insults to the islet cells may initiate the autoimmune reaction. This exposure would commonly precede the diagnosis of clinical IDDM by many years. While the exact nature of the "trigger" is unknown, it is believed that it could be a specifically-timed, short-lived event that converts a non-diseased individual to a pre-diseased individual.

It is also possible that the exposure to some environmental factor prevents people from developing IDDM. In this sense, the environmental factor rather than acting as a "trigger" acts like a "vaccine" by somehow conferring future protection. If this is true, it is conceivable that IDDM would develop in individuals lacking the necessary protective exposure that non-diseased individuals experienced.

If environmental factors play an essential role in the etiology of IDDM as either causative or protective agents, then by what mechanism do these factors act? Two general mechanisms have been proposed: molecular mimicry and direct toxicity. The molecular mimicry hypothesis argues that the environmental factor (virus, chemical, etc.) contains specific peptides that share antigen epitopes with human cell surface proteins, thereby eliciting the production of autoreactive antibodies and T cells. The direct toxicity hypothesis holds that the environmental factor is directly toxic to β cells resulting in the release of β-cell antigens. Common to both hypotheses is the ultimate break in immune tolerance to a large number of islet antigens.

If environmental exposure provided protection this might be mediated by these exposures causing tolerance to certain antigens. The mechanism might involve antigen presentation to a T cell but without the necessary accessory signals like lymphokines. This could render the T cell tolerant to that antigen and thereby inhibit future autoimmunity.

It is also possible that environmental factors may interact directly with T cells and alter their function. Depending on the cell type affected a wide array of immune effects could occur with variable effects on the IDDM disease process.

Certain foods, viruses and chemicals have been associated with the onset of clinical Type 1 diabetes. For example, there is evidence that IDDM occasionally develops after mumps. Group B coxsackievirus can infect pancreatic β cells and coxsackie viral infection has been reported prior to the abrupt onset of diabetes. Children and young adults who were infected in utero with rubella virus occasionally develop diabetes.

Some chemicals such as alloxan and streptozotocin specifically destroy β cells in experimental animals and produce acute diabetes. A rodenticide, Vacor, caused diabetes in humans who consumed it.

It has also been suggested that certain proteins in cow's milk serve as a trigger for IDDM. Epidemiologic data suggest that breast-fed children have a lower incidence of IDDM than do those nurtured on cow's milk formula. Moreover, various dietary changes including the elimination of these proteins have been shown to alter the incidence of diabetes in both the NOD mouse and the BB rat[19,20].

Further evidence for the impact of environmental factors in the pathogenesis of IDDM is the fact that there are major geographic differences in the incidence of IDDM[21]. For instance, a child born in Finland has a 10 times greater risk of developing diabetes than a child born in northern Greece[22].

As mentioned previously, there is evidence that environmental factors might also have a protective effect. Exposure to certain foods, viruses and chemicals has been shown to confer protection against IDDM in animal models[23]. It has been demonstrated that the frequency of IDDM in the NOD mouse and BB rat is increased by raising the animals under pathogen-free conditions. The exposure or lack of exposure can be thought of as simply one additional stage in a disease process with many such stages (Figure 1.3).

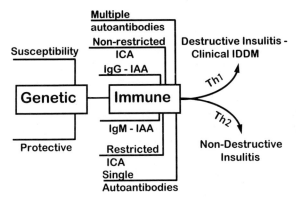

Figure 1.3. The genetic component of this disease enhances the likelihood of autoimmune β-cell destruction either by conferring autoimmunity or by decreasing the protection against autoimmune formation. The break in immune tolerance to certain antigens can cause a variety of immune responses. The nature and extent of the response is related to the IDDM disease process. It is unclear why, but certain antigens may initiate a Th1 response. This response is associated with clinical IDDM

INSULITIS

In children who die shortly after the acute onset of IDDM, the most characteristic lesion in the pancreas is an infiltrate of lymphocytes in the islets, sometimes accompanied by macrophages and neutrophils. The majority of infiltrating lymphocytes found in the islets of a patient who died at diagnosis were CD8+T cells[24]. The term insulitis has been applied to these changes. As the disease becomes chronic the β cells of the islets are progressively depleted and, in many long-standing cases, are no longer discernible.

During the initial stages of insulitis there appears to be increased expression of class I MHC molecules by the cells making up the islet of Langerhans. This enhanced expression of class I MHC has been observed in the NOD mouse, BB rat and humans. In addition to enhanced expression of class I MHC, there is evidence that the β cells may also be expressing class II MHC [24-26]. There has been much debate over the existence and possible significance of class II expression by these cells in vivo. Some have speculated that during the pre-clinical course of the disease, the pancreatic β cells may be presenting their own surface antigens to potentially autoreactive T lymphocytes. Others argue that the expression of class II molecules may in fact be protective because without the appropriate accessory signals (cytokines) the T cells will become inactivated for that antigen.

The inflammatory cells that arrive in the vicinity of the islets may secrete cytokines into the microenvironment of the islets. In vitro studies have shown that IL-1, TNF, and interferon-γ when acting alone or in combination can alter the β cells' ability to secrete insulin. These cytokines can also be cytotoxic to the β cell. The effect of the cytokines on the β cell is dependent on the concentration of the cytokines, other cytokines which may alter the anticipated effect of the cytokine alone, and the metabolic state of the β cells.

The widely held estimate that clinical diabetes occurs only after 90% of the β cells have been destroyed is unlikely to be true. The baboon given sub-diabetogenic doses of streptozotocin provides a model for the study of β-cell dysfunction prior to clinical onset of IDDM. It has been demonstrated that the acute insulin response to glucose becomes undetectable even when 40–50% of the β cells are still present[27]. During the late pre-clinical period and soon after diagnosis, it is likely that much of the insulin deficiency present at these times is a cytokine-mediated functional inhibition of the β cells. Most patients experience some recovery of β-cell function as reflected by increased C peptide levels within six months after the initial diagnosis and subsequent treatment[28]. Studies using the NOD mouse also suggest that much of the early β-cell dysfunction is caused by a reversible lesion. Islets isolated from mice with severe insulitis show functional recovery with procedures that reverse or block the insulitis process in vivo or in vitro [29–31]. These observations argue that at onset of hypergelycemia there is probably a greater amount of -cell mass than previously thought.

It is likely that the final destruction of β cells results from the assault of multiple cell types (macrophages, CD4+ and CD8+ lymphocytes) and multiple mechanisms (free-radical damage, cytokines, CD8+T-cell-mediated toxicity). The β cell specific destruction is most likely influenced by the specific targeting of islet antigens by immunoglobulin and T-cell receptors and by the unique susceptibility of β cells to certain types of damage.

PROGRESSORS VERSUS NONPROGRESSORS

An important question not yet addressed is whether the IDDM disease process once started leads definitely to the onset of clinical disease or whether there may be individuals who begin the process but never complete it.

Only a small percentage of those carrying the known genetic susceptibility alleles develop clinical IDDM[32]. It is likely that the autoimmune attack passes through a series of steps. At each step there may be multiple genetic or environmental determinants that must be satisfied before progressing to the next step. In addition, the timing of certain events may prove to be of crucial importance in determining further progression or protection.

The Barts–Windsor family study provided evidence that the IDDM disease process may not always reach completion. Over half of the non-diabetic first degree relatives of IDDM children who had initially been positive for complement-fixing ICAs became negative in long-term follow-up without developing IDDM[33]. The Lyon study and Chase *et al.* observed the loss of ICA positivity during the follow-up of initial screens on a number of patients[11,34]. In another study, non-diabetic first degree relatives of IDDM patients were screened for ICA at 0, 6, 12, 24, 36, 48 and 60 months. While only 2.7% were positive for the duration of the study, approximately 13% of the subjects were positive for at least part of the five years. The instability of one's ICA status may be indicative of the activity of the IDDM disease process. In other autoimmune diseases like rheumatoid arthritis and Hashimoto's thyroiditis the antibody titer correlates with disease activity. A study of non-insulin-dependent patients who were initially ICA+ and later became ICA− offers support for the relationship between immune markers and disease activity. Those patients that lost their ICA positivity showed significantly improved C-peptide and 2 hour blood glucose levels compared to the patients that remained ICA+[35].

The twin data provide compelling evidence that the IDDM disease process can be more likened to an "attack–retreat" paradigm rather than a smooth gradual decline as previously proposed. Nearly one-half of the discordant twins show abnormal immune responses and abnormal β-cell function. Interestingly, as the length of discordance increases the abnormal immunological markers become less common and the risk of concordance decreases[36,37]. Although non-diabetic twins[38] and first degree relatives of IDDM probands[39] may present with subclinical β-cell dysfunction, many times this fails to progress. These findings clearly indicate that the process leading to diabetes may slow or remit altogether.

It seems likely that clinical IDDM is the consequence of a disease process that has periods of attack as well as calm. There are some cases where the disease process appears to occur at an unrelenting pace resulting in the early clinical onset of diabetes. This might be the norm in children. However, the "older" individuals who are newly IDDM may have finally succumbed to a disease that took many years to progress. In many genetically susceptible individuals the attack may begin, but be non-progressive, failing to result in clinical IDDM.

ACKNOWLEDGMENT

This work was supported in part by the Medical Research Service of the Department of Veterans Affairs and the National Institutes of Health grants DK17047 and DK02456.

REFERENCES

1 Platz P, Jakobsen BK, Morling N, Ryder LP, Svejgaard A, Thomsen M *et al.* HLA-D and DR antigens in genetic analysis of insulin-dependent diabetes mellitus. *Diabetologia* 1981; **21**: 108–15.

2 Wolf E, Spencer KM, Cudworth AG. The genetic susceptibility to type I (insulin-dependent) diabetes: analysis of the HLA-DR association. *Diabetologia* 1983; **24**: 224–30.

3 Baisch JM, Weeks T, Giles R, Hoover M, Stastny, P, Capra JD. Analysis of HLA-DQ genotypes and susceptibility in insulin dependent diabetes mellitus. *N Engl J Med* 1990; **322**: 1836–41.

4 Trowsdale J, Campbell RD. Physical map of the human HLA region. *Immunol. Today* 1988; **9**: 34–5.

5 Wicker LS, Miller BJ, Coker LZ, McNally SE, Scott S, Mullen Y, Appel MC. Genetic control of diabetes and insulinitis in the nonobese diabetic (NOD) mice. *Diab Metab Rev* 1987; **3**: 751–78.

6 Todd JA, Bell JI, McDevitt HO. HLA-DQ gene contributes to susceptibility and resistance to insulin-dependent diabetes mellitus. *Nature* 1987; **329**: 599–604.

7 Khalil I, d'Auriol L, Gobet M, Morin L, Lepage V, Deschamps I *et al.* A combination of HLA-DQ β Asp57-negative and HLA-DQ alpha Arg 52 confers susceptibility to insulin dependent diabetes mellitus. *J Clin Invest* 1990; **85**: 1315–19.

8 Nepom GT. A unified hypothesis for the complex genetics of HLA associations with IDDM. *Diabetes* 1990; **39**: 1153–7.

9 Atkinson MA, MacClaren NK, Scharp DW, Lacy Pe, Riley WJ. 64,000 Mr autoantibodies as predictors of insulin-dependent diabetes. *Lancet* 1990; **335**: 1357–60.

10 Ginsberg-Fellner F, Witt ME, Franklin BH, Yaghashi S, Togushi Y, Dobersen MJ, Rubinstein P, Notkins AL. Triad of markers for identifying children at high risk of developing insulin dependent diabetes mellitus. *JAMA* 1985; **254**: 1469–70.

11 Srikanta S, Eisenbarth GS. Disappearing anti-islet antibodies? *Lancet* 1984; **1**: 1176–7.

12 Barmeier H, McCulloch DK, Neifing JL, Warnock G, Rajottee RV, Palmer JP, Lernmark A. Risk for developing Type I (insulin dependent) diabetes mellitus and the presence of islet 46K antibodies. *Diabetologia* 1991; **34**: 727–33.

13 Baekkeskov S, Landin Olsson M, Kristensen JK, Srikanta S, Bruining GJ, Mandrup-Poulsen T *et al.* Antibodies to a Mr 64,000 human islet cell antigen precede the clinical onset of insulin dependent diabetes. *J Clin Invest* 1987; **79**: 926–34.

14 Lampeter EF, Homberg M, Quabeck K, Schaefer UW, Wernet P, Bertrams J *et al.* Transfer of insulin-dependent diabetes between HLA-identical siblings by bone marrow transplantation. *Lancet* 1933; **341**: 1243–4.

15 Christanson SW, Shultz LD, Leiter EH. Adoptive transfer of diabetes into immunodeficient NOD-scid/scid Mice: relative contributions of CD4+ and CD8+T-cells from diabetic versus prediabetic NOD. NON-Thy-1^a donors. *Diabetes* 1993; **42**: 44–55.

16 Street NE, Mosmann TR. Functional diversity of T lymphocytes due to secretion of different cytokine patterns. *FASEB J* 1991; **5**: 1171–7.

17 Parish CR. The relationship between humoral and cell-mediated immunity. *Transplant Rev* 1972; **13**: 35–66.

18 Harrison LC, Honeyman MC, Deaizpurua HJ, Schmidli RS, Coman PG, Tait BD, Cram DS. Inverse relation between humoral and cellular immunity to glutamic acid decarboxylase in subjects at risk of insulin-dependent diabetes. *Lancet* 1993; **341**: 1365–9.

19 Coleman DL, Kuzava JE, Leiter EH. Effect of diet on incidence of diabetes in nonobese diabetic mice. *Diabetes* 1990; **39**: 432–6.

20 Elliott RB, Martin JM. Dietary protein: a trigger of insulin-dependent diabetes in the BB rat? *Diabetologia* 1984; **24**: 297–9.

21 Diabetes Epidemiology Research International Group. Geographic patterns of childhood insulin-dependent diabetes mellitus. *Diabetes* 1988; **37**: 1113–9.

22 Green A, Gale EAM, Patterson CC, the EURODIAB Subarea A Study Group: Incidence of childhood-onset diabetes mellitus: The EURODIOAB ACE Study. *Lancet* 1992; **339**: 905–9.

23 Oldstone MBA. Prevention of Type I diabetes in nonobese diabetic mice by virus infection. *Science* 1988; **239**: 500–2.

24 Bottazzo GF, Dean BM, McNally J, Hackay EH, Swift PGF, Gamble DR. In situ characterization of autoimmune phenomena and expression of HLA molecules in the pancreas in diabetic insulitis. *N Engl J Med* 1985; **313**: 353–60.

25 Foulis AK, Farquharson MA. Aberrant expression of HLA-DR antigens by insulin containing beta-cells in recent onset type I diabetes mellitus. *Diabetes* 1986; **35**: 1215–24.

26 Foulis AK, Farquharson MA, Harman R. Aberrant expression of class II major histocompatibility complex molecules by B cells and hyperexpression of class I major histocompatibility complex molecules by insulin containing islets in type I (insulin-dependent) diabetes mellitus. *Diabetologia* 1987; **30**: 333–43.

27 McCulloch DK, Koerker MJ, Kahn SE, Bonner-Weir S, Palmer JP. Correlation of in vivo β cell function tests with B cell mass and pancreatic insulin content in streptozocin treated baboons. *Diabetes* 1991; **40**: 673–9.

28 Agner T, Damm P, Binder C. Remission in IDDM: prospective study of basal C-peptide and insulin dose in 268 consecutive patients. *Diabetes Care* 1987; **10**: 164–9.

29 Strandell E, Eizirik DL, Sandler S. Reversal of β cell suppression in vitro in pancreatic islets isolated from nonobese diabetic mice during the phase preceding insulin dependent diabetes mellitus. *J Clin Invest* 1990; **85**: 1944–45

30 Eizirik DL, Strandell E, Sandler S. Prolonged exposure of islets isolated from prediabetic nonobese diabetic mice to a high glucose concentration does not impair β cell function. *Diabetologia* 1991; **34**: 6–11.

31 Strandell E, Sandler S, Boitard, C, Eizirk DL. Role of infiltrating T cells for impaired glucose metabolism in pancreatic islets isolated from nonobese diabetic mice. *Diabetologia* 1992; **35**: 924–31.

32 Bingley PJ, Bonificio E, Shattock M, Gillmore HA, Sawtell PA, Dunger DB, Bottazzo GF, Gale EAM. Can islet cell antibodies predict IDDM in the general population? *Diabetes Care* 1933; **16**: 45–50.

33 Spencer KM, Dean BM, Tarn A, Lister J, Bottazzo GF. Fluctuating islet cell autoimmunity in unaffected relatives of patients with insulin dependent diabetes. *Lancet* 1984; **1**: 764–6.

34 Chase HP, Voss MA, Butler-Simon N, Hoops S, O'Brien D, Dobersen MJ. Diagnosis of pre-type I diabetes. *J Pediatrics* 1987; **III**: 807–12.

35 Kobayashi T, Itoh T, Kosaka K, Sato K, Tsuji K. Time course of islet cell antibodies

and B cell function in non-insulin dependent stage of type I diabetes. *Diabetes* 1987; **36**: 510–17.

36 Olmos P, A'Hern R, Heaton DA, Risley D, Pyke DA, Leslie RDG. The significance of the concordance rate of type I insulin dependent diabetes in identical twins. *Diabetologia* 1988; **31**: 747–50.

37 Millward BA, Alviggi L, Hoskings PJ, Johnston C, Heaton D, Bottazzo GF *et al.* Immune changes associated with insulin dependent diabetes may remit without causing the disease: a study in identical twins. *Br Med J* 1986; **292**: 793–6.

38 Heaton DA, Milward BA, Gray P, Tun Y, Hales CN, Pyke DA, Leslie RDG. Evidence of B cell dysfunction which does not lead on to diabetes: a study of identical twins of insulin dependent diabetes. *Br Med J* 1987; **294**: 145–6.

39 McCulloch DK, Klaff LJ, Kahn SE, Schoenfeld SL, Greenbaum CJ, Mauseth RS *et al.* Nonprogression of subclinical B cell dysfunction among first degree relatives of IDDM patients. *Diabetes* 1990; **39**: 549–55.

40 Atkinson MA, Maclaren NK. Islet cell autoantigens in insulin-dependent diabetes. *J Clin Invest* 1993; **92**: 1608–16.

41 Rabinovitch A. Immunoregulatory and cytokine imbalances in the pathogenesis of IDDM. *Diabetes* 1994; **43** 613–21.

Part 2

PREDICTION

2

Genetic Markers in IDDM: the MHC

GERALD T. NEPOM
Virginia Mason Research Center, Seattle, USA

HLA CLASS II GENES

The human major histocompatibility complex (MHC), known as the HLA region, occupies approximately 4000 kb of DNA on choromosome 6 (6p21.2). HLA molecules encoded by these genes are the primary determinants of self–non-self recognition by the immune system. How they accomplish this—and how they predispose to diabetes—is the subject of this chapter.

There are two classes of related, but structurally distinct, HLA genes, known as class I and class II. Most of the HLA-encoded genetic susceptibility to IDDM localizes in the class II region, which is illustrated in Figure 2.1. Over 20 genes are known in this region; however, as summarized in the figure, the major class II molecules are encoded by three loci, known as DR, DQ and DP. Each locus contains an *A1* gene and at least one *B1* gene which encode the class II α and β polypeptide molecules, respectively.

The most remarkable feature of the HLA class II genes is their extraordinary polymorphism. In other words, multiple alleles exist at each locus, so that different individuals carry distinct HLA genes. Over 80 alleles are known at some class II loci, indicating strong evolutionary pressures to maintain diversity of HLA structure and function. The most common alleles are listed in Figure 2.1, grouped according to HLA "type", such as DR1, DR2, DR3, etc. As is apparent from the figure, an HLA "type" can correspond to multiple genes, each with a unique four digit numerical designation. Multiple nomenclature systems have evolved for HLA genes as genetic typing

Prediction, Prevention and Genetic Counseling in IDDM. Edited by Jerry P. Palmer.
© 1996 John Wiley & Sons Ltd.

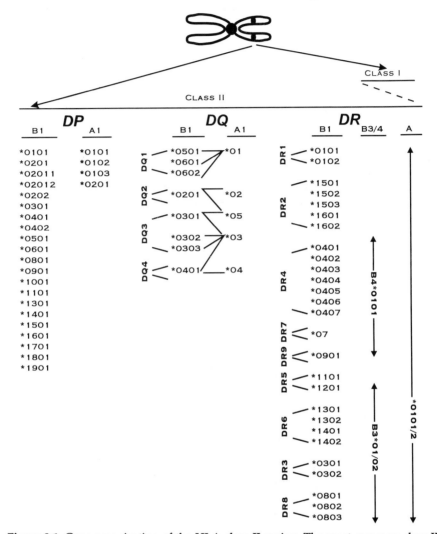

Figure 2.1. Gene organization of the HLA class II region. The most common class II alleles and associated HLA "types" are listed for the major loci. A more complete map of the MHC can be found in Towsdale et al.,[17] and a listing of additional alleles in Nepom[18]

methods have improved. Currently, based on recommendations of the World Health Organization Nomenclature Committee, HLA gene typing is based on individual allelic designations (DRB1 *0404, DRB1 *0404, etc.) in which the locus name is followed by the unique sequence identifier[1].

CLASS II MOLECULES, STRUCTURE AND FUNCTION

Class II molecules are heterodimers, with one α chain paired with one β chain to form a membrane-bound glycoprotein, schematically illustrated in Figure 2.2. The main function of class II molecules is to bind small peptides, and it is the recognition by T lymphocytes of this class II-peptide complex on the surface of antigen-presenting cells which is the primary activation event in antigen-specific T-cell responses.

The peptide bound by class II molecules may be derived from normal cellular or serum proteins or it may be derived from exogenous proteins from bacteria, viruses, tumors, or degraded self-tissues. As the class II molecule is synthesized and transported inside a cell on the way to the membrane, it encounters such peptides, primarily in endosomal compartments[2]. Specialized molecular chaperone proteins, known as Ii and DM, facilitate this pathway so

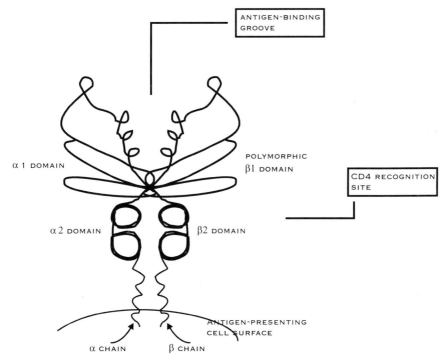

Figure 2.2. Domain structure of HLA class II molecules. The α_1 and β_1 domains of the class II α and β polypeptides, respectively, form a specialized peptide-binding groove on the class II molecule. Nucleotide polymorphisms among different class II genes encode variable amino residues which shape this groove to form an array of differing binding specificities

that, in normal immune responses, class II molecules bind appropriate foreign peptides and signal for protective immune responses.

Not all class II molecules bind all peptides. Indeed, different class II molecules may recognize largely non-overlapping sets of peptides derived from a single foreign or self-protein. This is because the shape of the peptide-binding pocket on the class II molecule, as shown in Figure 2.2, is determined by the precise sequence of amino acid residues encoded by each specific class II gene[3].

Viewed from this perspective, the probable reason for HLA genetic polymorphism becomes clear—different HLA molecules can bind different peptides so that genetic diversity ensures the ability of the species to immunologically recognize diverse pathogens.

This selective pressure for diversity in HLA structure and function comes with a price, however. Some class II molecules appear to bind peptides which lead to deleterious immune activation—autoimmunity. Specific class II genes predispose to specific autoimmune diseases. Identification of these genes and understanding their role in pathogenesis provide new opportunities for use in clinical diagnosis and therapy[4].

CLASS II GENES IN IDDM

HLA class II genes markedly influence susceptibility to IDDM. Different class II genes confer different degrees of risk, and many studies have been performed to fine-tune this analysis[5]. The different class II genes associated with IDDM form a hierarchy of genetic risk, complicated by both synergistic and protective genetic aspects[6]. A summary of these relationships is shown in Table 2.1.

The highest genetic risk attributed to the HLA complex is in individuals who are heterozygous at the HLA DQB1 locus, and carry both an *0302 and a *0201 allele. These individuals are more than 15 times as likely to get IDDM before the age of 30 compared to individuals who do not carry this genotype.

Table 2.1. HLA class II genes associated with IDDM

Risk	HLA-DQB1	Linked DR type	Ethnic group
Highest	*0302/*0201	4/3 heterozygous	Caucasian, Black
	*0302	4	Caucasian, Black
	*0201	3	Caucasian, Black, Oriental
	*0303	9	Oriental
	*0401	4	Oriental
Lowest	*0201	7	Black
Protective	*0602	2	Caucasian, Black

Each of these HLA genes alone also confers susceptibility, so that a DQB1 *0302-positive individual has an eight-fold relative risk, and a DQB *0201 positive individual a three-fold risk[7].

It is important to recognize, however, that many individuals carry these same genes and do not have clinical IDDM. Thus, the presence of a susceptibility gene confers *risk*, but not necessarily disease.

In Caucasian populations, approximately 75% of IDDM patients carry one or both of these genes. Many of the remaining patients carry one of the "minor" HLA susceptibility genes associated with DR1-, DR6-, or DR8-positive haplotypes. Interestingly, in non-Caucasian populations, a similar hierarchy is seen, although the overall prevalence of specific susceptibility genes depends on the population frequency of the specific gene. Thus, in American Blacks, the indigenous DRB *0201 gene is more prevalent than DQB1 *0302, and is also found in most diabetics, although the relative risks conferred by these genes are similar to those found in Caucasians[8]. In oriental populations, the indigenous DQB1 *0303 and *04 genes predominate in IDDM, along with DQB *0201, rather than the DQB *0302 gene, which is rare in Asia[9].

The primary genetic associations with IDDM occur among genes of the DQB1 locus, although other HLA genes may influence the degree of relative risk. For example, since the class II molecule is a heterodimer of an α chain and a β chain, the DQA1 locus plays a modifying, or "epistatic" genetic role. This may be part of the explanation for the genetic synergy between DR3 and DR4 haplotypes in heterozygotes, since it has been shown that DQA1 gene from the DR3 haplotype encodes an α chain that will pair with the DQβ chain from the DR4 haplotype, encoded by DQB1 *0302[10]. Other weak HLA associations, such as DR7 in American Blacks, may also be due to the linked DQA1 polymorphisms, since the DQα chain encoded on this haplotype is often the same as the DQA1 allele on Caucasian DR4 haplotypes. In addition, in some cases the specific DRB1 gene present in linkage with a DQB1 susceptibility gene may influence the relative risk, as is seen among different DR4-related haplotypes[11,12].

The most surprising feature of HLA associations with IDDM is the observation that a specific HLA haplotype, positive for DQB1 *0602, is actually *protective* of disease. This has been called "dominant protection", since a single copy of DQB1 *0602, is protective for IDDM[13].

This complex hierarchical set of HLA susceptibility and protective genes can best be interpreted in the context of HLA class II structure and function. As described in the previous section, different HLA molecules bind different sets of peptides; indeed, the relative affinity of an HLA–peptide interaction is itself a hierarchical array depending on the polymorphic peptide-binding site residues on each HLA molecule. This has important consequences for understanding the role of HLA in IDDM.

MOLECULAR MECHANISMS OF HLA CLASS II GENES IN IDDM

The precise molecular pathway by which HLA susceptibility genes confer risk for IDDM is not yet known. However, the function of class II molecules as a peptide-binding triggering factor for T-cell recognition suggests an obvious pathogenic link.

The class II-peptide complex is known to be critical at two different stages of T-cell development. On the one hand, when CD4+T cells mature in the immune system, their differentiation and development is dependent on signaling by a class II–peptide complex. In most cases, this recognition takes the form of a self-peptide bound to class II molecules in the thymic environment where T cells mature, and the consequence of recognition—for an immature T cell—is apoptosis, or cell death, to protect the individual from autoreactive lymphocyte development[14]. It is possible to speculate that, in some cases, specific HLA molecules might be inefficient at this self-peptide presentation, and thereby contribute to an immune repertoire biased toward autoimmunity.

On the other hand, when a mature CD4+T lymphocyte recognizes a class II–peptide complex, its activation response can lead to the development and amplification of cellular and humoral immunity directed against targets which contain that peptide. The hierarchical nature of HLA molecules associated with IDDM, and the concept of dominant protection, fit well with the notion that genetic susceptibility to IDDM is simply a function of which class II molecules bind and present pathogenic peptides. In this context, the HLA susceptibility genes are "permissive" for disease, and become pathogenic when they bind diabetes-associated peptides—peptides which themselves presumably derive from islet β cell self-proteins.

One implication of this proposed disease activation mechanism is that the permissive role of the IDDM susceptibility gene(s) is only manifest when a functional threshold is passed. In other words, sufficient peptide antigen needs to be present, along with the correct class II molecule, in an environment capable of T-cell triggering. Thus, levels of class II expression as well as antigen density may be crucial for pathogenesis. In this regard, it is interesting that different DQB1 alleles have different levels of transcriptional control, due to nucleotide polymorphisms in regulatory elements associated with the gene promoter[15].

CLINICAL UTILITY

As outlined in Figure 2.3, understanding HLA genes in IDDM leads to two types of clinical applications—in prediction and in therapy. The primary role

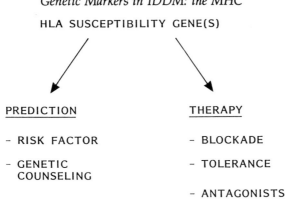

HLA SUSCEPTIBILITY GENE(S)

PREDICTION

- RISK FACTOR
- GENETIC
  COUNSELING

THERAPY

- BLOCKADE
- TOLERANCE
- ANTAGONISTS

Figure 2.3. Clinical application of HLA genetic analysis in IDDM

for HLA genetics in IDDM prediction is to ascertain a risk ratio for an individual at potential risk of disease. Thus, the risk of IDDM varies from approximately 1 in 1500 in someone with a protective DQBI *0602 allele to 1 in 60 for an individual with DBQ1 *0302, to 1 in 4 for someone heterozygous for *0302/*0201 who also has a family history of diabetes[7]. In conjunction with other genetic, immunologic, and metabolic markers of disease, this HLA genotyping can thus be a significant predictor of risk.

A future role for HLA genetics lies in the realm of IDDM therapeutics. Based on the concept that specific class II–peptide recognition events are critical for pathogenesis, new forms of immunotherapy are being developed to attempt to block the MHC–peptide interaction, block T-cell recognition, or substitute non-immunogenic signals through an altered, recognition process[16]. Although the descriptive era of HLA associations with IDDM is now at an end, the clinical era is just beginning.

REFERENCES

1 Bodmer JG, Marsh SGE, Albert ED, Bodmer WF, Dupont B, Erlich HA *et al.* Nomenclature for factors of the HLA system, 1991. *Human Immunol* 1992; **34**: 4–18.
2 Braciale TJ, Braciale VL. Antigen presentation structural themes and functional variations. *Immunol Today* 1992; **12**: 124–9.
3 Stern LJ, Brown JH, Jardetzky TS, Gorga JC, Urban RG, Strominger JL *et al.* Crystal structure of the human class II MHC protein HLA-DR1 complexed with an influenza virus peptide. *Nature* 1994; **368**: 215–21.
4 Nepom GT. Reverse immunogenetics: investigations of HLA-associated disease based on the structural and genetic identification of candidate susceptibility genes. In Melchers F (ed), *Progress in Immunology*, Vol VII. New York: Springer-Verlag, 1989, pp. 805–12.
5 Thomson G, Robinson WP, Kuhner MK, Joe S, MacDonald MJ, Gottschall JL *et al.* Genetic heterogeneity, modes of inheritance, and risk estimates for a joint study of

Caucasians with insulin-dependent diabetes mellitus. *Am J Hum Genet* 1988; **43**: 799–816.

6 Nepom GT. A unified hypothesis for the complex genetics of HLA associations with IDDM I diabetes. *Diabetes* 1990; **39**: 1153–7.

7 Nepom GT. Immunogenetics and IDDM. *Diabetes Rev* 1993; **1**: 93–103.

8 Mijovic CH, Jenkins D, Jacobs KH, Penny MA, Fletcher JA, Barnett AH. HLA-DQA1 and -DQB1 alleles associated with genetic susceptibility to IDDM in a Black population. *Diabetes* 1991; **40**: 748–53.

9 Awata T, Kuzuya T, Matsuda A, Iwamoto Y, Kanazawa Y, Okuyama M *et al*. High frequency of aspartic acid at position 57 of HLA-DQ β-chain in Japanese IDDM patients and nondiabetic subjects. *Diabetes* 1990; **39**: 266–9.

10 Nepom BS, Schwarz D, Palmer JP, Nepom GT. Transcomplementation of HLA genes in IDDM. HLA-DQ alpha- and beta-chains produce hybrid molecules in DR3/4 heterozygotes. *Diabetes* 1987; **36**: 114–17.

11 Erlich HA, Zeidler A, Chang J, Shaw S, Raffel LJ, Klitz W *et al*. HLA class II alleles and susceptibility and resistance to insulin dependent diabetes mellitus in Mexican-American families. *Nature Genetics* 1993; **3**: 358–64.

12 Sheehy MJ, Scharf SJ, Rowe, JR, Neme de Gimenez MH, Meske LM, Erlich HA *et al*. A diabetes-susceptible HLA haplotype is best defined by a combination of HLA-DR and -DQ alleles. *J Clin Invest* 1989; **83**: 830–5.

13 Baisch JM, Weeks T, Giles T, Hoover M, Stastny P, Capra JD. Analysis of HLA-DQ genotypes and susceptibility in insulin-dependent diabetes mellitus. *N Engl J Med* 1990; **322**: 1836–41.

14 Kappler JW, Roehm N, Marrack P. T cell tolerance by clonal elimination in the thymus. *Cell* 1987; **49**: 273–80.

15 Andersen LC, Beaty JS, Nettles JW, Seyfried CE, Nepom GT, Nepom BS. Allelic polymorphism in transcriptional regulatory regions of HLA-DQB genes. *J Exp Med* 1991; **173**: 181–92.

16 Nepom GT. Class II antigens and disease susceptibility. *Ann Rev Med* 1995; **46**: 17–25.

17 Trowsdale J., Ragoussis J, Campbell RD. Map of the human MHC. *Immunol Today* 1991; **12**: 443–6.

18 Nepom BS and Nepom GT. Immunogenetics and the rheumatic diseases. In Kelly WN, Harris ED, Ruddy S and Sledge CB (eds), *Textbook of Rheumatology*. Philadelphia: WB Saunders Co., 1992; 89–107.

3

Genetic Markers in IDDM: non-MHC

FLEMMING POCIOT and JØRN NERUP
Steno Diabetes Center, Gentofte, Denmark

INTRODUCTION

Genetic susceptibility to IDDM is not due to a single gene or gene defect, but rather several genes are of importance. No IDDM-specific gene(s) or gene polymorphisms have been identified and probably do not exist, and no single locus is obligatory for the development of the disease. The inheritance of IDDM appears most consistent with a single major locus providing the major part of the genetic susceptibility in combination with several contributing loci each of them with equally important and additive and/or synergistic effects.

The polygenetic nature of IDDM was suggested several years ago, and is experimentally supported by data from the NOD mouse[1], as well as the BB rat[2], and most recently from studies on human IDDM[3,4]. Of the known susceptibility genes, the HLA class II alleles show the strongest association to IDDM, although the pathogenetic mechanism underlying this association is not fully understood. Thus, HLA class II specificities are important for conferring genetic susceptibility to IDDM, but they are neither sufficient nor necessary for IDDM to occur[4]. The difference in concordance rates of IDDM between genetically identical twins (30–50%) and HLA-identical siblings (15%) underlines this point. Hence, in the search for new susceptibility genes, attention should be given to the identification of genes *outside* the HLA region.

Non-HLA genes have previously been studied in relation to IDDM susceptibility using a candidate gene approach[4–9]. Recently, a random marker approach which takes advantage of the most recent linkage maps from the

Prediction, Prevention and Genetic Counseling in IDDM. Edited by Jerry P. Palmer.
© 1996 John Wiley & Sons Ltd.

Human Genome Project has been applied to the search for new susceptibility genes. The preliminary data provided evidence to suggest that 20 different chromosomal regions show some evidence of linkage to IDDM[3] (Table 3.1). However, no new susceptibility genes were identified by this study.

Table 3.1. Identified chromosomal regions demonstrating evidence for linkage to IDDM and putative candidate genes identified through the pathogenetic model of IDDM[19]

IDDM susceptibility loci	IDDM candidate gene
IDDM1 (Chr.6p)	HLA region[a]
IDDM2 (Chr.11p)	(INS locus)
IDDM3 (Chr.15q)	—
IDDM4 (Chr.11q)	ICE[c], CD3[c]
IDDM5 (Chr.6q)	SOD2[a], γ-IFN-R[c]
IDDM7 (Chr.2q)	IL-1 gene cluster[a], bcg[c], GAD67[a], HOX[c]
? (12p)	CD4[a]
? (12q)	γIFN[a,b]
? (17q)	iNOS[c]

[a] Candidate genes which have been studied using the "candidate gene" approach (see text).
[b] Reference 81.
[c] Candidate genes which have not yet been studied.

Estimation of the degree of familial clustering of IDDM, may represent another powerful method to evaluate the importance of specific non-MHC markers. The degree of familial clustering of a disease (λ_s) can be estimated from the ratio of the risk to siblings of patients and the population prevalence[10]. For Caucasian, Danish IDDM $\lambda_s = 6\%/0.4\% = 15$. The contribution of a single disease locus to the total λ_s can be estimated from the ratio of the expected proportion of affected sibpairs sharing alleles IBD (identical by descent) and the observed proportion. For the major IDDM susceptibility locus, the HLA region, λ_s has been calculated as 3.1[3].

A number of loci within the MHC region have been studied and evidence exists to suggest that MHC-region genes other than -DR and -DQ are involved in susceptibility to IDDM. The best studied markers include the loci for tumor necrosis factor (TNF), heat shock protein 70 (hsp 70), TAP/LMP and C4[4,7,8,11-14]. These MHC class III and new class II genes will not be further detailed in this chapter. Rather we will discuss the markers outside the HLA region which are likely to be susceptibility genes.

THE INTERLEUKIN-1 GENE CLUSTER

There is increasing consensus that β-cell destruction is the result of a chronic inflammatory lesion in the islets of Langerhans (insulitis)[15], and that macrophages (Mø) and CD4+ lymphocytes are essential for the initiation and perpetuation, respectively, of this process[16,17]. The exact cellular and molecular mechanisms that lead to β-cell destruction are not completely understood. There is growing evidence that inflammatory mediators (cytokines), in particular IL-1 are involved as outlined in the model of Figure 3.1[18,19].

Apart from a role of high local concentrations of cytokines acting as effector molecules directly on β-cells in the insulitis process, there is increasing evidence that cytokines have important immunoregulatory properties affecting the immune system and thereby the development of IDDM in animal models[20]. Evidence from human studies to support the role of cytokines in

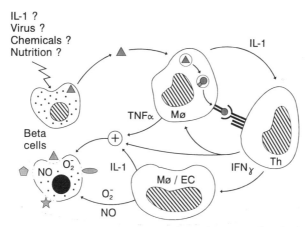

Figure 3.1. The model predicts that anything from the external or internal environment which can destroy a beta cell (nutrients?, virus?, chemical?, IL-1?) will lead to the release of beta cell proteins. These proteins will be taken up by residing antigen-presenting cells (Mø, MO, DC) in the islets, will be processed to antigenic peptides and as such be presented by MHC class II molecules on the cell surface. This activates the antigen-presenting cells (APC) to produce and secrete monokines (IL-1, TNF) and co-stimulatory signal(s) which, if T-helper lymphocytes with receptors specifically recognizing the antigenic peptide are present in the islet, induce the transcription of a series of lymphokine genes. One of these, IFN, will feed back stimulate the APC to increase expression of MHC class II molecules and IL-1 and TNF. In addition, other cells of the Mø/Mø/DC lineage present in the islet are also induced to secrete monokines. IL-1, potentiated by TNF and IFN is cytotoxic to beta cells through the induction of free radical (FR: NO, O_2) formation in the islet. As part of the beta cell destructive mechanism some beta cell proteins are damaged ("denatured") by FR and in more antigenic forms (linear epitopes) are presented to the immune system, thereby closing the loop in a self-perpetuating and self-limiting fashion. The magnitude of beta cell destruction will depend upon: (a) the velocity of the feedback circuit between the APC and the T-helper lymphocyte, i.e. on the efficacy of antigen transport presentation/recognition; (b) the magnitude of cytokine production; and (c) the capacity of beta cell defense mechanisms during cytokine exposure

β-cell destruction in IDDM is scarce. However, IL-1 in synergy with TNF-α or β and/or IFN-γ is cytotoxic to human β- cells *in vitro*[21,22].

Stable, significantly inter-individual differences in induced secretory capacities of IL-1β of Mo (monocytes) *in vitro* exist[23] revealing "high" and "low" producer phenotypes. Production phenotype is likely to be determined by transcriptional and/or translational mechanisms. Alternatively, they may be the result of a structurally changed gene product. In either case, the presence of polymorphism within the gene may underlie the different producer phenotypes. This can be caused by variation in one or more of the genes within the IL-1 gene cluster due to the complex interaction of their products[24,25].

The term "the interleukin-1 (IL-1) gene cluster" is used to cover the genomic region on the long arm of chromosome 2 (q12–21) which contains the genes for IL-1α *(IL1A)* and IL-1β *(IL1B)*, the IL-1 receptor antagonist (ra) *(IL1RN)*, and the two IL-1 receptors (IL-1R), types I and II *(IL1RI and IL1RII)*.

Reported polymorphisms identified within the IL-1 gene cluster region are listed in Table 3.2.

Only the *IL1B* TaqI RFLP, the *IL1RN* insertion polymorphism, and the *IL1RI* PstI RFLPs have been evaluated as genetic markers for IDDM so far[4,6]. The *IL1B* TaqI RFLP was useful as a marker for genetic susceptibility to IDDM especially in IDDM patients negative for HLA-DR3 and -DR4, where the frequency of the 13.4 kb allele was significantly increased[6]. In addition, familial cases differed significantly (increased frequency of the 13.4 kb allele) from controls whereas sporadic cases (no first degree relatives with IDDM) were comparable to controls[4]. The functional significance of this polymorphism has been investigated. A significant difference was observed between the groups indicating an allele-dosage effect on the IL-1β response: individuals homozygous for the 13.4 kb allele secreted more IL-1β than 9.4/13.4 kb heterozygous individuals, and heterozygous individuals more than 9.4 kb homozygous individuals[6].

The *IL1RN* second intron polymorphism has also been evaluated as a genetic marker of IDDM and a significant disease association of this marker was reported[4]. Again, this was primarily due to the association in familial IDDM but not in sporadic IDDM[4]. The A1/A1 genotype of the *IL1RN* polymorphism, which was more frequent in familial cases than in sporadic cases[4], was associated with low circulating plasma levels of the IL-1ra[26].

As this difference between familial and sporadic IDDM cases was true also for the IL-1β TaqI RFLP, it was suggested that these markers of the IL-1 gene cluster may preferentially be markers of familial IDDM[4] (Table 3.3). In contrast, no difference between familial and sporadic cases was found at the *IL1RI* locus. However, a significant difference was found between patients and control subjects[4]. Very recently, the disease association of this polymorphism was confirmed in a UK population[27]. A possible functional significance of the *IL1RI* locus polymorphism has not yet been studied. The mapping of the

Table 3.2. Identified polymorphisms within the IL-1 gene cluster on chromosome 2

Gene	Position	Type	Alleles	IDDM association tested	Ref.
IL1A	Intron 6	46 bp tandem repeat	A1, A2,..., A6	NT	75
IL1A	Intron 5	Microsatellite [AC]$_n$	1,2,...,6	NT	76
IL1B	Exon 5	T→C transition (silent)	TaqI IL-1β 13.4 kb (IL1B*1), TaqI IL-1β 9.4 kb (IL1B*2)	YES	4,6
IL1B	Pos. 3962 −511	C→T transition		NT	77
IL1RI	5'-UTR	PstI RFLPs	1.2/3.2 kb and 4.8/6.8 kb	YES	4,78
IL1R		Microsatellite		NT	60
IL1RN	Intron 2	86 bp tandem repeat	A1, A2,..., A6	YES	4,79,80

Nucleotide numbers are adapted from cited references and/or from the GenBank Database. For further details of association studies see the text. UTR: untranslated region; NT: not tested

Table 3.3. IDDM association non-HLA "candidate genes" with respect to familial and sporadic IDDM. No differences between familial and sporadic IDDM have been reported for MHC-region markers[4]. The *INS* locus and *TCR* loci have not been analyzed in this respect

Chromosome	Locus	Significant disease association
2q	*IL1B*	Familial cases
	IL1RN	Familial cases
	IL1RI	Familial and sporadic cases
6q	*SOD2*	Sporadic cases

polymorphic restriction site to a region thought to be important for gene regulation makes it a likely candidate for affecting *IL1RI* gene expression.

The markers of the IL-1 gene cluster are, in addition to the markers of the insulin gene region (see below), the only candidate IDDM-susceptibility genes outside the HLA region that demonstrate significant disease association. The statistical correlation of polymorphisms within the *IL1B* and *IL1RN* loci with in vitro stimulated or circulating protein levels is intriguing. In relation to the pathogenesis the data suggest that familial cases may be more prone to immune (IL-1β) mediated β-cell destruction since both phenotypes, most frequently found in familial cases, may result in an enhanced IL-1 response. However, regarding the functional significance of the polymorphisms, caution should be exerted when interpreting these data, until more detailed studies are available.

Two recent studies have expanded the search for new susceptibility loci on the long arm of chromosome 2[28,29]. Both studies found by linkage disequilibrium mapping evidence for localization of disease susceptibility genes to 2q31–33. The gene for the IDDM autoantigen glutamate decarboxylase 67 (*GAD1*) is located in this region and so is the *HOXD* loci, which may be interesting candidate genes for IDDM susceptibility. The HOX genes encode proteins that function as transcription factors regulating the function of other genes. Interestingly, one of these studies[29] found linkage most pronounced in individuals with low-risk HLA specificities, i.e. non-DR3, non-DR4 individuals.

In an analysis of IDDM multiplex families from the UK, the US, France, Denmark, and Italy the degree of familial clustering, λ_s, for *IDDM7* (chromosome 2q) was calculated to 1.3[28].

MANGANESE SUPEROXIDE DISMUTASE (MnSOD)

Although the detailed mechanisms behind the immune-mediated β-cell destruction are not fully clarified, accumulating evidence suggests a pivotal role for free radicals (FR)[20,30]. These may be oxygen derived or nitric oxide, NO. β cells have been suggested to be particularly sensitive to the toxic effect of oxygen-derived FR (OFR) due to a limited repertoire of O_2^- scavengers[31,32] like the enzyme MnSOD, which may explain the β-cell specificity of the process.

Thus, genetic susceptibility to IDDM might be related to genetic variation(s) of the MnSOD locus (*SOD2*) reflecting inter-individual differences in scavenging potential rendering some individuals more susceptible to IL-1-mediated β-cell destruction and IDDM.

The *SOD2* locus is localized on the long arm of chromosome 6 (6q21). The genomic sequence of the gene has not been reported. Only one polymorphism of the SOD2 has been published[33]. This TaqI RFLP has been evaluated as a genetic marker for IDDM susceptibility[9]. In a large sample of randomly, unrelated IDDM patients and controls no support for this RFLP as a genetic marker of IDDM was found. In a subsequent study[4] evidence that this polymorphism might be associated with IDDM in patients with no first degree relatives (true sporadic cases) with IDDM was reported (Table 3.3). However, these observations need confirmation in independent samples. Interestingly, positive evidence for linkage to IDDM for a chromosomal region at 6q (*IDDM5*) was recently found and *SOD2* was suggested as a candidate gene of this region, *IDDM5*[3].

Structurally polymorphic MnSOD protein variants with altered activities have been reported[34]. Selection for MnSOD variants with reduced activity might be part of the predisposition for IDDM. This would parallel the observation that mutation at the *SOD1* locus is associated with altered function of the Cu/Zn SOD protein and with amyotrophic lateral sclerosis[35].

THE T CELL RECEPTOR (TCR)

Since few MHC molecules are capable of presenting a wide range of antigens, the specificity of the MHC-antigen–TCR complex most likely resides within the TCR, making the TCR genes obvious candidates for IDDM susceptibility genes. The TCR is expressed in the T-cell membrane as a heterodimer associated with the CD3 complex and either CD4 or CD8[36]. The most abundant form of the TCR for antigen recognition in the context of HLA presentation, is the $\alpha\beta$ heterodimer form. The genes that encode the α and β chains are located on the human chromosomes 14 and 7, respectively, and are composed of variable (V), diversity (D; β chain only), joining (J), and constant (C) gene segments. It has been estimated that there are more than 50 human $V\beta$ genes extending over at least 600 kb (depending on the haplotype) of DNA on the long arm of chromosome 7, and an even larger number of $V\alpha$ genes on the long arm of chromosome 14[37,38].

A large number of studies have addressed the involvement of TCR gene regions in susceptibility to IDDM. Several studies have revealed associations between IDDM and alleles of an RFLP detected with a Cβ-gene probe (which is likely to reflect Vβ region gene contribution to IDDM susceptibility) at the population level[39-41], whereas in other studies no association was observed [42-44]. The studies on TCRα associations also appear to be contradictory. In some reports no TCRα-chain gene associated polymorphism was found related to IDDM susceptibility[45,46], whereas in another study a positive associated was observed[42]. The reported associations between IDDM and certain TCRβ gene variants were in most, if not all, studies restricted to subsets of the data, e.g. certain HLA-DR genotypes[39-41]. Analysis of TCRα or TCRβ haplotype sharing in affected sibling pairs from 36 multiplex IDDM families provided no evidence for contribution of germ-line polymorphisms of these genes to susceptibility[47]. Hence, despite the plausibility of the hypothesis, the numerous studies in the field have not provided consensus for the existence of any genetically determined TCR-influenced susceptibility to IDDM.

CD4 AND CD3

The αβ heterodimers of the TCR on the surface of both helper and cytotoxic T cells associate non-covalently with the CD3 complex which is involved in the delivery of signals to the T cell during antigen presentation, and is required for activation of the T cell[36]. The TCR complex is further flanked by a CD4 or CD8 molecule[36]. The engagement by the TCR of the CD4 or CD8 coreceptor augments signaling via the TCR by up to 100-fold[36]. The gene for CD4 is located on the short arm of chromosome 12 (12pter)[48]. The CD3 gene maps to the long arm of chromosome 11 (11q23)[49]. The possible association of CD4 and CD3 polymorphisms with IDDM was recently assessed[50]. Significant disease association was observed for allelic variants of both loci. This needs, however, to be confirmed in new independent samples and family studies are clearly in demand. Furthermore, the functional significance of either of these polymorphisms has yet to be investigated. Interestingly, because of its localization to chromosome 11q the CD3 locus may be a candidate for the *IDDM4* region identified in recent linkage studies[3].

THE INSULIN (INS) GENE LOCUS

Several studies have demonstrated that the regions flanking the insulin (INS) gene on chromosome 11p15.5 confer susceptibility to IDDM. The IDDM association has been demonstrated for a locus that lies within an approximately

20 kb region[51] and includes the structural genes for tyrosine hydroxylase, insulin like growth factor II (IGF2), HRAS1 and insulin. Studies which have analyzed all these genes support a role for the flanking regions of INS gene for conferring susceptibility—not for any of the other genes[52,53]. A large number of polymorphisms have been demonstrated within this region and map either to the 3'-untranslated region or introns of the insulin gene, and to the 5'-region of the insulin gene. Strong linkage disequilibrium is observed for this region[52] and association to IDDM of RFLPs in the 3'-region was shown to be secondary to a susceptibility locus in the 5'-region[52,53].

An association between IDDM and a polymorphic region in the 5'-flanking region of the human INS gene was described in 1984[54], and it is the most studied, non-HLA locus which may contribute to the genetic susceptibility of IDDM. The polymorphism arises from a variable number of tandemly repeated (VNTR) 14 bp oligonucleotides located at position -363 from the transcriptional start site. The different repeat numbers of the oligonucleotides are grouped into three classes according to their lengths (class I: average: 570 bp; class II: average 1200 bp; and class III: average 2200 bp) as measured by standard Southern blotting.

A number of studies in the mid-1980s identified an association of IDDM with the class I alleles in Caucasoid populations[54-56]. More recent studies have confirmed these observations using additional polymorphic markers to this region[51-53,57]. Several studies have been unable to demonstrate linkage of these alleles to IDDM in families[56,58] probably due to the fact that the disease-associated allele is present at high frequency in the general population: in unaffected controls the frequency of the class I allele is approximately 0.70–0.75, while in IDDM patients the frequency is somewhat higher, 0.80–0.85. However, two recent studies[51,57] and a re-analysis of the Genetic Analysis Workshop 5 (GAW5) data[59] did demonstrate linkage in diabetic families of IDDM-associated alleles in the INS region. These discrepancies may reflect variation between different populations[60].

No genes which are thought to be involved in autoimmunity have so far been localized to this chromosomal region. Thus, the identity and mechanism of action of the susceptibility gene(s) on chromosome 11p15.5 remain to be elucidated. Identification of new polymorphisms and sequencing analysis was recently used to redefine the region of susceptibility to a 4.1 kb segment spanning the insulin gene and associated 5'-VNTR, including its regulatory sequences[52]. Several IDDM-associated polymorphisms have been identified in the region[51,52,57] but none is located within known coding or defined promoter and enhancer sequences of genes within this region.

It has been speculated that size variation of the VNTR within the region could have a direct effect on insulin gene regulation[61-64]. This is supported by recent studies describing an unusual quadriplex structure of a class I VNTR in vitro[65] which has generated the hypothesis that different VNTR lengths could affect the configuration of chromatin in vivo[66]. If the different number of repeats affect, for example, the binding of a nuclear protein important in insulin gene transcription, another functional significance of this repeat could exist. However, earlier studies have been conflicting, as some[61,63], but not others[62,64], showed an association between polymorphism of the 5'-flanking region and insulin secretory responses. Although it is not clear that insulin or the insulin gene itself plays a role in the pathogenesis of IDDM, the association has been found consistently in population studies[58]. Furthermore, markers of this region (INS 1127/PstI RFLP) have been calculated to add, independently of HLA class II markers, around 1% to the absolute risk of IDDM in Caucasoid populations[67].

Several groups[68–70] have consistently reported the lack of association of the polymorphisms of the 5'VNTR of the INS gene with IDDM in Japanese subjects. The high frequency of the class I alleles in Japanese (approximately 95% are homozygous for class I alleles) despite the low incidence of IDDM in Japan suggests that either the INS region has a relatively low effect on genetic susceptibility to IDDM in Japanese, or that other gene(s) in the region are responsible for conferring susceptibility. Most recently, by systematically excluding RFLP polymorphisms in the region as primarily disease determinants, and by demonstrating significant heterogeneity according to VNTR genotype, an international collaboration[60] fine-mapped the susceptibility locus to within the INS VNTR. This locus is designated *IDDM2*[3]. Furthermore, correlation between certain VNTR and differential INS expression suggested that some VNTR sequences indeed may confer disease predisposition by influencing transcriptional control[60]. If this reflects a biosynthetically hyperactive β cell this fits well with in vitro observations showing that metabolically active β cells are more vulnerable to immune-mediated (cytokine) destruction[71].

In an analysis of IDDM multiplex families from the UK, the US, France, Denmark, and Italy, the λ_s for *IDDM2* (the INS locus) and for *IDDM7* (chromosome 2q) was 1.3 for both, suggesting that the contribution of *IDDM2* and *IDDM7* to familial clustering of IDDM is equal and greater than that for other tested regions[3,72]. Thus, at present the INS locus and the chromosome 2q loci represent the only non-MHC susceptibility loci outside the MHC region for which convincing association and/or linkage have been demonstrated.

FUTURE STUDIES

Given the many problems of genetic dissection of complex traits, it is mandatory to restrict the study population, if possible, to one which is likely to be highly homogeneous. This may be of special relevance when studying non-HLA genes. Selection of certain subgroups of IDDM patients, e.g. non-DR3, non-DR4 (non-DQA1*0501-DQB1*0201, non-DQA1*0301-DQB1*0302) individuals, in whom the contribution from non-MHC susceptibility genes is likely to be strong, and the comparison of patients with and without a family history of IDDM may be useful for studying non-HLA susceptibility markers.

The main methods for identifying new non-MHC susceptibility loci include the candidate gene approach which has to be based on a model of the pathogenesis of IDDM (exemplified in Figure 3.1). Another feasible approach is the identification of β-cell-specific expression of genes. This can be studied in different ways. One can compare the expression of mRNA in islets with other tissues in order to identify islet-specific transcripts (differential mRNA display and subtraction cloning). These can then be cloned and sequenced. This approach may be taken one step further and related to the pathogenetic model, for example. Then mRNA or protein patterns can be compared between unstimulated and cytokine-exposed islets in order to identify cytokine-induced changes. This approach—at the protein level—has demonstrated that IL-1 reproducibly induces changes in the expression level of 33 proteins, as resolved by two-dimensional gel electrophoresis[73]. The genes encoding these 33 proteins are obvious candidates for cloning and further genetic and functional analysis. Finally, cDNA clones randomly isolated from human pancreatic libraries can be sequenced and related to sequences in existing databases[74].

The random marker approach used for linkage disequilibrium mapping in IDDM multiplex families is likely to identify new chromosomal regions with linkage to IDDM. Further studies will then have to identify the structural genes of those regions responsible for conferring the susceptibility.

CONCLUSIONS

It seems reasonable to suggest that a hierarchy of genetic susceptibility to IDDM exists. Familial cases have a higher number of susceptibility genes than sporadic cases, and individuals with the highest number of susceptibility genes have the lowest age at onset. This hypothesis is shown graphically in Figure 3.2.

Table 3.1 lists the recently identified IDDM susceptibility loci identified through whole-genome searches in IDDM multiplex families and candidate susceptibility genes corresponding to these chromosomal regions. These chromosomal regions are likely to include a number of yet unknown susceptibility genes to IDDM.

As suggested in Figure 3.2 and supported by experimental data, non-HLA susceptibility genes may have limited value as independent genetic *markers* for susceptibility to IDDM. This does not necessarily rule out a pathogenetic

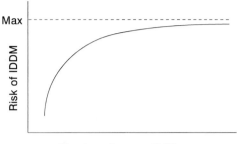

Figure 3.2. Graphic presentation of the hypothesis that a hierarchy of genetic susceptibility to IDDM exists. The implications of this hypothesis are that IDDM may develop in individuals with no known susceptibility markers, that the major part of the genetic susceptibility is conferred by few major loci (maybe only one), but that several minor loci may add to the risk of developing IDDM. The dotted line indicates the maximum genetic influence which is expressed best by the concordance rate of monozygotic twins, although it need not be equal to this

relevance of such genes, and in order to increase our understanding of the processes leading to β-cell destruction the search for new susceptibility genes should be continued.

REFERENCES

1 Ghosh S, Palmer SM, Rodrigues NR *et al.* Polygenic control of autoimmune diabetes in nonobese diabetic mice. *Nature Genet* 1993; 4: 404–9.
2 Jacob HJ, Pettersson A, Wilson D, Mao Y, Lernmark Å, Lander ES. Genetic dissection of autoimmune type I diabetes in the BB rat. *Nature Genet* 1992; 2: 56–60.
3 Davies JL, Kawaguchi Y, Bennett ST *et al.* A genome-wide search for human susceptibility genes. *Nature* 1994; 371: 130–6.
4 Pociot F, Rønningen KS, Bergholdt R *et al.* Genetic susceptibility markers in Danish patients with type 1 diabetes—accumulating evidence for polygenecity in man. *Autoimmunity* 1994; 19: 169–78.
5 Mølvig J, Pociot F, Baek L *et al.* Monocyte function in IDDM patients and healthy individuals. *Scand J Immunol* 1990; 32: 297–311.
6 Pociot F, Mølvig J, Wogensen L, Worsaae H, Nerup J. A TaqI polymorphism in the human interleukin-1β (IL-1β) gene correlates with IL-1β secretion in vitro. *Eur J Clin Invest* 1992; 22: 396–402.
7 Pociot F, Briant L, Jongeneel CV *et al.* Association of tumor necrosis factor (TNF) and class II MHC alleles with the secretion of TNFα and TNFβ by human mononuclear cells: A possible link to insulin-dependent diabetes mellitus. *Eur J Immunol* 1993; 23: 224–31.
8 Pociot F, Rønningen KS, Nerup J. Polymorphic analysis of the human MHC-linked heat shock protein 70 (HSP70-2) and HSP70-Hom genes in insulin-dependent diabetes mellitus (IDDM). *Scand J Immunol* 1993; 38: 491–5.

9 Pociot F, Lorenzen T, Nerup J. A manganese superoxide dismutase (SOD2) gene polymorphism in insulin-dependent diabetes mellitus. *Disease Markers* 1993; 11: 267–74.

10 Risch N. Assessing the role of HLA-linked and unlinked determinants of disease. *Am J Hum Genet* 1987; 40: 1–14.

11 Caplen NJ, Patel A, Millward A et al. Complement C4 and heat shock protein 70 (HSP70) genotypes and type I diabetes mellitus. *Immunogenetics* 1990; 32: 427–30.

12 Pugliese A, Awdeh ZL, Galluzzo A, Yunis EJ, Alper CA, Eisenbarth GS. No independent association between HSP70 gene polymorphism and IDDM. *Diabetes* 1992; 41: 788–91.

13 Rønningen KS, Undlien DE, Ploski R et al. Linkage disequilibrium between TAP2 variants and HLA class II alleles; no primary association between TAP2 variants and insulin-dependent diabetes mellitus. *Eur J Immunol* 1993; 23: 1050–6.

14 van Endert PM, Liblau R, Patel SD et al. Major histocompatibility complex-encoded antigen processing gene polymorphism in IDDM. *Diabetes* 1994; 43: 110–17.

15 Bach J-F. Insulin-dependent diabetes mellitus as an autoimmune disease. *Endocrine Reviews* 1994; 15: 516–42.

16 Hutchings P, Rosen H, O'Reilly L, Simpson E, Gordon S, Cooke A. Transfer of diabetes in mice prevented by blockade of adhesion-promoting receptor on macrophages. *Nature* 1990; 348: 639–42.

17 Peterson JD, Pike B, McDuffie M, Haskins K. Islet-specific T cell clones transfer diabetes to nonobese diabetic F_1 mice. *J Immunol* 1994; 153: 2800–7.

18 Nerup J, Mandrup-Poulsen T, Mølvig J et al. Pathogenesis of insulin-dependent diabetes mellitus (IDDM). In: Christiansen C, Riis, BJ (eds). *Highlights in Endocrinology*. Viborg, Denmark: Nørhaven 1987, pp 37–41.

19 Nerup J, Mandrup-Poulsen T, Andersen HU et al. On the pathogenesis of IDDM. *Diabetologia* 1994; 37 (Suppl 2): S82–S89.

20 Rabinovitch A. Immunoregulatory and cytokine imbalances in the pathogenesis of IDDM. *Diabetes* 1994; 43: 613–21.

21 Rabinovitch A, Sumoski W, Rajotte RV, Warnock GL. Cytotoxic effects of cytokines on human pancreatic islet cells in monolayer culture. *J Clin Endocrinol Metab* 1990; 71: 152–6.

22 Kawahara DJ, Kenney JS. Species differences in human and rat islet sensitivity to human cytokines. Monoclonal anti-interleukin-1 (IL-1) influences on direct and indirect IL-1-mediated islet effects. *Cytokine* 1991; 3: 117–24.

23 Mølvig J, Baek L, Christensen P et al. Endotoxin-stimulated human monocyte secretion of interleukin 1, tumour necrosis factor alpha, and prostaglandin E_2 shows stable interindividual differences. *Scand J Immunol* 1988; 27: 705–16.

24 Dinarello CA. Interleukin-1 and interleukin-1 antagonism. *Blood* 1991; 77: 1627–52.

25 Arend WP, Malyak M, Smith Jr MF et al. Binding of IL-1α, IL-1β and IL-1 receptor antagonist by soluble IL-1 receptors and levels of soluble IL-1 receptors in synovial fluids. *J Immunol* 1994; 153: 4766–74.

26 Mandrup-Poulsen T, Pociot F, Mølvig J et al. Monokine antagonism is reduced in patients with insulin-dependent diabetes mellitus. *Diabetes* 1994; 43: 1242–7.

27 Metcalfe KA, Pociot F, Hitman GA et al. A strong association of the interleukin-1 receptor type 1 gene with IDDM but not with ICA positivity. *Diabetic Med* 1995; 12 (Suppl 1): S13.

28 Copeman JB, Hearne C, Cornall RJ et al. Fine localisation of a type 1 diabetes susceptibility gene (IDDM7) to human chromosome 2q by linkage disequilibrium mapping. *Nature Genet* 1995; 9: 80–5.

29 Owerbach D, Gabbay KH. The HOXD8 locus (2q31) is linked to type I diabetes.

Interaction with chromosome 6 and 11 disease susceptibility genes. *Diabetes* 1995; **44**: 132–6.

30 Mandrup-Poulsen T, Helqvist S, Wogensen LD *et al*. Cytokines and free radicals as effector molecules in the destruction of the pancreatic β-cells. *Curr Topics Microbiol Immunol* 1990; **164**: 169–93.

31 Malaisse WJ, Malaisse-Lagae F, Sener A, Pipeleers DG. Determinants of the selective toxicity of alloxan to the pancreatic B cell. *Proc Natl Acad Sci USA* 1982; **79**: 927–30.

32 Asayama K, Kooy NW, Burr IM. Effects of vitamin E deficiency on insulin secretory reserve and free radical scavenging systems in islets. *J Lab Clin Med* 1986; **107**: 459–64.

33 Xiang K, Cox NJ, Hallewell RA, Bell GI. Multiple Taq I RFLPs at the human manganese superoxide dismutase (SOD2) locus on chromosome 6. *Nucl Acids Res* 1987; **15**: 7654.

34 Borgstahl GEO, Parge HE, Hickey MJ, Bayer WF, Hallewell RA, Tainer JA. The structure of human mitochondrial manganese superoxide dismutase reveals a novel tetrameric interface of two 4-helix bundles. *Cell* 1992; **71**: 107–18.

35 Rosen DR, Siddique T, Patterson D *et al*. Mutations in Cu/Zn superoxide dismutase gene are associated with familial amyotrophic lateral sclerosis. *Nature* 1993; **362**: 59–62.

36 Davis MM, Bjorkman PJ. T-cell antigen receptor genes and T-cell recognition. *Nature* 1988; **334**: 395–402.

37 Wilson RK, Lai E, Concannon P, Barth RK, Hood LE. Structure, organization and polymorphism of murine and human T-cell receptor α and β chain gene families. *Immunol Rev* 1988; **101**: 149–72.

38 Robinson MA, Mitchell MP, Wei S, Day CE, Zhao TM, Concannon P. Organization of human T-cell receptor β-chain genes: clusters of Vβ genes are present on chromosomes 7 and 9. *Proc Natl Acad Sci USA* 1993; **90**: 2433–7.

39 Millward BA, Welsh KI, Leslie RDG, Pyke DA, Demaine AG. T cell receptor beta chain polymorphisms are associated with insulin-dependent diabetes. *Clin Exp Immunol* 1987; **70**: 152–7.

40 Ito M, Tanimoto M, Kamura H *et al*. Association of HLA-DR phenotypes and T-lymphocyte-receptor β-chain-region RFLP with IDDM in Japanese. *Diabetes* 1988; **37**: 1633–6.

41 Hoover ML, Black KE, Ball E *et al*. Polymorphisms of the human T-cell receptor α and β chain genes and their relationship to insulin dependent diabetes mellitus. In New York: Springer-Verlag, *Immunobiology of HLA*. 1989, pp 411–12.

42 Boehm BO, Manfras BJ, Rosak C, Kuehnl P, Schöeffling K, Trucco M. TcR-alpha and TcR-beta diallelic RFLPs in insulin-dependent (type I) Caucasian diabetic patients. *Diabetes Res* 1990; **15**: 63–7.

43 Niven MJ, Caffrey C, Moore RH *et al*. T-cell receptor β-subunit gene polymorphism and autoimmune disease. *Hum Immunol* 1990; **27**: 360–7.

44 Martinez-Naves E, Coto E, Gutierrez V *et al*. Germline repertoire of T-cell receptor β-chain genes in patients with insulin-dependent diabetes mellitus. *Hum Immunol* 1991; **31**: 77–80.

45 Sheehy MJ, Meske LM, Emler CA *et al*. Allelic T-cell α complexes have little or no influence on susceptibility to type 1 diabetes. *Hum Immunol* 1989; **26**: 261–71.

46 Avoustin P, Briant L, de Préval C, Cambon-Thomsen A. Polymorphism study of TCRα and γ genes in insulin dependent diabetes mellitus (IDDM) multiplex families. *Autoimmunity* 1992; **14**: 97–100.

47 Concannon P, Wright JA, Wright LG, Sylvester DR, Spielman RS. T-cell receptor

genes and insulin-dependent diabetes mellitus (IDDM): no evidence for linkage from affected sib pairs. *Am J Hum Genet* 1990; **47**: 45–52.

48 Isobe M, Huebner K, Maddon PJ, Littman DR, Axel R, Croce CM. The gene encoding the T-cell surface protein T4 is located on the human chromosome 12. *Proc Natl Acad Sci USA* 1986; **83**: 4399–402.

49 Gold DP, van Dongen JJM, Morton CC *et al.* The gene encoding the ε subunit of the T3/T-cell receptor complex maps to chromosome 11 in humans and to chromosome 9 in mice. *Proc Natl Acad Sci USA* 1987; **84**: 1664–8.

50 Zamani Ghabanbasani M, Buyse I, Leguis E *et al.* Possible association of CD3 and CD4 polymorphisms with IDDM. *Clin Exp Immunol* 1994; **97**: 517–21.

51 Julier C, Hyer RN, Davies J *et al.* Insulin-IGF2 region on chromosome 11p encodes a gene implicated in HLA-DR4-dependent diabetes susceptibility. *Nature* 1991; **354**: 155–9.

52 Lucassen AM, Julier C, Beressi J-P *et al.* Susceptibility to insulin-dependent diabetes mellitus maps to a 4.1 kb segment of DNA spanning the insulin gene and associated VNTR. *Nature Genet* 1993; **4**: 305–10.

53 Owerbach D, Gabbay KH. Localization of a type I diabetes susceptibility locus to the variable tandem repeat region flanking the insulin gene. *Diabetes* 1993; **42**: 1708–14.

54 Bell GI, Horita S, Karam JH. A polymorphic locus of the human insulin gene is associated with insulin-dependent diabetes mellitus. *Diabetes* 1984; **33**: 176–83.

55 Owerbach D, Nerup J. Restriction fragment length polymorphism of the insulin gene in diabetes mellitus. *Diabetes* 1982; **31**: 275–7.

56 Hitman GA, Tarn AC, Winter RM *et al.* Type 1 (insulin-dependent) diabetes and a highly variable locus close to the insulin gene on chromosome 11. *Diabetologia* 1985; **28**: 218–22.

57 Bain SC, Prins JB, Hearne CM *et al.* Insulin gene region-encoded susceptibility to type 1 diabetes is not restricted to HLA-DR4-positive individuals. *Nature Genet* 1992; **2**: 212–15.

58 Cox NJ, Baker L, Spielman RS. Insulin-gene sharing in sib pairs with insulin-dependent diabetes mellitus: no evidence for linkage. *Am J Hum Genet* 1988; **42**: 167–72.

59 Spielman RS, McGinnis RE, Ewens WJ. Transmission test for linkage disequilibrium: the insulin gene region and insulin-dependent diabetes mellitus (IDDM). *Am J Hum Genet* 1993; **52**: 506–16.

60 Bennett ST, Lucassen AM, Gough SCL *et al.* IDDM2-encoded susceptibility to type 1 diabetes is determined by the insulin VNTR. *Nature Genet* 1995; **9**: 284–92.

61 Owerbach D, Poulsen S, Billesbølle P, Nerup J. DNA insertion sequence near the insulin gene affects glucose regulation. *Lancet* 1982; **i**: 880–2.

62 Permutt MA, Rotwein P, Andreone T, Ward WK, Porte D. Islet β-cell function and polymorphism in the 5'-flanking region of the human insulin gene. *Diabetes* 1985; **34**: 311–14.

63 Cocozza S, Riccardi G, Monticelli A *et al.* Polymorphism at the 5' end flanking region of the insulin gene is associated with reduced insulin secretion in healthy individuals. *Eur J Clin Invest* 1988; **18**: 582–6.

64 Weaver JU, Kopelman PG, Hitman GA. Central obesity and hyperinsulinaemia in women are associated with polymorphism in the 5'flanking region of the human insulin gene. *Eur J Clin Invest* 1992; **22**: 265–70.

65 Hammon-Kosack MCU, Dobrinski B, Lurz R, Docherty K, Kilpatick MW. The human insulin gene linked polymorphic region exhibits an altered DNA structure. *Nucl Acids Res* 1992; **20**: 231–6.

66 Hammond-Kosack MCU, Kilpatick MW, Docherty K. The human insulin gene-linked polymorphic region adopts a G-quartet structure in chromatin assembled in vitro.

J Mol Endocrinol 1993; **10**: 121–6.

67 Rønningen KS, Undlien D, Thorsby E. Genetic markers in IDDM prediction. *Autoimmunity* 1993; **15** (suppl): 37.

68 Awata T, Shibasaki Y, Hirai H, Okabe T, Kanazawa Y, Takaku F. Restriction fragment length polymorphism of the insulin gene region on Japanese diabetic and non-diabetic subjects. *Diabetologia* 1985; **28**: 911–13.

69 Takeda J, Seino Y, Fukumoto H *et al.* The polymorphism linked to the human insulin gene: its lack of association with either IDDM or NIDDM in Japanese. *Acta Endocrinologica (Copenh)* 1986; **113**: 268–71.

70 Matsumoto C, Awata T, Iwamoto Y, Kuzuya T, Saito T, Kanazawa Y. Lack of association of the insulin gene region with type 1 (insulin-dependent) diabetes mellitus in Japanese subjects. *Diabetologia* 1994; **37**: 210–13.

71 Palmer JP, Helqvist S, Spinas GA *et al.* Interaction of β-cell activity and IL-1 concentration and exposure time in isolated rat islets of Langerhans. *Diabetes* 1989; **38**: 1211–16.

72 Hashimoto L, Habita C, Beressi JP *et al.* Genetic mapping of a susceptibility locus for insulin-dependent diabetes mellitus on chromosome 11q. *Nature* 1994; **371**: 161–4.

73 Andersen HU, Larsen PM, Fey SJ, Karlsen AE, Mandrup-Poulsen T, Nerup J. Two-dimensional gel electrophoresis of rat islet proteins: interleukin-1β-induced changes in protein expression are reduced by L-arginine depletion and nicotinamide. *Diabetes* 1995; **44**: 400–7.

74 Takeda J, Yano H, Eng S, Zeng Y, Bell GI. A molecular inventory of human pancreatic islets: sequence analysis of 1000 cDNA clones. *Hum Mol Genet* 1993; **2**: 1793–8.

75 Bailly S, di Giovine FS, Blakemore AIF, Duff GW. Genetic polymorphism of human interleukin-1α. *Eur J Immunol* 1993; **23**: 1240–5.

76 Todd S, Naylor SL. Dinucleotide repeat polymorphism in the human interleukin 1 alpha gene (IL1A). *Nucl Acids Res* 1991; **19**: 3756.

77 di Giovine FS, Takhsh E, Blakemore AIF, Duff GW. Single base polymorphism at -511 in the human interleukin-1β gene (IL1β). *Hum Mol Genet* 1992; **1**: 450.

78 Bergholdt R, Karlsen AE, Johannesen J *et al.* Genetic characterization of polymorphisms of an interleukin-1 receptor type 1 gene (*IL1RI*) promotor region (P2) and their relation to insulin-dependent diabetes mellitus (IDDM). *Cytokine* 1995; **7**: 727–33.

79 Steinkasserer A, Koelble K, Sim RB. Length variation within intron 2 of the human IL-2 receptor antagonist protein gene (IL1RN). *Nucl Acids Res* 1992; **19**: 5095.

80 Tarlow JK, Blakemore AIF, Lennard A, Solari R, Hughes HN, Steinkasser A, Duff GW. Polymorphism in the human IL-1 receptor antagonist gene intron 2 is caused by variable numbers of an 86-bp tandem repeat. *Hum Genet* 1993; **91**: 403–4.

81 Awata T, Matsumoto C, Urakami T, Hagura R, Amemiya S, Kanazawa Y. Association of polymorphism in the interferon γ gene with IDDM. *Diabetologia* 1994; **37**: 1159–62.

4

Humoral Immune Markers: Islet Cell Antibodies

EZIO BONIFACIO

Department of Internal Medicine, Istituto Scientifico San Raffaele, Milan, Italy,

HISTORY

Substantial evidence supports the autoimmune pathogenesis of insulin-dependent diabetes mellitis (IDDM)[1]. The search for a disease-specific autoantibody in IDDM dates at least back to the late 1960s when, following the description of lymphocytic insulitis[2], the hypothesis of an autoimmune pathogenesis was proposed. For years this search had been unfruitful, so that in the early 1970s it was commonly believed that islet cell antibodies (ICAs) could only occasionally be found in diabetic patients and did not represent a marker of the disease. However, improvements in fluorescent microscopy, the availability of fresh frozen human pancreas, and a better classification of insulin-dependent (Type 1) and non-insulin-dependent (Type 2) diabetes, led to the discovery of ICAs and to their establishment as a marker of IDDM. Cytoplasmic ICAs were reported in 1974 in IDDM patients with associated autoimmune polyendocrine disease[3], and subsequently in the majority of IDDM patients at the time of disease onset[4,5]. This discovery provided a basis for the concept that IDDM is an organ-specific autoimmune disease. Since then, many studies have been performed on humoral autoimmunity associated with IDDM, and the list of putative autoantibodies continues to grow[6].

Prediction, Prevention and Genetic Counseling in IDDM. Edited by Jerry P. Palmer.

ICA CHARACTERIZATION

ICAs are demonstrated by indirect immunofluorescence on frozen pancreas (Figure 4.1). The antibodies are exclusively of the IgG class with a tendency toward IgG1 restriction[7,8], and are able to fix complement[9]. In early studies ICAs were shown to react with the cytoplasm of all the endocrine cells within islets (α, β, δ, and PP cells) suggesting that at least one of the antigen specificities is common to each of these cells. This antigen target remains unknown. Biochemical characterization suggested a glycolipid target[10] and a monosialoganglioside was proposed as a candidate[11]. Sulfatides have also been suggested as an antigen specificity of ICAs[12], and some ICAs contain reactivity to glutamic acid decarboxylase (GAD)[13,14].

At least two ICA staining patterns have been observed[13,15]. Some ICAs stain predominantly β cells with a granular appearance (β-selective or restricted ICAs), whereas a second pattern appears less granular and stains all the endocrine cells within the islets (whole-islet ICAs). ICAs giving rise to the β-selective pattern can be further distinguished by their unreactivity to mouse islets[16]. A major antigen specificity of the β-selective ICA is GAD[13,14], which is also the antigen specificity of the immunoprecipitable 64 kDa islet protein[17]. GAD has also been shown to contribute to the staining of whole islet ICAs[18], and presumably in these sera, the combination of antibodies to several islet autoantigens results in a whole islet staining appearance. In some patients ICAs disappear soon after clinical onset of IDDM, possibly reflecting a progressive decline of the residual β-cell mass, whereas in others they persist indefinitely at high titers long after onset of disease[19]. At onset of IDDM ICAs are predominantly seen as a whole islet pattern[13,14], while ICAs which persist long after disease onset appear to be the GAD-specific β-selective type[14].

ICA IN THE PATHOGENESIS OF IDDM

The possible pathogenetic role of ICAs has been considered since they were first reported. In vitro complement-dependent antibody-mediated islet

---

Figure 4.1. *Opposite* Islet staining patterns by immunofluorescence. (A) ICA associated with IDDM; (B) islet staining by a serum with mitochondrial antibodies; (C–F) staining of islets by sera with anti-nuclear antibodies. C and D are stained with the same serum and are from the same cryostat section. E and F are stained with another serum and are from the same cryostat section. While in D and in F nuclear staining in both the islets and in exocrine tissue is clear, in C and E the nuclear staining in the islets is almost absent and staining appears cytoplasmic and may result in false positive ICA results

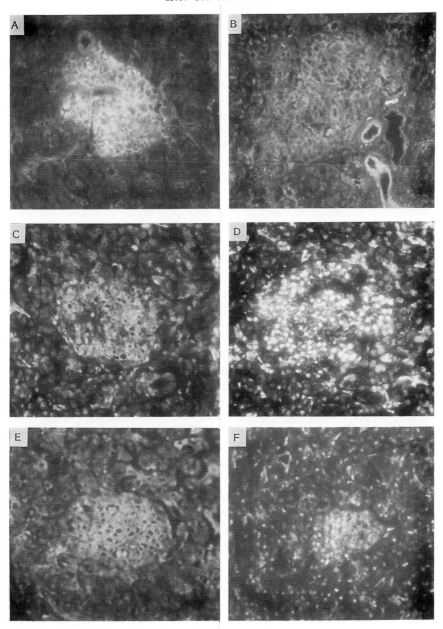

cytotoxicity[20-26], as well as antibody-dependent cell cytotoxicity[27,28] have been demonstrated in several experiments using human IDDM sera. In addition to cytotoxic effects, immunoglobulin from IDDM sera functionally affect β cells, interfering with the insulin response to glucose[29-34]. Purified immunoglobulin from the majority of patients was also shown to inhibit 3-O-methyl-glucose uptake by islet cells[35], and an IgM-mediated increased activity on β-cell calcium channels has been shown in sera from IDDM patients[36]. Despite these findings, and the demonstration of immunoglobulin and complement deposition within diabetic insulitis[37], it is now generally agreed that β-cell destruction is predominantly effected by cell-mediated immunity[38]. Supporting a lesser role of humoral activity is the lack of diabetes transfer by antibodies in experimental models, as well as the absence of diabetogenic effects on neonates from IDDM mothers with islet antibodies[39]. ICAs should, therefore, be considered markers of autoimmunity and not necessarily destructive immunity. This is important when considering the disease specificity of islet autoantibodies (see below).

MEASUREMENT OF ICA

THE ICA ASSAY

The standard assay used for the detection of ICAs is indirect immunofluorescence on cryostat sections of frozen unfixed human blood group O pancreas[40] The availability of suitable human pancreas substrate remains one of the intrinsic difficulties in the measurement of ICAs. Pancreata from other species, including rat and monkey, have been utilized, but since some interspecies differences have been demonstrated, the use of human pancreas remains almost obligatory. The tissue is best obtained from organ donors since experience shows that the longer the ischemia time the less suitable the pancreas is for use in the ICA assay. Pancreas obtained post-mortem is, therefore, usually unsuitable. Pancreas which has been subjected to chemical fixation is also unsuitable as the antigenicity of the ICA antigens is altered sufficiently to render them much less reactive with ICAs.

After removal, the pancreas should be kept ice-cold. Transport in a medium such as Collin's solution on ice is satisfactory. The tail of the pancreas is preferred as substrate, since it is the area containing the highest density of large islets. Therefore when processing the pancreas it is advisable to commence with the tail and proceed to the body of the pancreas, in order to keep ischemia time of the most suitable pancreas blocks to a minimum. A suggested procedure for processing is to slice approximately 1 cm from the beginning of the tail. While the remainder of the pancreas is kept in ice-cold solution, this slice is processed into blocks of around 5 mm cubes and each block frozen in a beaker of isopentane immersed in a dry ice/acetone slurry. At least 5 minutes after the last block is placed in isopentane should be allowed before the blocks are transferred to a −80°C freezer. The remainder of the pancreas can be processed in sequential 1 cm slices. For laboratories which do not have access to suitable material, at least one institute in Europe provides pre-tested pancreas blocks.

Unfortunately, not all pancreata processed immediately will be satisfactory for ICA measurement. Their suitability can be assessed by islet morphology, the number of islets per field, the detection limit using dilutions of ICA standard sera, background islet and exocrine staining of several normal sera, and the degree of islet autofluorescence which can interfere with the interpretation of islet staining. A further useful guide to preservation can be obtained by testing a serum with intermediate titers of antinuclear antibodies (ANAs), since variations in what is probably tissue preservation between different pancreata, different blocks and, strikingly, often different areas within the same section can be visualized by differences in ANA staining (Figure 4.1). Cutting of sections is best performed with a cryostat temperature of −18 to −2°C, an ambient temperature of around 20°C, and in an environment with little or no humidity. Summer, when laboratory temperature and humidity increase, can be a major source of poor tissue morphology and ICA reactivity. Cryostat sections should be 4–5 μm thick. They should be air dried for 15–30 minutes, preferably with a fan, to avoid further ice crystal artefact, and slides stored at −80°C. Upon removal from the freezer they should be air dried in front of a fan before use.

Several modifications to the originally described method have been reported[40]. Most of these have been in the type of secondary detection system used. A workshop aimed at determining whether these modifications altered assay performance found that apart from serum incubation time, methodologic differences between assays could not be correlated to eventual results[40]. Indirect immunofluorescence using a fluorescein-conjugated anti-human IgG remains the most commonly used method for ICA detection. Serum is often used undiluted in a screening assay and the incubation time can be divided into those assays with a short incubation time of around 30 minutes at room temperature, and those which use an overnight incubation at 4°C in the presence of a protease inhibitor such as aprotinin[41]. The latter method increases the analytical sensitivity of the assay and allows sera to be used diluted, thereby reducing background staining. When sera are used undiluted, longer washing times prior to the addition of fluoresceinated antibodies should be used to reduce background fluorescence. Anti-human IgG conjugates can vary substantially, and it is recommended that several be tried at varying dilutions before choosing the most suitable one.

Since ICAs are measured by immunofluorescence, they have been criticized, not unjustifiably, as being subject to reader bias. It is therefore important to render the reading and interpretation of results as objective as possible. Essential is the reading of slides in a "blinded" fashion. Systematic and uniform reading of the whole of each section and not just a few islets will also reduce reader bias. To reduce false negatives, islets must be recognized in each section, even if there is no islet staining. The use of a graded islet fluorescence intensity score rather than an assessment of positivity may also render results more objective. Quality control sera including replicates of more than one serum around the designated positive threshold, and negative sera should be tested randomly in each assay, and these can be used to interpret "positivity" of test sera after results have been unblinded. Most of the variability will be at low levels of antibody, and it is important that adequate quality control is applied around the threshold of positivity in order to avoid non-reproducibility and changes in assay performance over time. Assay validity will depend upon the experience of the reader, and the ability of the reader to be as objective as possible. It remains to be determined what makes a good reader, but color blindness is an obvious disadvantage.

Apart from variability in interpreting low levels of ICAs, false positives can occur due to interfering antibodies. The most common are ANAs and mitochondrial antibodies (Figure 4.1). Some ANAs can be particularly difficult as some of the nuclear antigens appear to leach into the cytoplasm. Cells within islets are more prone to this, and the ANAs may appear as a definite cytoplasmic islet cell staining with negative nuclei (Figure 1C and E). ICA in the presence of ANA can sometimes be confirmed by absorption of ANA from the serum with liver powder. Mitochondrial antibodies will appear as a general granular cytoplasmic staining throughout the section with islets staining more strongly. Their presence can be confirmed on liver and kidney sections. Islet fluorescence in the presence of mitochondrial antibodies cannot be interpreted unless it is considerably stronger than that in the exocrine cells. Some ICAs selectively stain glucagon or somatostatin cells within islets[42]. These are referred to as ICA2, and are not considered to be associated with IDDM. False negatives can arise when a serum gives high exocrine staining, since assessment of islet fluorescence is often made by comparison to that of exocrine cells. Excessive variability of exocrine staining between sera can be reduced by testing diluted serum.

INTERNATIONAL WORKSHOPS AND ICA QUANTIFICATION

Several international workshops aimed at the standardization of ICA measurement have been held[40, 43–46]. Initially they showed poor concordance between laboratories, particularly in sera with low titer ICAs, and wide scatter of titers reported in different laboratories[43]. It was subsequently demonstrated that these differences were contributed to by some laboratories having poor reproducibility, and by large systematic differences between laboratories due to variation in the detection limits[44]. It was concluded that laboratories with poor precision should not measure ICA until assay of replicates showed that they had improved, and that the systematic differences between laboratories with satisfactory precision could be reduced by comparison to a common standard.

The proposal, introduction, evaluation and eventual use of a reference Juvenile Diabetes Foundation (JDF) standard and JDF units has perhaps been the most significant step forward in ICA standardization[43,44]. Scatter of results between laboratories was reduced, and laboratories reported ICA in common units rather than gradations of positivity or titers which could not be compared between different studies. Several reference ICA standard preparations have now been evaluated and are available to the scientific community.

Workshop recommendations for ICA quantification in JDF units is by the use of a standard curve (Figure 4.2). Dilutions of the reference 80 JDF unit standard in negative serum to levels of 40, 20, 10, 5 and 2.5 JDF units and titration of each of these to end-point in the ICA assay allows construction of a standard curve by plotting the $\log_2$ of the JDF units versus the $\log_2$ of the reciprocal of the end-point titer[43]. The ICA titer of each test serum is interpolated into JDF units from the standard curve derived from the plot. Ideally, a standard curve should be included in each assay to minimize

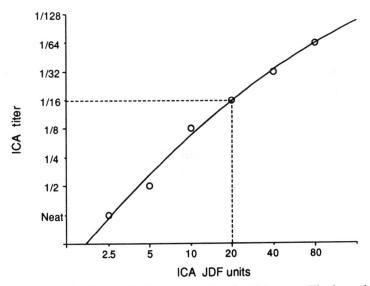

Figure 4.2. Example of a standard curve used in the ICA assay. The $\log_2$ of the JDF units for each standard are plotted against the $\log_2$ of the reciprocal ICA titer for each standard. A standard curve of best fit is calculated and the ICA titer of test samples is interpolated into JDF units from this curve. In the example shown, an ICA titer of 1/16 interpolates to 20 JDF units

between-assay systematic variation. Again, all standards and samples should be tested in a blinded fashion. To avoid depletion of reference standards, each laboratory must calibrate its own working standards against the reference preparation.

External validation of assay performance has also continued in the form of an ICA proficiency program (N Maclaren, Gainesville, Florida). Although there has been considerable improvement in the international measurement of ICA, there remains scatter between results from different laboratories, and as has been suggested[47], the inherent variability of pancreas substrate used may not allow such differences to be overcome.

ICA AND IDDM RISK ASSESSMENT

The onset of IDDM is usually preceded by a period in which several evidences for ongoing islet immunity, including ICA, are found[48]. This period is variable between patients but is commonly found to be several years. It remains unknown whether destruction of the β cells is ongoing during the whole of this pre-clinical phase of IDDM or whether this is restricted to certain periods. Studies of islet function suggest a variable rate of destruction during this phase[49]. Regardless of this, the pre-clinical phase is important since it gives the opportunity to identify individuals prior to insulin dependence, and at a time when their β-cell mass is sufficient to maintain physiological glucose metabolism. Clearly this gives rise to the possibility of intervention in order to halt further β-cell damage and prevent or delay clinical diabetes.

ICA AND RISK ASSESSMENT WITHIN FAMILIES

The earliest reports of ICAs preceding the onset of IDDM were in first degree relative of IDDM patients prospectively followed to disease[50,51]. The risk of IDDM is increased 10–20-fold within first degree relatives of IDDM patients resulting in an estimated risk before age 20 of around 3%[52]. The detection of ICA in first degree relatives is associated with substantially increased risk for disease[53]. ICAs are detected in around 5% of siblings, being more frequently detected in HLA- and haplo-identical siblings[54]. All prospective studies of first degree relatives have reported an increased risk in the presence of ICAs. The introduction of JDF units has allowed comparison between studies. The three largest reported population-based family studies which include quantified ICA—the Barts-Windsor/Barts-Oxford study[53], the Gainesville study[55], and the Finnish DiMe study[56]—show similar risks and a correlation of risk with the titer of ICA. High titer ICA (>80 JDF units) confers a risk for developing IDDM within 10 years of >50%, while the risk conferred by ICA <10 JDF units is less than 25%. The Finnish study has shown that the risk conferred by ICA >80 JDF units is high even in the absence of susceptible HLA haplotypes, while the risk conferred by lower titer ICAs is increased when susceptible haplotypes are also present[57]. Age has also been shown to modify risk, the highest risk being in younger relatives[55].

Recently, data from several family studies have been pooled in the ICA register user study (ICARUS) in order to more precisely define the risk of IDDM in first degree relatives with ICA, and to identify factors which may modify risk[58]. This ambitious effort has amassed data on over 500 relatives with ICAs. Quantification of ICAs in reference laboratories and life table analysis have produced risk estimates for developing IDDM within 5 years of 26% for any ICA >5 JDF units, rising to 34% for ICA >20 JDF units and 43% for ICA >80 JDF units.

The measurement of ICAs in first degree relatives of IDDM patients is now an established screening test used to identify persons at risk for developing IDDM, and therefore eligible to enter into clinical trials designed to evaluate therapies for IDDM prevention. The importance given to ICA measurement is exemplified by its use in the European Nicotinamide Diabetes Intervention Trial (ENDIT), where eligibility is based on the detection of ICA >10 JDF units on at least two occasions (EAM Gale, personal communication), and in the Diabetes Prevention Trial in the USA (DPT-1), where ICA ≥10 JDF units and low first phase insulin are prerequisites for eligibility. Often we consider the implications and trauma associated with the finding of positivity in family members, but sometimes overlooked is the benefit of the absence of detectable ICAs, which, provided the threshold for positivity is low, is associated with a risk similar to that of the general population. This is important when counseling family members participating in prospective studies.

ICA AND IDDM RISK ASSESSMENT IN THE GENERAL POPULATION

Since the majority of cases of IDDM occur before age 20, screening in the general population implies testing the childhood population. Large studies are few and consequently it remains controversial whether the risk conferred by ICA in the absence of a family history of IDDM will be the same as in first degree relatives of IDDM patients. Two studies in which school children have been prospectively followed for 8–10 years suggest that detection of ICAs in school children is as predictive of IDDM as in the higher risk first degree relatives[59,60]. In particular, the Gainsville study directly compared the predictive value of ICA >10 JDF units found in 57 of 9696 school children screened with that in 103 of 2959 age matched first degree relatives screened. Ten of the school children and 31 of the relatives developed IDDM. The estimated risk in the school children with ICA was 28% at 5 years follow-up compared to 38% in the relatives[60].

The controversy is not whether the detection of ICA in children without a family history of IDDM is associated with increased risk for disease, but how high is the risk in these children, and arises from other studies which have determined ICA prevalences in the general school age population. Unlike that of the Gainesville study, where ICA was found at a frequency around twice the prevalence of IDDM, several studies have reported ICA prevalences much higher than IDDM prevalence. In particular, 4% of 1218 Finnish school children[61], 2.9% of 2925 English school children[62] and 1.8% of 8363 French school children[63] had ICA. These are around 10-fold the IDDM risk in those countries[64]. The differences in ICA prevalences may reflect true population differences, but are also likely to be due to different thresholds of detection used in the studies. Indeed, if a similar threshold of >10 JDF units on two occasions was used in our own study in the Oxford region, we find 30 (1%) of the school children positive (unpublished observations). This is closer to that of the Gainesville study, but the estimated risk of developing IDDM before age 20 is less than 20% which is less than half that in first degree relatives from the same region[65]. Differences may also reflect the difficulty of measuring low level ICAs and raise the possibility of non-specific interfering antibodies which may be more readily detected in some ICA assays or populations. We should consider that ICAs have more than one specificity, and that some of these may not be IDDM specific.

Despite the differences, it is clear that ICAs will be a valuable screening test to at least pre-select an at risk population which can be further assessed with other markers[66]. How good a screening test ICA will be in the general childhood population requires more large studies. Again, pooling of data in an ICARUS-like effort should more precisely define this risk assessment.

THRESHOLD FOR POSITIVITY

The predictive value of a test directly correlates with its sensitivity and specificity, and the prevalence of the disease in the population studied. Since the prevalence of IDDM in the general population is at least 10 times lower than in persons with a family history of the disease, mathematically, the predictive value of ICA for development of IDDM should be decreased when used to screen the general population. As we have seen, this may not always be the case, and will depend upon the specificity and sensitivity of ICA in that population.

The indirect relationship between sensitivity and specificity of markers is well established, as is the dependence of these parameters on the threshold selected for positivity. Threshold does not distinguish the presence or absence of antibodies, but represents a point which maximizes the clinical utility of results. This will vary, depending upon the purpose of the test. For example, selection of individuals for clinical trials is more likely to require a low false positive rate and therefore high specificity. This is most easily achieved by raising the threshold for positivity. Clearly, however, sensitivity will be reduced[66], and in order to recruit sufficient individuals for clinical trials, substantially more individuals will need to be screened. Furthermore, if a successful intervention therapy becomes available, its application to the general population will have a significant impact on public health only if sufficient cases are treated, and therefore high sensitivity will be required. We can, of course, improve sensitivity and specificity by the use of several markers in parallel and series (see below and subsequent chapters).

The question at hand is: What threshold should be used for the ICA test? The answer is whatever level provides the user with the sensitivity and predictive value required for his or her purposes. In the case of screening in the DPT-1 trial, the required predictive value or risk assessment was >50% in 5 years. As mentioned, several criteria and thresholds for ICA can be used. A threshold of 80 JDF units will give sufficient risk regardless of the presence or absence of other markers. A threshold of 10 JDF units was chosen to select those eligible based on ICA plus low first phase insulin response. In the European insulin trial, a risk assessment of 75% was chosen, and several thresholds are applied depending upon whether ICA alone (>40 JDF units) or ICA (>10 JDF units) plus low first phase insulin response is used to select eligible children.

These are examples of screening in first degree relatives. Let us examine the case when screening the general population. In the Gainesville study, the predictive value of ICA >10 JDF units on two occasions for developing IDDM within 7 years was 45%. This is, however, an estimate. The 95% confidence interval (CI) of this estimate is 15–74%. Although the estimate appears the same as that in first degree relatives with ICA (43%; 95%CI 22–63%), the large confidence intervals make any comparison statistically weak. In essence, the Type 2 error (probability of not detecting a difference, when in fact there is one) is high. The Gainesville study, however, is by no means small, but more precise risk estimates can only be achieved by screening even larger numbers.

Recently we made an estimate of how many need to be screened[67]. If a test which had a sensitivity of around 80% was applied to the general childhood population in the UK where the overall risk for developing IDDM before age 20 is around 0.3%, the positive predictive value of the test would rise to above 50% only if it was positive in less than 0.5% of those screened. To be 95% certain that the prevalence of a marker is <0.5%, we need to test around 3000 subjects if it is detected in 0.2%, and around 40 000 if it is found in 0.4%. In order to set our threshold for 95% certainty that the prevalence is less than

0.5%, we would test our population of 3000, and find the point where only six (0.2%) remain positive. In our study, a threshold of >80 JDF units identifies seven (0.24%) of 2925 school children. This comes close, but we must remember the inverse relationship between sensitivity and specificity. A threshold of >80 JDF units identifies less than 20% of those who develop IDDM in the UK, and therefore the predictive value would be substantially reduced[67]. We are therefore forced to test much larger numbers. Interestingly, only one of these seven has developed IDDM in 4 years of follow-up. Elliot and colleagues recently communicated ICA screening in over 30 000 New Zealand children[68]. Around 0.2% had ICA >40 JDF units. Such a threshold in their population appears, therefore, to define a risk for IDDM which may be >50%. Without laboring the point further, the message is that 100 controls is adequate for establishing association, but not for estimating risk.

THRESHOLD FOR POSITIVITY VERSUS DETECTION LIMIT

A further criterion for the selection of thresholds is the detection limit of the assay used. Many laboratories have the habit of setting their threshold very close to the detection limit of their assay. This, however, is dangerous, since normal between-assay variation is likely to change the detection limit, and hence threshold, and dramatically affect specificity and sensitivity. Secondly, interpretation of non-specific or interfering islet fluorescence may substantially affect the number of false positives. Therefore, for "safety" it is wise to use a threshold sufficiently far from the results of the majority of normals so as to minimize the risk of false positives due to interfering antibodies and, importantly, "drift". This is particularly so when screening populations where disease prevalence is very low, since a very small decrease in specificity will markedly reduce the predictive value.

The same argument applies to other antibody assays including the measurement of IAAs and GAD antibodies (GADAs). Our own GADA data illustrate this well. The upper first percentile of controls corresponds to a readout of 217 cpm. A drift of only 20 cpm would reduce the specificity from 99% to 95%, and a drift of 40 cpm to 80%. Clearly, quality control needs to be heavily directed at maintaining precision and accuracy at the chosen threshold(s) for positivity.

Although the issue has long been debated, the question of how low a level of ICA the assay should detect is less ambiguous than what threshold should be used? The answer is as low as possible. I will go as far as to suggest that an assay that cannot detect at least 5 JDF units is not suitable for ICA measurement. The principal reason is that, as we have discussed, one of the critical factors in assay detection limit is the "quality" of the pancreas substrate used. An assay which has a detection limit of 20 JDF units, may in all probability do so because of poor tissue substrate which is equivalent to a poor antigen preparation. An assay which detects very low levels of ICAs does not necessarily have low specificity as the user has the possibility to adjust the detection limit by increasing the serum dilution, or more appropriately, increase the threshold for positivity far away from the detection limit of the assay by quantification in JDF units.

ICA IN COMBINATION WITH OTHER MARKERS

Testing for other markers in ICA-positive individuals to increase the specificity has been suggested in many forms and is now used in screening strategies for clinical trials. As long as the marker(s) used are associated with IDDM and found in only a subset of those with ICAs, specificity will be increased. The most commonly used are a family history of IDDM, the additional detection of IAAs, and low first phase insulin response (see revue in reference 66). These are discussed in other chapters. Again, it should be remembered that while the specificity will be increased, a number of cases will be lost, since not all those who develop IDDM will have the combination of markers.

We have recently examined the value of using other islet antibody markers to improve risk assessment in relatives with ICA >10 JDF units. Not unexpectedly, what is clearly apparent is that the greater the number of antibody specificities, the greater the risk for developing IDDM[65]. In a separate study[69], we confirm that the ICA screening test can identify around 90% of newly diagnosed patients and first degree relatives progressing to disease. Interestingly, all cases with ICA, including those with very low levels, also had either antibodies to GAD and/or to 37 000/40 000 M_r islet tryptic fragments (anti-37K)[70] (Figure 4.3). In contrast, only 17 (49%) of 35 first degree relatives with ICA >10 JDF units who have not developed IDDM in over 5 years of follow-up (unpublished observations) and 6 (15%) of 40 school children with ICA >10 JDF units also had at least one of these other antibodies[71]. We are tempted to conclude, therefore, that ICAs in the absence of both GADA and anti-37K are not associated with disease, again emphasizing that not all ICA specificities may be strongly associated with IDDM. The very strong link of anti-37K with ICA also suggests that this is one of the relevant ICA specificities.

FUTURE

Probably since the discovery of ICAs, investigators have been searching for a replacement, either through the identification of ICA antigen specificities or

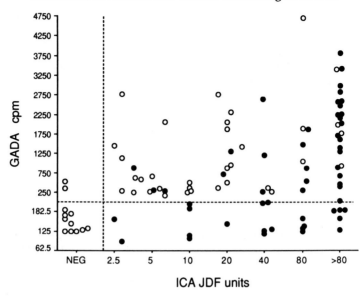

Figure 4.3. Islet autoantibodies in sera from 100 newly diagnosed IDDM patients. The filled symbols represent those in which antibodies to islet 37 000/40 000 M_r tryptic fragments were detected. The upper percentile of 83 control sera are represented by the broken lines at 2 JDF units for ICA and 217 cpm for GADA

another marker. The fact is that the ICA assay is not favored by all. As we have discussed, it relies on semi-quantitative titration, the interpretation of islet fluorescence is subject to reader bias, results are dependent upon pancreas substrate and remain difficult to standardize, many laboratories cannot measure low levels consistently, and ICAs contain more than one specificity, not all of which may be associated with IDDM. Furthermore, its application to the screening of the general population is relatively laborious. As a replacement, GADAs are an obvious candidate and will be discussed in subsequent chapters. Our own studies using recently developed assays show very high sensitivity in adult onset cases of IDDM, but sensitivity appears significantly lower than that of ICA in childhood onset cases of IDDM[69]. Clearly, however, the recently described GADA assays have enormous potential, allow mass screening, and do not suffer from many of the difficulties associated with the ICA assay. Their value should be further improved when other relevant antigens, such as the 37K antigen[72], are identified and can be incorporated into the GADA assay thereby offering a single rapid screening test for IDDM risk assessment[73]. One suspects, however, that identification of antibodies down the microscope still has a substantial amount to offer in improving risk assessment of IDDM.

NOTE

Since writing this chapter, the islet 37/40 Kda autoantigen has been identified as the protein tyrosine phosphatase-like IA2 (islet cell antigen 512) and as one of the targets of cytoplasmic ICAs[73].

REFERENCES

1 Eisenbarth GS. Type 1 diabetes mellitus: a chronic autoimmune disease. *N Engl J Med* 1986; **314**: 1360–8.
2 Gepts W. Pathologic anatomy of the pancreas in juvenile diabetes mellitus. *Diabetes* 1965; **14**: 619–33.
3 Bottazzo GF, Florin-Christensen A, Doniach D. Islet cell antibodies in diabetes mellitus with autoimmune polyendrocrine deficiency. *Lancet* 1974; ii: 1279–83.
4 Lendrum R, Walker IG, Gamble DR. Islet cell antibodies in juvenile diabetes mellitus of recent onset. *Lancet* 1975; I: 880–2.
5 Landin-Olsson M, Karlsson A, Dahlquist G, Blom L, Lernmark A, Sundkvist G. Islet cell and other organ-specific autoantibodies in all children developing Type I (insulin-dependent) diabetes mellitus in Sweden during one year and in matched control children. *Diabetologia* 1989; **32**: 387–95.
6 Bosi E, Bonifacio E. Autoantibodies in insulin-dependent diabetes mellitus. *J Endocrinol Invest* 1994; **17**: 521–31.
7 Schatz DA, Barrett DJ, Maclaren NK, Riley WJ. Polyclonal nature of islet cell antibodies in insulin-dependent diabetes. *Autoimmunity* 1989; **1**: 45–50.
8 Dozio N, Belloni C, Girardi AM, Genovese S, Sodoyez JC, Bottazzo GF, Pozza G, Bosi E. Heterogeneous IgG subclass distribution of islet cell antibodies. *J Autoimmun* 1994; **7**: 45–53.
9 Bottazzo GF, Dean BM, Gorsuch AN, Cudworth AG, Doniach D. Complement-fixing islet-cell antibodies in Type I diabetes: possible monitors of active beta-cell damage. *Lancet* 1980; i: 668–72.
10 Nayak RS, Omar MAK, Rabizadeh A, Srikanta S, Eisenbarth GS. "Cytoplasmic" islet cell antibodies: evidence that the target antigen is a sialoglycoconjugate. *Diabetes* 1984; **34**: 617–19.
11 Colman PG, Nayak RC, Campbell IL, Eisenbarth GS. Binding of 'cytoplasmic' islet cell antibodies is blocked by human pancreatic glycolipid extracts. *Diabetes* 1988; **37**: 645.
12 Buschard K, Josefsen K, Horn T, Fredman P. Sulphatide and sulphatide antibodies in insulin dependent diabetes mellitus. *Lancet* 1993; **342**: 840.
13 Genovese S, Bonifacio E, McNally JM, Dean BM, Wagner R, Bosi E, Gale EAM, Bottazzo GF. Distinct cytoplasmic islet cell antibodies with different risks for type 1 (insulin-dependent) diabetes mellitus. *Diabetologia* 1992; **35**: 385–8.
14 Atkinson MA, Kaufman DL, Newman D, Tobin AJ, Maclaren NK. Islet cell cytoplasmic autoantibody reactivity to glutamate decarboxylase in insulin-dependent diabetes. *J Clin Invest* 1993; **91**: 350–6.
15 Timsit J, Caillat-Zucman S, Blondel H, Chédin P, Bach JF, Boitard C. Islet cell antibody heterogeneity among Type 1 (insulin-dependent) diabetic patients. *Diabetologia* 1992; **35**: 792–5.
16 Gianani R, Pugliese A, Bonner-Weir S, Shiffrin AJ, Soeldner JS, Erlich H, Awdeh Z,

Alper CA, Jackson RA, Eisenbarth GS. Prognostically significant heterogeneity of cytoplasmic islet cell antibodies in relatives of patients with type I diabetes. *Diabetes* 1992; **41**: 347–53.

17 Baekkeskov S, Aanstoot HJ, Christgau S, Reetz A, Solimena M, Cascalho M, Folli F, Richter-Olesen H, de Camilli P. Identification of the 64K autoantigen in insulin-dependent diabetes as the GABA-synthesizing enzyme glutamic acid decarboxylase. *Nature* 1990; **347**: 151–6.

18 Marshall MO, Moyer PE, Petersen JS, Hejnaes KR, Genovese S, Dyrberg T, Bottazzo GF. Contribution of glutamate decarboxylase antibodies to the reactivity of cytoplasmic islet cell antibodies. *J Autoimmun* 1994; **7**: 497–508.

19 Lendrum R, Walker IG, Cudworth AG, Theophanides C, Pyke DA, Bloom A, Gamble DR. Islet cell antibodies in diabetes mellitus. *Lancet* 1976; **ii**: 1273–6.

20 Dobersen MJ, Scharff JE, Ginsberg-Fellner F, Notkins AL. Cytotoxic autoantibodies to beta-cells in the serum of patients with insulin dependent diabetes mellitus. *N Engl J Med* 1980; **303**: 1493–8.

21 Lernmark A, Sehlin J, Taljedal IB, Kromann H, Nerup J. Possible toxic effects of normal and diabetic patient serum on pancreatic B-cells. *Diabetologia* 1978; **14**: 25–31.

22 Rittenhouse HG, Oxender DL, Pek S, Ar D. Complement mediated cytotoxic effects on pancreatic islets with sera from diabetic patients. *Diabetes* 1980; **29**: 317–22.

23 Eisenbarth GS, Morris MA, Scearce RM. Cytotoxic antibodies to cloned rat islet cells in serum of patients with diabetes mellitus. *J Clin Invest* 1981; **67**: 403–8.

24 Kanatsuna T, Freedman ZR, Rubenstein AH, Lernmark A. Effect of islet cell surface antibodies and complement on the release of insulin and chromium from perifused β cells. *Clin Exp Immunol* 1982; **47**: 85–92.

25 Dobersen MJ, Scharff JE. Preferential lysis of pancreatic β-cells by islet cell surface antibodies. *Diabetes* 1982; **31**: 459–62.

26 Toguchi Y, Ginsberg-Fellner F, Rubinstein P. Cytotoxic islet cell surface antibodies (ICSA) in patients with type I diabetes and their first degree relatives. *Diabetes* 1985; **34**: 855–60.

27 Maruyama T, Takei I, Matsuba I, Tsuruoka A, Taniyama M, Ikeda Y, Kataoka K, Abe M, Matsuki S. Cell-mediated cytotoxic islet cell surface antibodies to human pancreatic beta cells. *Diabetologia* 1984; **26**: 30–3.

28 Michaelis D, Rjasanowski I, Helmke B, Kohnert KD, Hildman W, Keilacker H, Richter KV. Lack of strong association between residual human C-peptide secretion and islet cell antibodies, complement-dependent antibody-mediated cytotoxicity and HLA antigens in newly diagnosed type I diabetics. *Biomed Biochim Acta* 1985; **44**: 99–105.

29 Kanatsuna T, Lernmark A, Rubenstein AH, Steiner D. Block in insulin release from column-perfused pancreatic beta cells induced by islet cell surface antibodies and complement. *Diabetes* 1981; **30**: 231–4.

30 Sai P, Boitard C, Debray-Sachs M, Pouplard A, Assan R, Hamburger J. Complement-fixing islet cell antibodies from some diabetic patients alter insulin release in vitro. *Diabetes* 1981; **30**: 1051–7.

31 Kanatsuna T, Baekkeskov S, Lernmark A, Ludvigsson J. Immunoglobulin from insulin dependent diabetic children inhibits glucose-induced insulin release. *Diabetes* 1983; **32**: 520–4.

32 Sensi M, Zuccarini O, Spencer KM, Beales P, Pujol-Borrell R, Pozzilli P. In vitro inhibition of insulin release mediated by sera with complement-fixing islet cell antibodies belonging to normal first degree relatives of patients with type I diabetes. *Diabetes Res* 1985; **2**: 1–6.

33 Svenningsen A, Dyrberg, T, Gerling, I, Lernmark A, Mackay P, Rabinovitch A.

Inhibition of insulin release after passive transfer of immunoglobulin from insulin dependent diabetic children to mice. *J Clin Endocrinol Metab* 1983; **57**: 1301–4.

34 Boitard C, Sai P, Debray-Sachs M, Assan R, Hamburger J. Anti-pancreatic immunity. In vitro studies of cellular and humoral immune reactions directed towards pancreatic islets. *Clin Exp Immunol* 1984; **55**: 571–80.

35 Johnson JH, Crider BP, McCorki K, Alford M, Unger RH. Inhibition of glucose transport into rat islet cells by immunoglobulins from patients with new-onset insulin-dependent diabetes mellitus. *N Engl J Med* 1990; **322**: 653–9.

36 Juntti-Berggren L, Larsson O, Rorsman P, Ammala C, Bokvist K, Wahlander K, Nicotera P, Dypbukt J, Orrenius S, Hallberg A, Berggren PO. Increased activity of L-type Ca^{2+} channels exposed to serum from patients with type I diabetes. *Science* 1993; **261**: 86–90.

37 Bottazzo GF, Dean BM, McNally JM, Mackay EH, Swift PGF, Gamble DR. In situ characterization of autoimmune phenomena and expression of HLA molecules in the pancreas in diabetic insulitis. *N Engl J Med* 1985; **313**: 353–60.

38 Bach JF. Insulin-dependent diabetes mellitus as an autoimmune disease. *Endocrine Rev* 1994; **15**: 516–42.

39 Tingle AJ, Lim G, Wright VJ, Dimmick JE, Hunt JA. Transplacental passage of islet cell antibody in infants of diabetic mothers. *Pediatr Res* 1979; **13**: 1323–7.

40 Gleichmann H, Bottazzo GF. Progress towards standardization of cytoplasmic islet-cell antibody assays. *Diabetes* 1987; **36**: 578–84.

41 Pilcher C and Elliot RB. Improved sensitivity of islet cell cytoplasmic antibody assay in diabetes. *Lancet* 1984; **i**: 1352.

42 Bottazzo GF, Lendrum R. Separate antibodies to human pancreatic glucagon and somatostatin cells. *Lancet* 1976; **ii**: 873–6.

43 Bottazzo GF, Gleichmann H. Immunology and Diabetes Workshops: report of the first international workshop on the standardisation of cytoplasmic islet cell antibodies *Diabetologia* 1986; **29**: 125.

44 Bonifacio E, Lernmark A, Dawkins RL et al. Serum exchange and use of dilutions have improved precision of measurement of islet cell antibodies. *J Immunol Methods* 1988; **106**: 83–8.

45 Bonifacio E, Boitard C, Gleichmann H, Shattock MA, Molenaar JL, Bottazzo GF. Assessment of precision, concordance, specificity and sensitivity of islet cell antibody measurement in 41 assays. *Diabetologia* 1990; **33**: 731–6.

46 Greenbaum CJ, Palmer JP, Nagataki S, Yamaguchi Y, Molenaar JL, Van Beers WAM, Maclaren NK, Lernmark A, and participating laboratories. Improved specificity of ICA assays in the Fourth International Immunology of Diabetes Serum Exchange Workshop. *Diabetes* 1992; **41**: 1570–4.

47 Landin-Olsson M. Precision of the islet cell antibody assay depends on the pancreas. *J Clin Lab Anal* 1990; **4**: 289–94.

48 Colman PG, Eisenbarth GS Immunology of type 1 diabetes: 1987. In Alberti KGGM, Krall LP (eds), *Diabetes Annual*, Vol 4. Amsterdam: Elsevier, 1988, pp 17–45.

49 McCulloch DK, Klaff LJ, Kahn SE, Schoenfield SL, Greenbaum CJ, Mauseth RS, Benson EA, Nepom GT, Shewey L, Palmer JP. Nonprogression of subclinical β-cell dysfunction among first degree relatives of IDDM patients: 5-yr follow-up of the Seattle family study. *Diabetes* 1990; **39**: 549–56.

50 Gorsuch AN, Spencer KM, Lister J, McNally JM, Dean BM, Bottazzo GF, Cudworht AG. Evidence for a long prediabetic period in type 1 (insulin-dependent) diabetes mellitus. *Lancet* 1981; **ii**: 1363–5.

51 Srikanta S, Ganda OP, Rabizideh A, Soeldner JS, Eisenbarth GS. First-degree relatives of patients with type 1 diabetes mellitus: islet-cell antibodies and

abnormal insulin secretion. *N Engl J Med* 1985; **313**: 462–4.
52 Bingley PJ, Gale EAM. The incidence of insulin-dependent diabetes in England: a study in the Oxford region 1985–6. *Br Med J* 1989; **298**: 558–60.
53 Bonifacio E, Bingley PG, Shattock M, Dean BM, Dunger D, Gale EAM, Bottazzo GF. Quantification of islet cell antibodies and prediction of insulin-dependent diabetes. *Lancet* 1990; **335**: 147–9.
54 Tarn AC, Thomas JM, Dean BM, Ingram D, Scharz G, Bottazzo GF, Gale EAM. Predicting insulin-dependent diabetes *Lancet* 1988; **i**: 845–50.
55 Riley WJ, Maclaren NK, Krischer J, Spillar RP, Silverstein JH, Desmond A, Schatz DA, Schwartz S, Malone J, Shar S, Vadheim C, Rotter JI. A prospective study of the development of diabetes in relatives of patients with insulin-dependent diabetes. *N Engl J Med* 1990; **323**: 1167–72.
56 Knip M, Vahasalo P, Karjalainen J, Lounamaa R, Akerblom HK, and the Childhood Diabetes in Finland Study Group. Natural history of preclinical IDDM in high risk siblings. *Diabetologia* 1994; **37**: 388–93.
57 Reijonen H, Vahasalo P, Ilonen J, Knip M, Akerblom HK, The Childhood Diabetes in Finland Study Group. HLA-DQB1 genotyping and islet cell antibodies in identification of siblings at IDDM risk. (Abstract) 13th International Immunology and Diabetes Workshop, 1994.
58 Bingley PJ. Interaction of risk markers in ICA + family members: the first analysis of the ICARUS dataset. (Abstract) 13th International Immunology and Diabetes Workshop, 1994.
59 Bruining GJ, Molenaar JL, Grobee D, Hoffman A, Scheffer SJ, Bruining HA, de Bruyn AM, Valkenburg HA. Ten year follow up study of islet cells antibodies and childhood diabetes mellitus. *Lancet* 1989; **i**: 1100–3.
60 Schatz D, Krischer J, Horne G, Riley W, Spillar R, Silverstein J, Winter W, Muir A, Derovanesian D, Shah S, Malone J, Maclaren N. Islet cell antibodies predict insulin-dependent diabetes in United States school age children as powerfully as in unaffected relatives. *J Clin Invest* 1994; **93**: 2403–7.
61 Karjalainen J. Islet cell antibodies as predictive markers for IDDM in children with high background incidence of disease. *Diabetes* 1990; **39**: 1144–50.
62 Bingley PJ, Bonifacio E, Shattock M, Gillmor HA, Sawtell PA, Dunger DB, Scott RDM, Bottazzo GF, Gale EAM. Can islet cell antibodies predict IDDM in the general population? *Diabetes Care* 1993; **16**: 45–50.
63 Levy-Marchal C, Tichet J, Fajardy I, Gu XF, Dubois F, Czernichow P. Islet cell antibodies in normal French school-children. *Diabetologia* 1992; **35**: 577–82.
64 Green A, Gale EAM, Patterson CC, the EURODIAB Subarea A Study Group. Incidence of childhood-onset diabetes mellitus: The EURODIAB ACE Study. *Lancet* 1992; **339**: 905–9.
65 Bingley PJ, Christie MR, Bonifacio E, Bonfanti R, Shattock M, Fonte MT, Bottazzo GF, Gale EAM. Combined analysis of autoantibodies improves prediction of IDDM in islet cell antibody positive relatives. *Diabetes* 1994; **43**: 1304–10.
66 Bingley PJ, Bonifacio E, Gale EAM. Can we really predict IDDM? *Diabetes* 1993; **42**: 213–20.
67 Bingley PJ, Bonifacio E, Gale EAM. Antibodies to glutamic acid decarboxylase as predictors of insulin-dependent diabetes mellitus. *Lancet* 1994; **344**: 266.
68 Elliot RB, Pilcher CC, Mcgregor M. Predictive value of islet cell antibodies in a population of 'normal' schoolchildren. (Abstract) 13th International Immunology and Diabetes Workshop, 1994.
69 Bonifacio E, Genovese S, Braghi S, Bazzigaluppi E, Lampasona V, Bingley PJ, Rogge L, Pastore MR, Bognetti E, Bottazzo GF, Gale EAM, Bosi E. Islet autoantibody

markers in insulin dependent diabetes: identification of screening strategies yielding high sensitivity Diabetologia 1995; **38**: 816–22.

70 Christie MR, Vohra G, Champagne P, Daneman D, Delovitch TL. Distinct antibody specificities to a 64-kD islet cell antigen in Type 1 diabetes as revealed by trypsin treatment. *J Exp Med* 1990; **172**; 789–95.

71 Genovese S, Bingley PJ, Bonifacio E, Christie MR, Shattock M, Bonfanti, R, Foxon R, Gale EAM, Bottazzo GF. Combined analysis of IDDM-related autoantibodies in healthy schoolchildren. *Lancet* 1994; **344**: 756.

72 Payton MA, Hawkes CJ, Christie MR. Relationship of the 37,000- and 40,000-M2 tryptic fragments of islet antigens in insulin-dependent diabetes to the protein tyrosine phosphatase-like molecule 1A-2 (ICA512). *J Clin Invest* 1995; **96**: 1506–11.

73 Bonifacio E, Lampasona V, Genovese S, Ferrari M, Bosi E. Identification of protein tyrosine phosphatase-like 1A2 (islet cell antigen 512) as the insulin-dependent diabetes-related 37/40 kDa autoantigen and a target of islet cell antibodies. *J Immunol* 1995; **155**: 5419–26.

5

Humoral Immune Markers: Insulin Autoantibodies

CARLA J. GREENBAUM[1] and JERRY P. PALMER[2]

[1]Department of Medicine, University of Washington, Seattle, USA and [2]Division of Endocrinology, Metabolism and Nutrition, Seattle Veterans Affairs Medical Center, Seattle, USA

DISCOVERY AND DEFINITION

Antibodies that bind to insulin in subjects that are insulin-naive are termed insulin autoantibodies (IAAs). By definition, these antibodies are distinguished from insulin antibodies (IAs) which are seen after insulin administration. First described in a 1963 report, IAAs were found in 34% of a group of insulin untreated Type 1 and Type 2 patients and 4% of controls[1]. Both this initial finding and several subsequent case reports in the early 1970s were largely dismissed. In 1983, however, we published data demonstrating that at least 18% of newly diagnosed, untreated, subjects with Type 1 diabetes had insulin autoantibodies[2].

Since our report, many papers have appeared not only confirming the presence of IAA in newly diagnosed Type 1 subjects, but also demonstrating that these autoantibodies are present in non-diabetic subjects and have predictive power in determining who will subsequently develop clinical disease.

METHODS

Nonetheless, the past decade has seen the publication of conflicting reports regarding the prevalence of IAAs in various subject groups and the value of IAAs in predicting the development of clinical IDDM. It is now apparent that

Prediction, Prevention and Genetic Counseling in IDDM. Edited by Jerry P. Palmer.
© 1996 John Wiley & Sons Ltd.

many of the differences in these papers were due to the methods used to measure IAA. IAA has been measured by either a fluid-phase radioimmunoassay (RIA) or a solid-phase, enzyme-linked immunoabsorbent assay (ELISA). There are several theoretical reasons why these assays may be measuring different populations of antibodies. In a fluid-phase assay, most of the epitopes on the insulin molecule are available for binding; in contrast, in the solid-phase assay since insulin is bound to the plates some epitopes are inaccessible (Figure 5.1). Additionally, a RIA technique generally measures high affinity antibodies, while the ELISA measures antibodies of lower affinity.

The prediction that these inherent differences in antibody measurement technique in fact result in measurements of different populations of antibodies has now been confirmed. Early international immunology workshops on the standardization of IAA demonstrated that each method obtained different results when measuring the same sera[3,4]. Subsequent workshops compared results from RIA and ELISA laboratories on sera from newly diagnosed patients, non-diabetic subjects who subsequently developed IDDM, first degree relatives of IDDM patients and normal controls. Both techniques had a very low frequency of IAA in control sera. However, the laboratories using RIA methods found a much higher percentage of sera to be IAA positive among both newly diagnosed patients and individuals who later developed diabetes than laboratories using ELISA methods. Interestingly, there was considerable overlap in the percentage of sera from first degree relatives found positive by both assays and each assay type found different sera

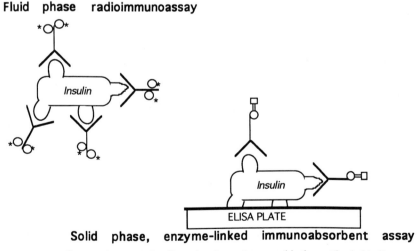

Some epitopes on insulin molecule are inaccessible for antibody binding

Figure 5.1. Possible explanation for differences in insulin autoantibody measurements between RIA and ELISA assays

positive among the first degree relatives. This workshop data strongly suggest that IAA measured by RIA methods are more disease related than those measured by ELISA and therefore should be used in studies to predict subsequent IDDM or in assigning individual risk[5] (Figure 5.2). These differences do not appear to be accounted for by iodination site for the RIA method[6]. The fact that the ELISA laboratories still were very specific in their measurements (i.e. very few controls were positive), and that they are clearly measuring antibodies in relatives of IDDM subjects leaves open the possibility that these assays may provide useful information in future studies.

The 5th international immunology workshop tested whether the use of a standard serum or monoclonal antibody would improve the variation between RIA laboratories worldwide. The workshop report concluded that these standards did not improve differences, and suggested that results could be reported either as raw data expressed as percent binding or as a standard deviation score[7].

One of at least two RIA methods is now generally used to determine IAA in association with IDDM. In one, 160 lambda of test serum is used. An acid charcoal extraction is performed to remove any insulin that may be bound to antibodies in the serum. The serum is then incubated overnight with about 20 000 cpm of labeled insulin. After washing twice with polyethylene glycol (PEG) the precipitate is counted in the gamma counter for 3 minutes. The count of precipitated bound insulin, divided by the total count, determines the percent binding for each sample. Data can also be expressed as number of standard deviations from the mean of a group of control sera. The other commonly used RIA method requires 600 lambda of test serum. No acid charcoal extraction is performed. About 10 000 cpm of labeled insulin is added to the sera and incubated for 7 days. After three washings with PEG, the precipitate is counted for 9 minutes. In general, there appears to be good correlation between these two methods using results expressed as standard deviations from a control population; however, work is continuing to analyze differences in results with selected serum. It appears that a major reason for concordance between these two methods is that both use a displacement step which allows measurement of specific versus non-specific binding. We have shown that when a cold displacement step is added to IAA determination, both sensitivity and specificity are improved[8].

ETIOLOGY

It is not known why insulin autoantibodies are found in association with the IDDM disease process. Insulin autoantibodies could be involved in autoimmune disease as initiators of the disease process, as effectors causing the actual immune destruction, or as a consequence of the β-cell destruction. When

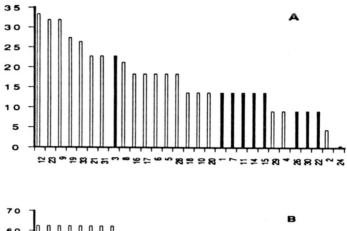

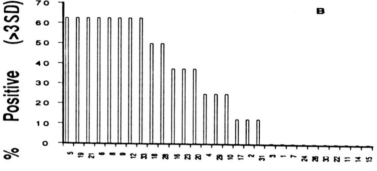

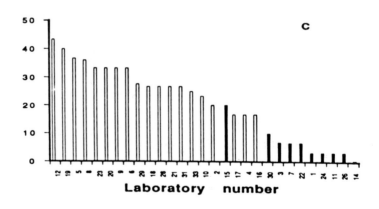

Figure 5.2. Percentage of IAA positive (>3 SD from mean of controls) sera from first degree relatives of IDDM patient probands (A; *n*=22), healthy subjects who later developed IDDM (B; *n*=8) and newly diagnosed IDDM patients (C; *n*=30) in 19 RIA (□) and 10 ELISA (■) laboratories[37]

autoimmune disease occurs, they may also be present as markers without being directly involved.

Initiation of autoimmunity occurs when the immune system loses tolerance and responds to a self-antigen as if it were foreign. One mechanism by which insulin autoantibodies may be involved in the initiation of autoimmunity involves structural or molecular alterations in the insulin molecule which make it newly recognizable to the immune system. It is also possible that the newly recognizable antigen is not insulin itself, but rather proinsulin or another early biosynthetic precursor. Recently, it has been shown that recombinant human preproinsulin reacts with insulin autoantibodies[9]. Alternatively, a foreign antigen which shares antigenic determinants with insulin could initiate an autoimmune reaction through molecular mimicry. This mechanism has been proposed for poststreptococcal rheumatic fever in which antibodies against streptococcal M-protein cross-react with cardiac myosin[10]. Suggestive evidence for molecular mimicry occurring in diabetes comes from murine diabetes which is frequently associated with increased expression of an endogenous retrovirus. Antibodies to a specific antigen (p73) of this endogenous retrovirus in diabetic mice also bind to insulin and are therefore indistinguishable from insulin autoantibodies[11]. In humans, approximately 65% of ELISA (+) IAA and IA subjects have antibodies which recognize both insulin and p73[12]. This raises the possibility that for some subjects who are IAA positive, the immunizing antigen may be antigenically similar to p73, rather than insulin, and that endogenous retroviruses may be involved in human IDDM.

Defects in the immune system regulatory process could also initiate an autoimmune disease. It is now believed that not all self-reactive T cells are deleted in the thymus prior to maturation, and thus, normal humans have T and B cells as well as antibodies in their peripheral blood with autoimmune potential. There are multiple, not fully understood mechanisms that suppress this low level autoimmune potential and keep the subject from developing autoimmune disease. In this regard it is interesting to note that in a normal healthy population, one can measure very low levels of insulin autoantibodies. It is only when using a standard cutoff of three standard deviations from the normal population that a serum is generally called insulin autoantibody positive, and it is these positives that are related to the diabetes disease process. The presence of positive insulin autoantibodies may thus represent a defect in the regulatory process whereby IAAs develop as part of an idiotype and anti-idiotype cascade with varying affinity antibodies keeping the immune system in check or accelerating the destruction of self-tissue. The development of insulin autoantibodies after clinical hypoglycemia due to anti-insulin receptor antibodies[13], and an anti-idotype antibody which reacts with both insulin autoantibodies and the insulin receptor causing increased insulin requirement have both been reported[14].

Insulin autoantibodies theoretically could be effectors in the autoimmune process, actually causing the immune killing or giving specificity to natural killer (NK) cells. Potential mechanisms include binding to receptors and thereby altering a physiologic response, formation of antigen–antibody complex which directly damages tissue, or antibody binding to tissue antigens and damage via activation of complement-mediated mechanisms. By binding to receptors, antibodies cause disease in both Graves' disease (in which an autoantibody stimulates the TSH receptor causing hyperthyrodism[15]) and in myasthenia gravis (in which autoantibodies to the acetylcholine receptor block transmission of nerve impulses causing muscle weakness[16]). Though some forms of insulin-resistant diabetes are caused by antibodies to the insulin receptor[17] and Kloppel reported insulitis after immunizing sheep, rabbits and cattle with crystallized insulin and Freund's adjuvant[18], there is no evidence of insulin antibody binding causing IDDM. In fact, the pancreas of people with insulin autoimmune syndrome demonstrates β-cell hypertrophy but no insulitis. Similarly, though present in other autoimmune diseases (SLE, polyarteritis nodosa[19]), deposition of insulin/insulin antibody immune complexes in the islet has never been demonstrated. Finally, insulin autoantibodies could cause tissue damage after binding via complement-mediated lysis or opsonization and phagocytosis. There is also no evidence for this effect of insulin autoantibodies. Additionally, insulin antibodies cannot experimentally transfer IDDM. Thus it appears very unlikely that insulin autoantibodies are involved as primary effectors of the autoimmune destructive process.

If the evidence is poor that insulin autoantibodies are initiators of disease, and they do not appear to be primary in the destructive process itself, it remains possible that IAAs develop as markers, without really being involved in the autoimmune process. They may be occurring secondarily as a result of β-cell damage from other mechanisms. When the pancreas is damaged by iron from repeated transfusions, insulin autoantibodies can be found[20]. Alternatively, they may serve as a general marker of susceptibility to autoimmune disease. Since autoreactive clones appear to be normally present in healthy individuals, polyclonal activation (?loss of suppression) could result in elevated levels of IAAs. Potentially supporting this mechanism are the reports of IAAs in non-diabetic subjects with autoimmune thyroid disease, SLE, and rheumatoid arthritis.

ANTIBODY CHARACTERISTICS

One report has compared the binding characteristics of insulin autoantibodies (found at diagnosis) and insulin antibodies (measured after patients have received insulin therapy). They noted that IAAs had a similar affinity but reduced binding capacity as compared to IAs[21]. Other information regarding binding characteristics of insulin autoantibodies noted that they were of high affinity and low capacity. These authors found no antibody affinity differences when tested with insulins from different species. Investigation of IAAs from relatives of IDDM patients demonstrated that binding of these antibodies to intact insulin could be inhibited by human proinsulin, insulin containing Gln in position 17, and desoctapeptide insulin, suggesting that the IAAs from different subjects share a common epitope[22]. Insulin autoantibodies appear to be able to cross the placenta, as they have been found in the cord blood of offspring of mothers with diabetes[23].

CLINICAL USE

Despite the unresolved questions regarding why insulin autoantibodies occur, there is now a large amount of data describing their prevalence and predictive value for the course of the IDDM disease process during the pre-clinical period.

Data from many laboratories worldwide indicate that about 40–50% of subjects newly diagnosed with IDDM have insulin autoantibodies as measured by RIA methods[24–26]. These autoantibodies may be more prevalent when clinical diabetes is diagnosed at an early age[27–29]. Interestingly, a subgroup of subjects diagnosed with Type 2 diabetes have been reported to have glutamic acid decarboxylase (GAD) autoantibodies or ICAs. These patients appear to have a clinical course requiring insulin treatment at an earlier stage than typical Type 2 subjects[30]. The presence of these autoantibodies may imply destruction of pancreatic β cells and may be more accurately described as "slowly evolving Type 1". Whether IAAs are also prevalent in these subjects is unknown.

The finding that insulin autoantibodies are often present in people prior to the onset of clinical disease led to hope that these antibodies could serve as markers to predict which subjects would develop clinical disease. Cross-sectional studies of first degree relatives of patients with IDDM have indicated that about 1–3% have insulin autoantibodies. Prospective evaluation of first degree relatives who are IAA positive alone (i.e. ICA and GAD antibody negative) indicates that these subjects are at very low risk for development of clinical disease[31]. Indeed, prospective evaluation of this group's pancreatic β-cell function demonstrates no functional abnormalities as compared to controls, reinforcing the concept that IAAs themselves are neither initiators nor effectors in the immune destructive process[31]. Perhaps the presence of IAAs in these subjects who never developed other antibodies represents the group of people who have successfully fought off the immune attack. In this regard it is important to note a lack of consensus as to whether

IAAs are associated with high risk HLA types. Some investigators have noted an association[32,33], whereas our data and those of others have failed to demonstrate a relationship[27,34-36]. In contrast, the presence of IAA in association with either ICA or GAD antibodies in first degree relatives confers a higher risk than ICA or GAD antibodies alone[37,38] (Figure 5.3). Among ICA or GAD antibody positive first degree relatives, about 30-40% will also be IAA positive[39]. While it appears to be true that the presence of a severely abnormal first phase insulin secretion in response to an IVGTT is the most predictive measurement of subsequent development of clinical IDDM among ICA positive first degree relatives, if one is measuring antibodies alone, the combination of ICA and IAA is the most highly predictive combination.

Though ICAs certainly have more predictive value than IAAs as markers for development of IDDM, several aspects of insulin autoantibodies emphasize the continued need to investigate their role in the diabetes disease process. First, while we remain ignorant of the antigen(s) resulting ICAs, for IAAs and GAD antibodies the antigen is known, and in the case of IAAs the antigen is β-cell specific like the disease itself. Secondly, IAAs appear to develop early in the disease process. Studies in animal models and small studies in very young children have claimed the presence of IAAs (and GAD antibodies) prior to the development of ICAs[23].

Studies evaluating the predictive value of antibodies for development of IDDM have largely concentrated on family members, since the "at risk" genetic background is already present. However, since most people who

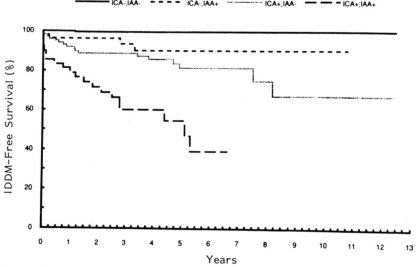

Figure 5.3. Probability of remaining IDDM free stratified by the appearance of insulin (IAA) and islet cell (ICA) autoantibodies[37]

develop IDDM do not have a first degree relative with the disease, it is important to assess the prevalence and predictive value of autoantibody measurements in the general population as well. In a large study of Swedish children from ages 0 to 14 who were controls for subjects with IDDM, 1% were positive for IAA (positive value=mean+3SD). The cumulative incidence rate of diabetes for children up to age 15 in Sweden is only 0.38%, indicating that over half of the subjects who are IAA positive would not be expected to develop clinical disease. In the 3–5 year follow-up for this study, none of the IAA positive control children developed disease.[40] In Washington State, a study of a population of healthy school children aged 12–18 without any family history of IDDM demonstrated that 1.7% were ICA positive. Of the ICA positive students (n=69), 10% were also IAA positive[41]. Prospective evaluation of these antibody positive subjects is underway.

Aside from diabetes, insulin autoantibodies have been found in at least two other clinical situations. In a rare disease, termed insulin autoimmune syndrome, high levels of insulin autoantibodies are found in association with high insulin and C-peptide levels and at times severe clinical hypoglycemia. The hypoglycemia presumably occurs secondary to inappropriate release of insulin from the insulin–insulin autoantibody complex[42]. IAAs are also found in association with other autoimmune diseases even when diabetes does not occur. Most frequently described in association with thyroid disease, IAAs have also been found in patients with SLE and rheumatoid arthritis. After removal of non-specific binding using a cold displacement step, specific IAA binding was still present in about 8% of our thyroid subjects[8], and others have reported up to 15% of insulin-specific binding in this group[43]. The association of rheumatoid arthritis with IAAs may be related to treatment with penicilliamine (a sulfhydryl containing drug)[44]. Specific IAAs have not been found in subjects with Addison's disease, pernicious anemia, or increased gamma globulin[45].

As strategies for predicting the development of IDDM become more precise, trials of numerous therapeutic agents to delay or prevent the onset of clinical disease have begun. It is possible that a new clinical use of IAA may develop during analysis of these trials; measurement of change in IAA may serve as an indicator of success of therapy. When subjects with autoimmune thyroiditis are treated successfully, decreases in thyroid antibodies are seen. Interestingly, however, though many of these subjects have IAAs, treatment of thyroid disease results in no change in insulin autoantibody levels, suggesting specificity[43]. In a pilot study, five first degree relatives at high risk of development of IDDM within the next 3 to 5 years were treated with parenteral insulin administered every 9 months for 5 days via continuous intravenous infusions and outpatient injections. After their initial treatment with insulin, in two subjects insulin antibody levels rose moderately and then leveled off. These subjects have remained on treatment without development of diabetes. In two subjects who developed IDDM despite treatment, the insulin antibody levels were higher on their initial measurement, and then increased markedly (5–10-fold) prior to diagnosis of IDDM. The fifth subject had only a moderate elevation of antibody at initial evaluation which subsequently increased 20-fold, though that subject remains without diabetes[46]. Whether these interesting observations will be helpful in predicting treatment success or failure when applied to a large-scale randomized trial remains to be seen. Insulin antibody levels will be measured regularly in the multicentered randomized trial of parenteral insulin in the US., termed Diabetes Prevention Trial-1.

SUMMARY

Insulin autoantibodies measured by RIA are associated with the IDDM disease process. It is not known why they develop. Cross-sectional evaluation of IAAs alone does not predict development of disease. However, measurements of IAAs over time, and in association with other autoantigens or abnormalities of insulin secretion does correlate with clinical disease. It is possible that in the future IAAs will be helpful in evaluating response to intervention trials in which alterations in the IDDM disease process may be induced.

ACKNOWLEDGMENT

This work was supported in part by the Medical Research Service of the Department of Veterans Affairs and the National Institutes of Health grants DK17047 and DK02456.

REFERENCES

1 Pav J, Prague MD, Jexokova Z, Skrha F. Insulin antibodies. *Lancet* 1963; ii: 221 2.
2 Palmer JP, Asplin CM, Clemons P. Insulin autoantibodies in insulin-dependent diabetes before insulin treatment. *Science* 1983; **222**: 1337–9.
3 Wilkin T, Schoenfeld S, Diaz J-L, Kruze V, Bonifacio E, Palmer J. Systematic variation and differences in insulin-autoantibody measurements. *Diabetes* 1989; **38**: 172–81.
4 Wilkin T, Palmer J, Kurta A, Bonifacio E, Diaz J-L. The Second International Workshop on the Standardization of Insulin Autoantibody (IAA) Measurement. *Diabetologia* 1988; **31**: 449–50.
5 Greenbaum CJ, Palmer JP, Kuglin B, Kolb H *et al*. Insulin autoantibodies measured by radioimmunoassay methodology are more related to insulin-dependent diabetes mellitus than those measured by enzyme-linked immunosorbent assay: results of

the Fourth International Workshop on the Standardization of Insulin Autoantibody Measurement. *J Clin Endocrinol Metab* 1992; **74**: 1040–4.

6 Stumpo RR, Llera AS, Cardoso AI, Poskus E. Solid versus liquid phase assays in detection of insulin antibodies. Influence of iodination site on labelled insulin binding. *J Immunol Methods* 1994; **169**: 241–9.

7 Greenbaum C, Palmer J. No improvement in interassay precision using a standard curve with each assay to determine ICA JDF titers. *Autoimmunity* 1993; **15**: 72.

8 Hegewald MJ, Schoenfeld SL, McCulloch DR, Greenbaum CJ, Klaff LJ, Palmer JP. Increased specificity and sensitivity of insulin autoantibody measurements in autoimmune thyroid disease and type I diabetes. *J Immunol Methods* 1992; **154**: 61–8.

9 Berg H, Walter M, Mauch L, Seissler J, Northemann W. Recombinant human preproinsulin. Expression, purification and reaction with insulin autoantibodies in sera from patients with insulin-dependent diabetes mellitus. *J Immunol Methods* 1993; **164**: 221–31.

10 Dale JB, Beachey EH. Epitopes of streptococcal M proteins shared with cardiac myosin. *J Exp Med* 1985; **162**: 583–91.

11 Serreze DV, Leiter EH, Kuff EL, Jardieu P, Ishizaka K. Molecular mimicry between insulin and retroviral antigen p73. Development of cross-reactive autoantibodies in sera of NOD and C57BL/KsJ db/db mice. *Diabetes* 1988; **37**: 351–8.

12 Hao W, Serreze DV, McCulloch DK, Neifing JL, Palmer JP. Insulin (auto)antibodies from human IDDM cross-react with retroviral antigen p73. *J Autoimmun* 1993; **6**: 787–98.

13 Elias D, Cohen I, Schechter Y, Spirer A, Golander A. Antibodies to insulin receptor followed by anti-idiotype. *Diabetes* 1987; **36**: 348–54.

14 Shoelson S, Marshall S, Horikoshi H, Kolterman O, Rubenstein A, Olefsky J. Antiinsulin receptor antibodies in an insulin-dependent diabetic may arise as autoantiidiotypes. *J Clin Endocrinol Metab* 1986; **63**: 56–61.

15 Abbas AK, Lichtman AH, Pober JS. Diseases caused by humoral and cell-mediated immune reactions. In Wonsiewixz M (ed), *Cellular and Molecular Immunology*. Philadelphia, PA: W.B. Saunders Company, Harcourt Brace Jovanovich, Inc., 1991, pp 353–76.

16 Lindstrom J, Shelton D, Fujii Y. Myasthenia gravis. *Adv Immunol* 1988; **42**: 233–84.

17 Grigorescu F, Flier JS, Kahn CR. Characterization of binding and phosphorylation defects of erythrocyte insulin receptors in the type A syndrome of insulin resistance. *Diabetes* 1986; **35**: 127–38.

18 Kloppel G. "Insulin" induced insulitis. *Acta Endocrinol Suppl Copenh* 1976; **205**: 107–21.

19 Rose N, Mackay I. The immune response in autoimmunity and autoimmune disease. In Rose N, Mackay I (eds) *The Autoimmune Diseases*, Vol II. San Diego, CA: Academic Press, 1992, pp 1–26.

20 Shah S, Benaim E, Benaim E, Hvizdala E, Griggs S. Insulin autoantibodies may be an indicator of beta cell destruction rather than autoimmunity in insulin dependent diabetes (Abstract). *Autoimmunity* 1993; **15**: 80.

21 Vahasalo P. Autoantibodies to insulin have insulin have similar affinity to that of antibodies to exogenous insulin but lower binding capacity. *Eur J Clin Invest* 1992; **22**: 772–6.

22 Castano L, Ziegler AG, Ziegler R, Shoelson S, Eisenbarth GS. Characterization of insulin autoantibodies in relatives of patients with type I diabetes. *Diabetes* 1993; **42**: 1202–9.

23 Ziegler AG, Hillebrand B, Rabl W, Mayrhofer M, Hummel M, Mollenhauer U *et al.* On the appearance of islet associated autoimmunity in offspring of diabetic mothers: a prospective study from birth. *Diabetologia* 1993; **36**: 402–8.

24 Lendrum R, Walker JG, Gamble DR. Islet cell antibodies in juvenile diabetes mellitus of recent onset. *Lancet* 1975; **1**: 880–2.
25 MacCuish AC, Irvine WJ, Barnes EW, Duncan LJ. Antibodies to pancreatic islet cells in insulin-dependent diabetics with coexistent autoimmune disease. *Lancet* 1974; **2**: 1529–31.
26 Ludvigsson J, Binder C, Mandrup-Poulsen T. Insulin autoantibodies are associated with islet cell antibodies; their relation to insulin antibodies and B-cell function in diabetic children. *Diabetologia* 1988; **31**: 647–51.
27 Karjalainen J, Salmela P, Ilonen J, Surcel H-M, Knip M. A comparison of children and adult type I diabetes. *N Engl J Med* 1989; **320**: 881–6.
28 Vardi P, Ziegler AG, Mathews JH, Dib S, Keller RJ, Ricker AT *et al*. Concentration of insulin autoantibodies at onset of type I diabetes. Inverse log-linear correlation with age. *Diabetes Care* 1988; **11**: 736–9.
29 Vardi P, Dib SA, Tuttleman M, Connelly JE, Grinbergs M, Radizabeh A *et al*. Competitive insulin autoantibody assay. Prospective evaluation of subjects at high risk for development of type I diabetes mellitus. *Diabetes* 1987; **36**: 1286–91.
30 Tuomi T, Groop LC, Zimmet PZ, Rowley MJ, Knowles W, Mackay IR. Antibodies to glutamic acid decarboxylase reveal latent autoimmune diabetes mellitus in adults with a non-insulin-dependent onset of disease. *Diabetes* 1993; **42**: 359–62.
31 Neifing JL, Greenbaum CJ, Kahn SE, McCulloch DK, Barmeier H, Lernmark A *et al*. Prospective evaluation of B-cell function in insulin-autoantibody-positive relatives of insulin-dependent diabetic patients. *Metabolism* 1993; **42**: 482–6.
32 Atkinson MA, MacLaren NK, Riley WJ, Winter WE, Fisk DD, Spillar RP. Are insulin autoantibodies markers for insulin-dependent diabetes mellitus? *Diabetes* 1986; **35**: 894–8.
33 Ziegler AG, Standl E, Albert E, Mehnert H. HLA-associated insulin autoantibody formation in newly diagnosed type I diabetic patients. *Diabetes* 1991; **40**: 1146–9.
34 Goday A, Motana E, Ercilla G, Fernandez J, Gomis R, Vilardell E. HLA antigens in Spanish type 1 diabetic population. Correlations with clinical, biological and autoimmune markers. *Acta Diabetol Lat* 1990; **27**: 215–22.
35 L'evy-Marchal C, Tichet J, Fajardy I, Gu XF, Dubois F, Czernichow P. Islet cell antibodies in normal French schoolchildren. *Diabetologia* 1992; **35**: 577–82.
36 Robert J, Deschamps I, Chevenne D, Roger M, Mogenet A, Boitard C. Relationship between first-phase insulin secretion and age, HLA, islet cell antibody status, and development of type I diabetes in 220 juvenile first-degree relatives of diabetic patients. *Diabetes Care* 1991; **14**: 718–23.
37 Krischer JP, Schatz D, Riley WJ, Spillar RP, Silverstein JH, Schwartz S *et al*. Insulin and islet cell autoantibodies as time-dependent covariates in the development of insulin-dependent diabetes: a prospective study in relatives. *J Clin Endocrinol Metab* 1993; **77**: 743–9.
38 Dean B, Becker F, McNally J. Insulin autoantibodies in the prediabetic period. Correlation with islet cell antibodies and development of diabetes. *Diabetologia* 1986; **29**: 339–42.
39 Roll U, Christie MR, Standl E, Ziegler AG. Associations of anti-GAD antibodies with islet cell antibodies and insulin autoantibodies in first-degree relatives of type I diabetic patients. *Diabetes* 1994; **43**: 154–60.
40 Landin-Olsson M, Palmer JP, Lernmark A, Blom L, Sundkvist G, Nystrom L *et al*. Predictive value of islet cell and insulin autoantibodies for type 1 (insulin-dependent) diabetes mellitus in a population-based study of newly-diagnosed diabetic and matched control children. *Diabetologia* 1992; **35**: 1068–73.
41 Rowe RE, Leech NJ, Nepom GT, McCulloch DK. High genetic risk for IDDM in the

Pacific Northwest. First report from the Washington State Diabetes Prediction Study. *Diabetes* 1994; **43**: 87–94.

42 Ichihara K, Shima K, Saito Y, Nonaka K, Tarui S, Nichikawa M. Mechanism of hypoglycemia observed in a patient with insulin autoimmune syndrome. *Diabetes* 1977; **26**: 500–6.

43 Vardi P, Modan-Mozes D, Ish-Shalom S, Soloveitzik L, Barzilai D *et al.* Low titer, competitive insulin autoantibodies are spontaneously produced in autoimmune diseases of the thyroid. *Diabetes Res Clin Pract* 1993; **21**: 161–6.

44 Vardi P, Brik R, Barzilai D, Lorber M, Scharf Y. Frequent induction of insulin autoantibodies by D-penicillamine in patients with rheumatoid arthritis. *J Rheumatol* 1992; **19**: 1527–30.

45 Harrop M, Caudwell J, Stojanovski C, Colman PG. Insulin autoantibodies in patients with autoimmune diseases. *Diabetes Res Clin Pract* 1992; **18**: 107–12.

46 Jackson R. Personal communication.

6

Humoral Immune Markers: Antibodies to Glutamic Acid Decarboxylase

MICHAEL R. CHRISTIE
Department of Medicine, King's College Hospital, London, UK

INTRODUCTION

Circulating antibodies to islet components (islet cell antibodies; ICAs) in insulin-dependent diabetes were first detected by immunofluorescence on frozen sections of pancreatic tissue in 1974. The subsequent realization that ICAs appear several years before the onset of insulin-dependent diabetes provided evidence that development of the disease could be predicted by screening for antibodies to islet components. It is now recognized that ICAs are heterogeneous[1,2] and that the disease is associated with the presence of autoantibodies to multiple islet components[3]. Identification of these islet cell autoantigens gives the potential to develop simple but accurate assays for screening large populations for individuals at risk for disease. In this chapter, I review recent advances in our knowledge of one such autoantigen, glutamic acid decarboxylase (GAD).

DETECTION OF A 64K-ANTIGEN IN INSULIN-DEPENDENT DIABETES

The first successful attempts to identify islet components recognized by antibodies in IDDM were published by Baekkeskov and co-workers in 1982[4].

Prediction, Prevention and Genetic Counseling in IDDM. Edited by Jerry P. Palmer.
© 1996 John Wiley & Sons Ltd.

This group used an immunoprecipitation protocol to detect antibody binding to islet cell proteins. Detergent-solubilized extracts of human islet proteins radiolabeled with [35][S] methionine were incubated with sera from recent-onset diabetic patients and immune complexes formed in the incubation purified on protein A sepharose. Islet proteins in the immune complexes were separated by gel electrophoresis and detected by autoradiography. The major protein(s) specifically recognized by antibodies in diabetic patients' sera using this procedure had a relative molecular mass (M_r) of 64 000 (Figure 6.1) and was referred to as the "64K-antigen". Antibodies have been shown to bind the protein in monkey, dog and rat pancreatic islets, as well as human islets, indicating that epitopes recognized by the autoantibodies are not species specific. Approximately 80% of Type 1 diabetic patients possessed antibodies that recognized the 64K-antigen at the time of disease onset[5,6]. In studies on samples from first degree relatives of diabetic patients who later developed the disease themselves, antibodies to the 64K-antigen were found to appear several years before disease onset[5,6]. The presence of these antibodies was considered to be relatively diabetes -specific, since they were not detected in normal control individuals or patients with a number of other endocrine autoimmune disorders[6]. These studies provided early evidence that antibodies to the 64K-antigen are highly specific markers for later development of insulin-dependent diabetes.

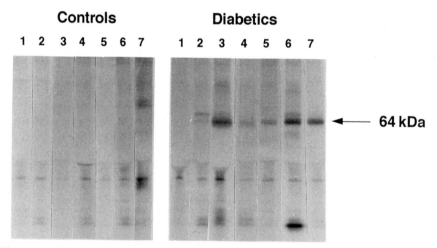

Figure 6.1. Immunoprecipitation of islet 64K-antigen by antibodies in IDDM. The figure shows proteins immunoprecipitated from detergent extracts of [35S]methionine-labeled islets by antibodies in sera from normal control individuals or IDDM patients. The 64K-antigen represents the major islet protein specifically immunoprecipitated by sera from diabetic, but not from control, individuals

PROPERTIES OF THE 64K-ANTIGEN

The 64K-antigen was found to possess hydrophobic properties consistent with a membrane localization within islet cells. Thus, the antigen partitioned into a detergent phase on phase separation in Triton X-114[6], a property typical of amphiphilic membrane proteins. Furthermore, in subcellular fractionation studies on density gradients, the protein was recovered in a fraction containing plasma membranes and other light membrane vesicles[7]. At that time, specific antibodies to the antigen were not available to define the specific membrane compartment in which the antigen was expressed.

Within the heterogeneous population of the pancreatic islet, the 64K-antigen was detected predominantly in the insulin-secreting β cells, and at much lower levels in other islet cell types[7]. The antigen was not detected in a number of other normal endocrine and non-endocrine tissues. There is therefore a degree of tissue specificity to the antigen expression, which may have relevance to the selective destruction of the pancreatic β cells in diabetes.

IDENTIFICATION OF THE 64K-ANTIGEN AS GLUTAMIC ACID DECARBOXYLASE

In 1990, the 64K-antigen was identified as the enzyme, glutamic acid decarboxylase (GAD). Clues to the identification of the antigen came not directly from studies in diabetes, but from observations in a rare neurological disorder, Stiff-man syndrome. Stiff-man syndrome (SMS) is characterized by progressive rigidity of the musculature accompanied by painful spasms and is considered to be a result of impairment of inhibitory neuronal systems that act through gamma amino butyric acid (GABA). Symptoms of the disease are alleviated by administration of drugs that enhance GABA-mediated neuro-transmission. Importantly, SMS is associated with a number of autoimmune disorders, including insulin-dependent diabetes[8].

A study on patients with SMS revealed the presence of high levels of IgG antibodies in the cerebrospinal fluid and in the serum[8]. These antibodies produced intense staining on sections of brain tissue; in particular regions of the brain rich in GABA-ergic neurons. Western blotting studies indicated that the predominant brain antigen recognized by these antibodies co-migrated on gel electrophoresis with GAD, the enzyme responsible for the synthesis of GABA in these neurons. Antibodies to GABA-ergic neurons and GAD were detectable in around 60% of patients with Stiff-man syndrome, consistent with SMS being an autoimmune disease with GAD as a major autoantigen. All SMS patients with GAD antibodies were also found to possess ICA, and 30% of these patients also had IDDM. The strong association of SMS with islet autoimmunity and IDDM, together with the similarity in M_r of GAD

(60 000–67 000) and the 64K-antigen (64 000) prompted studies to determine whether the 64K-antigen in IDDM was related to the GAD antigen detected in SMS.

A collaborative study between the groups of Baekkeskov and DeCamilli produced strong evidence that the 64K-antigen is equivalent to pancreatic islet GAD[9]. Polyclonal antibodies to GAD, as well as antibodies in sera from IDDM and SMS patients, were shown to immunoprecipitate islet proteins that co-migrate on one- and two-dimensional gel electrophoresis with islet 64K-antigen. Furthermore, sera from diabetic patients were able to immunoprecipitate a GAD enzyme activity from extracts of both islets and brain. Subsequent studies demonstrated a strong correlation between the presence of antibodies to 64K-antigen and antibodies to GAD[10] and unlabeled recombinant GAD was shown to block the binding of antibodies to the islet 64K-antigen in immunoprecipitation reactions. A high proportion of patients with recent-onset IDDM have now been shown to possess antibodies that immunoprecipitate recombinant GAD, confirming that GAD is a major autoantigen in IDDM as well as in SMS[11].

PROPERTIES OF GAD

GAD is the enzyme responsible for the synthesis of the inhibitory neurotransmitter GABA by the pyridoxal-phosphate-dependent decarboxylation of glutamic acid. GAD is expressed in the GABA-ergic neurons of the central nervous system, in the pancreatic islets (predominantly in the pancreatic β cells), in the oviduct, ovary and testis[12]. Lower levels of GAD enzyme activity have been detected in a number of other peripheral tissues, including the liver and kidney. It is now known that GAD is expressed as multiple isoforms. Two major isoforms of 65 and 67 Kda (GAD-65 and GAD-67 respectively) have been cloned and sequenced and shown to be the products of two distinct genes. In humans, the gene for GAD-65 is found on chromosome 10 and that for GAD-67 on chromosome 2. The two isoforms show considerable sequence diversity in the first 100 amino acids at the N-terminus of the molecule but show a high degree of sequence similarity over the rest of the molecule (Figure 6.2). The junction between these two regions of differing sequence diversity is a major target for a number of different proteolytic enzymes (proteolytic "hot spot") and may be the boundary of distinct domains within the molecule. GAD from more primitive species such as *Drosophila* lack the N-terminal domain. The amino acid sequence shows little homology with other known proteins. However, both GAD-65 and GAD-67 show similarities in a region of the molecule (amino acids 250–273 for GAD-65 and 258–281 for GAD-67) with the P2-C protein of coxsackievirus[11]. A number of studies have reported an association of coxsackievirus B4 infection with development of

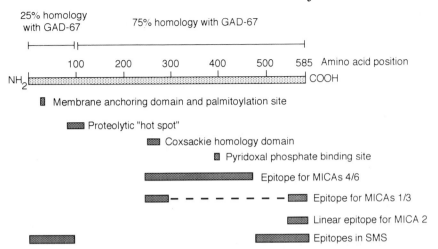

Figure 6.2. Features of GAD-65. GAD-65 is a protein of 585 amino acids in length that shares homology with GAD-67. The location of the major features of the protein sequence described in the text, together with the major epitopes recognized by antibodies, are illustrated on the figure

IDDM. It is possible that molecular mimicry between coxsackievirus P2-C protein and GAD may be involved in the induction of autoimmune responses to GAD. There are intraneuronal differences in the level of expression of the two isoforms: GAD-67 is found throughout the neuron whereas GAD-65 is detected predominantly in the axon terminals. Furthermore, there are species differences in the level of expression of the isoforms in the pancreatic β cells. Human islets express predominantly GAD-65 and the level of expression of GAD-67 is very low[13], although GAD-67 mRNA can be detected in islets by polymerase chain reaction. In mouse islets, GAD expression is low and the major isoform is GAD-67. Rat islets express higher levels of both isoforms.

GAD-67 is a hydrophilic, soluble molecule. In contrast, GAD-65, in its mature form, is hydrophobic and can associate with membranes; in neuronal cells the enzyme associates with synaptic vesicles and in pancreatic β cells with synapatic-like vesicles. The sequence diversity within the first 100 amino acids of GAD-65 and GAD-67 may be responsible for the different compartmentalization of the two isoforms. The amino acid sequence of GAD-65 does not reveal any hydrophobic domains indicative of membrane spanning regions; rather there is evidence that post-translational modification of the GAD-65 molecule is critical for membrane anchoring[14]. The nature of the membrane anchor is not clear, but site directed mutagenesis has implicated residues 24–31 as a critical region in membrane binding. It is known that GAD is palmitoylated on cysteine residues 30 and/or 45; palmitoylation of proteins has been shown to be important in membrane anchoring. However, palmitoylation of GAD only seems to promote the association of the protein with the synaptic-like vesicle membrane, and does not appear to be essential for membrane anchoring.

Despite the high degree of sequence homology between the GAD-65 and GAD-67, there are clear differences in the ability of autoantibodies to bind the two isoforms. In human IDDM, GAD-65 is the major isoform recognized; GAD-67 is recognized by antibodies from a minority of IDDM patients (less than 20%) and a considerable portion of GAD-67 binding is likely to be due to partial cross-reactivity with GAD-65[15]. Nevertheless, GAD-67 specific antibodies have been described in IDDM, and GAD-67 is clearly recognized by immuno-precipitating antibodies in the majority of patients with autoimmune SMS.

IDENTIFICATION OF A 64 000 M_r ANTIGEN DISTINCT FROM GAD

There is no doubt that GAD is a major target for autoantibodies in IDDM and that the enzyme is the predominant component of the protein originally identified as the "64K-antigen". However, there is evidence that there are proteins of similar molecular weight (M_r 60 000–70 000) that are also autoantigens in IDDM. Thus, the 65 kDa heat shock protein (hsp 65) has been implicated in the pathogenesis of diabetes in the NOD mouse animal model for IDDM[16], although the involvement of the protein in human IDDM is less clear. A 69 kDa protein (ICA69) has been identified as a target for autoantibodies in IDDM by screening of cDNA expression libraries with sera from IDDM patients[17]. However, neither hsp 65 nor ICA69 can be immunoprecipitated by antibodies in IDDM patients' sera and these proteins are unlikely to be components of the protein(s) identified as the "64K-antigen". Nevertheless, my own laboratory has evidence that 64 000 M_r proteins other than GAD may be immunoprecipitated by antibodies in IDDM. By studying the ability of antibodies to bind proteolytic fragments, two distinct antibody specificities to components of the islet 64K-antigen have been detected[18]. Partial tryptic proteolysis of immunoprecipitated 64K-antigen was shown to generate three major fragments of M_r 50 000, 40 000 and 37 000. Analysis of antibody binding to the fragments revealed the presence of at least two antibody specificities associated with IDDM that bound different fragments. One antibody specificity ound 50 000 M_r fragments of antigen and the second 37 000 and 40 000 M_r fragments. Antibodies that bound the 50 000 M_r fragment also recognized GAD enzyme activity from brain, suggesting that this fragment is derived from islet GAD. In contrast, antibodies that bound the 37 000 and 40 000 M_r fragments did not immunoprecipitate GAD[10].

Further characterization of the 37 000 and 40 000 M_r antigenic fragments indicated that these are derived from a 64K-antigen that is distinct from

GAD[18]. Thus, polyclonal antibodies raised to purified GAD, or to synthetic GAD peptides, bound to 50 000 M_r fragments but failed to recognize the 37 000 and 40 000 M_r fragments. Recombinant GAD-65 competed for auto-antibody binding to 50 000 M_r fragments, but neither GAD-65 nor GAD-67 affected antibody binding to 37 000 or 40 000 M_r fragments. These results indicate that the 50 000 M_r fragment is derived from islet GAD-65, whereas the 37 000 and 40 000 M_r fragments are derived from different proteins (37K- and 40K-antigens). The 37K- and 40K- antigens have now been identified as two distinct proteins related to the tyrosine phosphatase-like protein, 1A-2[19].

GAD AS A TARGET FOR ICAs

Although ICAs were first described 20 years ago, the nature of the antigen or antigens recognized by these antibodies is still not defined. It is now apparent that ICAs are heterogeneous, binding multiple autoantigens on the pancreas section. Evidence for this has come from detailed analysis of the staining pattern of antibody binding on pancreatic sections, and from analysis of species specificity of ICA reactivity[1,2]. Thus, studies of ICAs in sera from IDDM patients, diabetic and non-diabetic subjects with other endocrine autoimmunity and first degree relatives of patients with IDDM revealed two distinct staining patterns on pancreas sections. One gave a diffuse staining of all islet cells (whole islet ICAs), whereas the other stained predominantly the islet β cells (β-cell selective ICAs). Sera with β-cell selective ICAs failed to stain islets on mouse pancreas, in contrast to those with whole islet ICAs. The two ICA staining patterns were found to confer different risks for diabetes development. Thus, IDDM patients, and relatives or autoimmune patients who progressed to IDDM, were found to have predominantly the whole islet staining pattern, whereas those relatives and autoimmune patients who had not developed IDDM after prolonged follow-up possessed the β-cell selective ICA pattern. Clearly, identification of the targets for these two ICA staining patterns would aid identification of ICA positive individuals at highest risk for IDDM. The β-cell selective ICA was found to be blocked by the addition of a rat brain extract, suggestive of common antigens in islets and brain. Furthermore, the blocking activity was removed by pre-clearing with an antibody raised to GAD, and addition of recombinant GAD-65 and GAD-67 was also found to prevent β-cell selective ICA staining[20]. Thus, GAD appears to be a major target for the β-cell selective ICA, an ICA sub-specificity which paradoxically confers low risk of IDDM development. This GAD–ICA specificity fails to react with islets on mouse pancreas, probably as a result of the low levels of GAD, particularly GAD-65, expressed in islets of this species.

The degree to which GAD is a target for ICA in IDDM patients is not clear. The majority of patients with IDDM have a whole islet, rather than β-cell selective ICA staining. Nevertheless, a weak correlation has been observed between ICA titers and levels of antibodies to 64K-antigen or antibodies to GAD in recent onset IDDM patients[21]. Furthermore, recombinant GAD has been shown to block or reduce ICA staining in approximately one-quarter of new-onset IDDM patients. Monoclonal antibodies to GAD have also been generated by screening Epstein–Barr virus transformed B lymphocytes for secretion of antibodies reactive in an ICA assay[22]. It is therefore likely that GAD antibodies in IDDM patients' sera do, to some degree, contribute to ICA reactivity in the sera. However, it is probable that islet cell antigens other than GAD are the major targets of ICA in recent-onset IDDM patients.

GAD ANTIBODIES AND DEVELOPMENT OF IDDM

METHODS FOR DETECTION OF GAD ANTIBODIES

After GAD was identified as a major target for antibodies in Type 1 diabetes, it was anticipated that simple, accurate, high capacity assays would very quickly be developed that would allow assessment of the value of GAD antibodies as predictive markers for IDDM. GAD autoantibodies in human autoimmune disease were first reported in SMS by Western blotting[8]. In this technique, SDS-solubilized (and denatured) GAD is separated by electrophoresis, transferred to an appropriate membrane and autoantibody binding to GAD on the membrane detected with an enzyme conjugated second antibody linked to production of a colored product. When this technique was applied to serum samples from IDDM, it became apparent that very few patients were positive, in contrast to the high proportion of antibody-positive patients with SMS[8,9]. Western blotting procedures are thus unsuitable for detection of most GAD antibodies that develop in IDDM. GAD antibodies are present at lower levels in IDDM than in SMS and IDDM antibody may be more highly dependent on protein conformation that may be disrupted during the denaturing conditions of SDS gel electrophoresis. This places a restriction on the type of procedures that can be used to detect GAD antibodies associated with IDDM and has complicated the development of suitable large-scale assay procedures. Solid phase assays such as ELISA would be most convenient for large-scale screening of populations, being relatively easy to automate. Unfortunately, to date ELISA assays have also proved relatively insensitive for the detection of GAD antibodies in IDDM patients. Most studies have therefore employed liquid phase assays, being variants on the original immunoprecipitation assays for antibodies to islet 64K-antigen, but using GAD at varying purities isolated from brain or recombinant expression systems.

The first analyses of GAD autoantibodies in sera from IDDM patients relied on the detection of GAD enzymatic activity associated with immunoprecipitates from extracts containing GAD. GAD enzyme activity is usually measured by the release of $^{14}CO_2$ from 1-[^{14}C]glutamic acid. These studies were useful in demonstrating that GAD is a major autoantigen in IDDM, but the technique is not suitable for routine screening. Detection of the small amount of enzyme activity immunoprecipitated by the low levels of antibodies in IDDM has not proved easy and the enzyme assay is subject to interference. Furthermore, antibody binding to GAD can influence the activity of the enzyme, so the enzyme activity associated with immunoprecipitates may not be a true reflection of the quantity of GAD precipitated. More recently, radiometric assays using ^{125}I-iodinated or [^{35}S]methionine-labeled antigen have been developed and these assays are more appropriate for antibody detection. The availability of purified recombinant GAD isoforms for use in antibody assays allows one to distinguish antibodies to GAD-65 and GAD-67, which is difficult with GAD purified from natural sources. Most assays are still based on the original immunoprecipitation protocol, which involves laborious washings of immunoprecipitates. Attempts are being made to simplify the washing steps by using vacuum filtration devices in a 96-well format. This should greatly increase the capacity of these assays. To date, however, information on GAD-antibody associations with disease have been on rather small study groups and it is too early to be confident of the true value of GAD antibodies as a predictive marker for IDDM.

Experience from the measurement of ICAs and insulin autoantibodies in sera has demonstrated that there can be large differences in the detection of IDDM-associated autoantibodies by different laboratories using apparently similar techniques. Even subtle differences in assay protocols might influence the detection of GAD antibodies in human sera. It is clearly important that GAD antibody assays are standardized to allow comparison of data between different groups. Serum exchange through GAD antibody workshops organized by the Immunology and Diabetes Workshops (IDW) will be valuable in identifying the most accurate procedures for antibody detection and ensuring that data from different centers can be compared.

PREVALENCE OF GAD ANTIBODIES IN IDDM

Analysis of autoantibodies to the islet 64K-antigen in IDDM patients indicated that approximately 80% of patients with recent onset IDDM possess these antibodies[4-6]. A similar proportion of first degree relatives of patients with IDDM who were initially non-diabetic, but who subsequently developed IDDM were found to be positive for antibodies to the 64K-antigen. These antibodies were detected up to 13 years before IDDM onset. From these studies it was concluded that antibodies to the 64K-antigen are early and sensitive markers for the later development of the disease.

Following the identification of the 64K-antigen as GAD, a number of investigators reported that a considerably lower proportion of recent onset IDDM patients immunoprecipitated a GAD enzyme activity from crude rat brain extracts than recognized the islet 64K-antigen. The low frequency of antibodies detected in these experiments is almost certainly due to poor sensitivity in detecting the GAD immunoprecipitated, rather than a lack of GAD antibodies in the sera. More recent studies, using recombinant GAD as substrate, have confirmed that around 80% of recent-onset IDDM patients possess antibodies to GAD, a frequency similar to that reported for antibodies to the islet 64K-antigen.

Many immune abnormalities associated with IDDM decline or disappear shortly after diagnosis. In contrast, antibodies to GAD appear to persist for many years. Thus, in a prospective study, there was little change in the level of GAD antibodies (measured as antibodies to 64K-antigen) during the first three years after diabetes onset, and antibodies to the enzyme can be detected as long as 40 years after diagnosis. This persistence in the GAD antibody response in IDDM contrasts with the rapid decline in ICA titers during the first two years of diabetes, which occurs in parallel to the decline in circulating C-peptide levels and continuing loss of functional β cells after disease onset. The antibody response to GAD appears less dependent on residual β cells than the ICA response. GAD from extra-pancreatic sources, or GAD released from the few remaining β cells, may be sufficient to drive the GAD antibody response for many years.

A proportion of patients with non-insulin-dependent diabetes mellitus (NIDDM) also possess antibodies to GAD. On follow-up, it was found that a high proportion of these GAD antibody positive NIDDM patients eventually required insulin to maintain glucose homeostasis. The presence of GAD antibodies may therefore identify a subgroup of patients who present with NIDDM but who have a slowly progressing form of autoimmune diabetes. GAD antibody analysis may be particularly useful in identifying these NIDDM patients who will eventually become insulin dependent.

HLA AND THE GAD ANTIBODY RESPONSE

IDDM is strongly associated with the expression of particular HLA alleles. In Caucasians expression of HLA-DR 3 and HLA-DR 4 and the associated alleles DQw2 and DQw8 confer susceptibility to IDDM. It has been proposed that HLA gene products might confer susceptibility through the preferential binding, and presentation to autoreactive T cells, of processed peptide from autoantigens. One might therefore expect to find an association between the expression of particular HLA gene products and immune responses to β-cell antigens. Indeed, insulin autoantibody responses have been shown to be dependent on the expression of HLA-DR4, or associated alleles. Similar searches for HLA associations between HLA genotypes and antibody responses to GAD have been performed. Serjeantson *et al.*, reported that GAD antibody responses are most prevalent in IDDM patients with the high risk genotype HLA-DR 3/4; DQ 2/8 than in patients with other genotypes and HLA-DQ2 was significantly increased in GAD antibody positive IDDM patients, compared to those who were GAD antibody negative[23]. The HLA association was most evident in IDDM patients with disease onset after the age of 14. In our own studies we failed to detect an HLA association with GAD antibodies in sera from young, recent-onset IDDM patients (Table 6.1). Thus, HLA may play only a minor role in determining the prevalence and strength of the GAD antibody response by the time of disease onset.

GAD ANTIBODIES IN FAMILIES OF IDDM PATIENTS

First degree relatives of patients with IDDM have an increased risk of developing the disease through the inheritance of disease susceptibility genes. The estimated risk of diabetes development in these relatives is around 3%, some 10-fold higher than that in the general population. Risk increases further when there is expression of diabetes susceptibility HLA alleles (12% for HLA heterozygous relatives), or genetic identity (30% risk in identical twins). These populations have proved useful in studying the appearance of anti-islet immunity in the pre-diabetic period and in assessing the value of different immune markers for the prediction of IDDM.

Table 6.1. HLA antigens and GAD antibodies in IDDM patients. GAD antibodies were determined in HLA-typed recent-onset IDDM patients aged 6 months to 16 years at diagnosis. No significant association of GAD-antibody positivity with expression of specific HLA alleles, or combinations of alleles, was detected

HLA antigens	*n*	Number (%) GAD-antibody positive
DR1, DQ1	12	7 (58%)
DR2, DQ1	3	2 (67%)
DR3, DQ2	31	21 (68%)
DR4, DQ8	37	26 (70%)
DR4, DQ7	5	4 (80%)
DR7, DQ2	7	6 (86%)
DR9, DQ9	2	2 (100%)
DR13, DQ1,7	3	3 (100%)
DR3/4,DQ2/8	20	14 (70%)
DR3/non-4	11	7 (64%)
DR4/non-3	22	17 (77%)
Other	2	1 (50%)

Analysis of GAD antibodies in non-diabetic relatives and identical twins has shown that these antibodies appear early in the pre-diabetic period, in some cases > 10 years prior to disease onset, and GAD antibodies have been detected before the appearance of other immune markers such as ICAs[5,6,24]. It is also established that the presence of GAD antibodies is associated with ICA in first degree relatives, suggesting that both of these markers identify subgroups of relatives who have anti-islet immunity and are at highest risk for disease. However, neither ICAs nor GAD antibodies are entirely predictive of IDDM in relatives. Studies with identical twins of IDDM patients have shown that 15–20% of twins who are long-term (>6 years) discordant with their diabetic co-twin are positive for GAD antibodies[24]. Since 90% or more of twins who develop IDDM do so within 6 years of their co-twin, most of these GAD antibody positive non-diabetic twins are unlikely to become diabetic. Furthermore, ICA in relatives is acknowledged to be heterogeneous, with sub-specificities conferring different risks for IDDM. A target for the ICA specificity with the lowest risk may be GAD. Thus, GAD antibodies can clearly appear in relatives who have a relatively low risk for IDDM.

Studies of islet antigens in IDDM have identified a number of other promising antibody markers that are associated with IDDM. Antibodies to the islet 37K- and 40K-tyrosine phosphatase-like antigens appear to be particularly useful in identifying identical twins who later develop disease[24]. However, it is possible that no single immune marker used on its own will have sufficient sensitivity and specificity to accurately identify individuals at risk for disease. An alternative approach is to analyse multiple immune and/or genetic markers to develop a strategy for disease prediction based on the possession of multiple markers. This approach has been tested by analysing antibodies to GAD, insulin and 37/40K-antigens in a group of ICA-positive first degree relatives who have been followed for up to 15 years for the development of IDDM[25]. The distribution of antibodies in this population is shown in Figure 6.3. The proportion of relatives with each combination of antibodies who developed IDDM, which is likely to give an indication of diabetes risk, is also illustrated. The results of this study showed clearly that relatives who were positive for multiple antibodies were most likely to develop disease. It is anticipated such an analysis can be refined, perhaps by including additional or alternative immune and genetic markers, to provide an accurate screening strategy for identification of individuals who will develop IDDM.

GAD ANTIBODIES IN ENDOCRINE AUTOIMMUNE DISEASE

Early studies on antibodies to GAD, detected as 64K-antigen, indicated that the majority of patients with autoimmune diseases other than IDDM were negative[6]. However, recently it has become clear that a small proportion of patients with endocrine autoimmune diseases can possess very high levels of

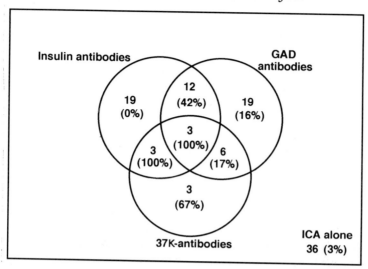

Figure 6.3. Distribution of antibodies to GAD, insulin and 37/40K-antigens in ICA positive relatives of IDDM patients. The numbers within each circle represent the number of relatives positive for the relevant antibody specificity; where circles overlap more than one antibody is detected. Numbers in parentheses indicate the proportion of individuals with the particular antibody combination who have progressed to IDDM

antibodies to GAD. A significant proportion of patients with Type 1 autoimmune polyglandular syndrome have been shown to possess high levels of GAD antibodies[26], as well as almost all patients with organ-specific endocrine autoimmune disease who are positive for ICAs[27]. Only a proportion of these GAD antibody positive polyendocrine patients develop IDDM, and the additional detection of antibodies to 37/40K-antigens and/or insulin identify most of those who become diabetic[27], consistent with the presence of multiple islet antibodies being indicative of diabetes progression. Individuals who have an immune response to one or more antigens expressed in endocrine tissues may be particularly prone to developing high levels of antibodies to GAD. However, this GAD antibody response is not necessarily indicative of later development of IDDM.

The detection of high levels of GAD antibodies in individuals with polyendocrine autoimmunity is of particular interest since most SMS patients, who themselves have strong GAD antibody responses, also have antibodies to other endocrine organs and/or other endocrine autoimmune diseases[8]. SMS is thought to be predominantly an antibody-mediated disease, whereas IDDM is T-cell mediated. GAD immune responses in individuals with polyendocrine autoimmunity may be directed primarily towards the production of antibodies, rather than a cellular immune response; hence the high levels of serum antibodies and relatively low incidence of IDDM. Patients with SMS may represent a special case where a high level of GAD antibody response has broken through to the central nervous system, resulting in the disruption of the functioning of those neurons expressing GAD.

GAD ANTIBODIES IN THE GENERAL POPULATION

Since the majority of new cases of IDDM have no family history of IDDM or other autoimmune disease, accurate assays to identify individuals at risk for IDDM in the general population are required if procedures to prevent IDDM in susceptible individuals are to be effectively introduced. There is therefore a need to assess the value of any potential immune marker for IDDM in a population that has a very low disease prevalence (around 0.2%). Analysis of markers in a relatively large sample of the population combined with long-term follow-up for disease is necessary to define accurately their predictive value. Such studies have started to be undertaken for ICA and preliminary results suggest that the prevalence of ICA in the general population is considerably higher than that of IDDM. ICA may be a poorer predictor of IDDM in the general population than in families of IDDM patients where there may be an inherited risk for disease. To date, no large-scale studies of GAD antibody frequency in the general population have been undertaken. In most small-scale studies with a population size <100, the individuals tested have usually been negative. However, a low prevalence (<5%) of GAD antibody positive individuals has been detected in samples of normal individuals in a few studies. Reports claiming a 100% specificity for GAD antibodies in predicting diabetes based on the absence of these antibodies in small numbers (100) of non-diabetic normal individuals may be unduly optimistic[28]. Clearly, antibody prevalence in a particular study depends on the assay procedures used and the definition of antibody positivity. Assessment of antibody prevalence in the background population must await larger scale studies using validated assays.

EPITOPES RECOGNIZED BY ANTIBODIES

Antibodies in IDDM react poorly with GAD that has been denatured, indicating that the conformation of the molecule is critical for antibody binding in most patients. This complicates the identification of epitopes recognized by antibodies in IDDM; analysis of antibody binding to proteolytic fragments, synthetic polypeptides or deletion mutants will detect preferentially antibodies recognizing linear epitopes. However, there is evidence that autoantibodies in IDDM may be directed to specific regions of the molecule. Firstly, the N-terminus of the molecule seems to play at most a minor role in autoantibody binding. Tryptic cleavage of the N-terminal 80–90 amino acids of GAD, to generate 50 kDa fragments, does not have a major influence on binding of IDDM- associated autoantibodies to the molecule. Kaufman *et al.*[11] analyzed the reactivity of four sera from IDDM patients, all strongly positive for GAD antibodies, with three segments of GAD-65 representing respectively the *N*-terminus (amino acids 1–224), the middle region (amino acids 224–398) and the *C*-terminus (amino acids 398–585) in immunoprecipitation reactions. One serum failed to bind any of the GAD segments, indicating that the integrity of a large part of the GAD molecule is essential for antibody reactivity in this serum. The other three all recognized the *C*-terminal segment and two also bound the middle segment. All sera failed to bind the *N*-terminal segment. This study provides further evidence that the middle and *C*-terminal domains of GAD are the most important regions for antibody binding of IDDM-associated GAD antibodies.

Richter *et al.*[29] have characterized the epitopes recognized by six human monoclonal antibodies (MICAs 1–6) to GAD, all generated from the same IDDM patient Epstein–Barr virus transformation. All antibodies were found to be specific for GAD-65 in immunoprecipitation experiments. Consistent with the findings discussed above, analysis of binding to deletion mutants of GAD-65 indicated that the *N*-terminal domain is not important in antibody binding since deletion of amino acids 1–244 did not affect reactivity of any of the monoclonal antibodies. Two monoclonal antibodies (MICAs 1, 3) recognized a similar conformational epitope at the *C*-terminus of the molecule (Figure 6.2). An additional conformational epitope located in the middle region of the molecule (residues 244–476) was recognized by MICAs 4 and 6. Only one monoclonal antibody (MICA 2) was positive in Western blotting and this antibody may recognize a linear epitope at the *C*-terminus of the molecule, localized predominantly between residues 545 and 585 (Figure 6.2). In another study, Mauch *et al.*[30] screened cDNAs representing small fragments of GAD-65 for epitopes recognized by autoantibodies in IDDM by Western blotting. A linear epitope, again at the *C*-terminus of the molecule, between residues 552 and 582, was identified by this approach. Although a similar epitope was identified independently by two different groups, this epitope is likely to be relatively rare in IDDM, since very few IDDM patients recognize GAD-65 in Western blotting.

Antibodies in SMS exhibit a number of differences compared to those in IDDM. Much higher levels of antibodies are detected in SMS patients and GAD antibodies in most SMS patients recognize GAD by Western blotting. It is therefore possible that different epitopes are recognized in the two diseases. Antibodies in SMS react with both GAD-65 and GAD-67 in immunoprecipitation experiments, but bind specifically to GAD-65 in Western blotting[31]. Thus, antibody recognition of GAD-67 in SMS appears to be highly conformation dependent. Analysis of antibody binding to deletion mutants of GAD-65 identified two major epitopes in Western blotting studies: a dominant epitope at the C-terminus encompassing residues 475–585 and an additional epitope at the N-terminus including residues 1–95 (Figure 6.2). Although both are located in the C-terminal domain, the dominant epitope in SMS appears to be distinct from the linear epitope identified in IDDM, since residues 475–484 are essential for antibody reactivity in SMS patients' sera. The studies described do not exclude the presence of common epitopes for autoantibodies in IDDM and SMS. Nevertheless, these studies on antibody binding to GAD are sufficiently encouraging to warrant a search for specific epitopes for autoantibodies that are characteristic of these two diseases.

GAD AUTOIMMUNITY IN ANIMAL MODELS OF IDDM

Antibodies to 64 000 M_r proteins have been detected in two animal models of IDDM, the BB rat and the NOD mouse. However, it remains to be established that the proteins recognized in these studies are related to GAD, as is the case in human IDDM, since the proteins may be distinct species of similar molecular weight. There have been reports of immunoprecipitating antibodies to GAD in the NOD mouse, but many attempts to immunoprecipitate GAD in the animal models have been unsuccessful. GAD might be expected to be less important as an autoantigen in mouse models of IDDM, in view of the very low expression of the enzyme, particularly GAD-65, in mouse pancreatic islets. However, recent studies have implicated GAD-65 as key autoantigen in the NOD mouse model, as well as in human IDDM. This finding may greatly assist in determining the precise role of GAD in the immunopathogenesis of IDDM.

Two independent groups analyzed T-cell reactivity to a number of potential β cell autoantigens, including GAD, during the period preceding development of diabetes in the NOD mouse[32,33]. Both groups reported that, of a number of antigens tested, T-cell proliferative responses to GAD appeared earliest, being detectable at 4 weeks of age, when inflammation of the pancreatic islet (insulitis) is first apparent. Induction of tolerance to GAD prevented development of IDDM, reduced the severity of insulitis and also blocked T-cell proliferative responses to other islet antigens. These studies suggest that T-cell responses to GAD are critical for the development of islet autoimmunity, and of diabetes, in the NOD mouse, whereas autoimmune responses to other antigens may be secondary and strongly dependent on the initiation of a T-cell response to GAD. One group was also able to detect autoantibody responses to both GAD-65 and GAD-67 in the period preceding diabetes in the NOD mouse. Antibodies were measured using an ELISA technique. The success of this technique is perhaps surprising, in view of the poor performance of ELISA assays in detecting GAD antibodies in human IDDM, and the difficulties many groups have experienced in detecting immunoprecipitating antibodies to GAD in the NOD mouse. Nevertheless,

GAD antibodies were first detectable at 4 weeks of age, preceding antibody responses to other islet autoantigens, and at a similar time to the first detection of GAD-reactive T cells and onset of insulitis. Antibody levels to all antigens tested, including GAD, peaked at 24 weeks of age, shortly before onset of diabetes.

Intrathymic injection of GAD at 3 weeks of age, although partially effective in blocking T-cell proliferative responses to GAD and protecting against diabetes, did not block antibody responses in the NOD mice[33]. Most antibody responses are dependent on antigen-specific helper T-cell activation and proliferation. Two classes of helper T (Th) cells have been classified according to their cytokine secretion; activated Th1 cells secrete interferon-γ and provide help for cell-mediated immunity, whereas activated Th2 cells secrete interleukin 4 and promote antibody-mediated immunity. IDDM is generally considered to be a T-cell (rather than antibody)-mediated disease and may therefore be dependent on the activation of Th1 cells. Tisch *et al.*[33] were able to demonstrate secretion of interferon-γ during the T-cell response to GAD, consistent with the proliferation of primed GAD-specific Th1 cells in the in vitro system. The tolerization protocol was apparently effective at blocking the Th1 response, but may not have inhibited Th2 responses to GAD that may be responsible for promoting antibody responses to the antigen. Th2 cells are known to inhibit Th1-mediated immunity in many systems. It is possible that this class of cells play a role in blocking Th1-cell reactivity to GAD and may protect against diabetes development. Thus, detection of an antibody response to GAD (or other islet antigens), perhaps promoted by antigen-specific Th2 cells, may not necessarily be indicative of the presence of a destructive autoimmune response against the islet.

CONCLUSIONS

The identification of GAD as an autoantigen in IDDM has made a considerable impact in the field of IDDM research. Evidence is accumulating from studies in humans and animal models that GAD may play a major role in the immunopathogenesis of IDDM, and also SMS. GAD autoimmunity is therefore a potential target for antigen-specific immune intervention to prevent these diseases. GAD autoantibodies are also likely to be useful in the prediction of IDDM. However, as discussed, GAD antibodies also develop, sometimes at high levels, in individuals with low risk for disease. The finding that the immune system can develop along predominantly cellular or humoral pathways may have relevance to this. IDDM is suggested to be a cell-mediated disease, and deviation of a GAD immune response along a humoral pathway may not result in β-cell destruction. It is therefore probable that detection of antibodies to the whole GAD molecule will not have sufficient specificity to identify accurately those individuals who have a pathogenic immune response. Dissection of the GAD antibody response may identify antibody sub-specificities, recognizing specific epitopes on GAD, that are most closely associated with IDDM development and that can be used to predict accurately IDDM. Alternatively, GAD antibodies may be used in combination with other immune markers to achieve high sensitivity and specificity of prediction. There is now an urgent need for large-scale population studies to define accurately the true predictive value of antibodies to GAD and other antigens, so that the best strategy for the prediction of IDDM can be defined.

REFERENCES

1 Genovese S, Bonifacio E, McNally JM, Dean BM, Wagner R, Bosi E, Gale EAM, Bottazzo GF. Distinct cytoplasmic islet cell antibodies with different risks for Type 1 (insulin-dependent) diabetes mellitus. *Diabetologia* 1992; **35**: 385–8.

2 Gianani R, Pugliesi A, Bonner-Weir S, Shiffrin AJ, Soeldner JS, Erlich H, Awdeh Z, Alper CA, Jackson RA, Eisenbarth GS. Prognostically significant heterogeneity of cytoplasmic islet cell antibodies in relatives of patients with type 1 diabetes. *Diabetes* 1992; **41**: 347–53.

3 Harrison LC. Islet cell autoantigens in insulin-dependent diabetes: Pandora's box revisited. *Immunol Today* 1992; **13**: 348–52.

4 Baekkeskov S, Nielsen JH, Marner B, Bilde T, Ludvigsson J, Lernmark Å. Autoantibodies in newly diagnosed diabetic children immunoprecipitate pancreatic islet cell proteins. *Nature* 1982; **298**: 167–9.

5 Atkinson MA, Maclaren NK, Sharp DW, Lacy, PE, Riley WJ. 64000 Mr antibodies as predictors of insulin-dependent diabetes. *Lancet* 1990; **335**: 1357–60.

6 Baekkesov S, Landin M, Kristensen JK, Srikanta S, Bruining GJ, Mandrup-Poulsen T, de Beaufort C, Soeldner JS, Eisenbarth G, Lindgren F, Sundquist G, Lernmark A. Antibodies to a 64000-Mr human islet cell protein precede the clinical onset of insulin-dependent diabetes. *J Clin Invest* 1987; **79**: 926–34.

7 Christie MR, Pipeleers DG, Lernmark A, Baekkeskov S. Cellular and subcellular localization of an Mr 64,000 protein autoantigen in insulin-dependent diabetes. *J Biol Chem* 1990; **265**: 376–81.

8 Solimena M, Folli F, Aparisi R, Pozza G, De Camilli P. Autoantibodies to GABA-ergic neurons and pancreatic beta cells in stiff-man syndrome. *New Engl J Med* 1990; **322**: 1555–60.

9 Baekkeskov S, Aanstoot HJ, Christgau S, Reetz A, Solimena M, Cascalho M, Folli F, Richter-Olesen H, De Camilli P. Identification of the 64k autoantigen in insulin-dependent diabetes as the GABA-synthesizing enzyme glutamic acid decarboxylase. *Nature* 1990; **347**: 151–6.

10 Christie MR, Brown TJ, Cassidy D. Binding of antibodies in sera from type 1 (insulin-dependent) diabetic patients to glutamate decarboxylase. Evidence for antigenic and non-antigenic forms of the enzyme. *Diabetologia* 1992; **35**: 380–4.

11 Kaufman DL, Erlander MG, Clare-Salzer M, Atkinson MA, Maclaren NK, Tobin AJ. Autoimmunity to two forms of glutamate decarboxylase in insulin-dependent diabetes mellitus. *J Clin Invest* 1992; **89**: 283–92.

12 Erdo SL, Wolff JR. γ-Aminobutyric acid outside the mammalian brain. *J Neurochem* 1990; **54**: 363–72.

13 Karlsen AE, Hagopian WA, Petersen JS, Boel E, Dyrberg T, Grubin C, Michelsen B, Madsen OD, Lernmark Å. Recombinant glutamic acid decarboxylase representing the single isoform expressed in human islets detects IDDM-associated 64k autoantibodies. *Diabetes* 1992; **41**: 1335–9.

14 Shi Y, Veit B, Baekkeskov S. Amino acid residues 24–31 but not palmitoylation of cysteines 30 and 45 are required for membrane anchoring of glutamic acid decarboxylase, GAD65. *J Cell Biol* 1994; **124**: 927–34.

15 Hagopian WA, Michelsen B, Karlsen AE, Larsen F, Moody A, Grubin CE, Rowe R, Petersen J, McEvoy R, Lernmark Å. Autoantibodies in IDDM primarily recognize the 65,000-M_r rather than the 67,000-M_r isoform of glutamic acid decarboxylase. *Diabetes* 1993; **42**: 631–6.

16 Elias D, Markovits D, Reshev T, van der Zee R, Cohen IR. Induction and therapy of autoimmune diabetes in the non-obese diabetic (NOD/Lt) mouse by a 65-kDa heat shock protein. *Proc Natl Acad Sci* 1990; **87**: 1576–80.

17 Pietropaolo M, Castano L, Babu S, Buelow R, Kuo Y-LS, Martin S, Martin A. Powers AC, Prochada M, Naggert J, Leiter EH, Eisenbarth GS. Islet cell autoantigen 69kD (ICA 69). Molecular cloning and characterization of a novel diabetes-associated autoantigen. *J Clin Invest* 1993; **92**: 359–71.

18 Christie MR, Hollands JA, Brown TJ, Michelsen BK, Delovitch TL. Detection of pancreatic islet 64,000 Mr autoantigens in insulin-dependent diabetes distinct from glutamate decarboxylase. *J Clin Invest* 1993; **92**: 240–8.

19 Payton MA, Hawkes CJ, Christie MR. Relationship of the 37,000- and 40,000-M_r tryptic fragments of islet antigens in insulin-dependent diabetes to the protein tyrosine phosphatase-like molecule 1A-2 (ICA512). *J Clin Invest* 1995; **96**: 1506–11.

20 Atkinson MR, Kaufman DL, Newman D, Tobin AJ, Maclaren NK. Islet cell cytoplasmic autoantibody reactivity to glutamate decarboxylase in insulin-dependent diabetes. *J Clin Invest* 1993; **91**: 350–6.

21 Hagopian WA, Karlsen AE, Gottsäter A, Landin-Olsson M, Grubin CE, Sundkvist G, Petersen JS, Boel E, Dyrberg T, Lernmark Å. Quantitative assay using recombinant human islet glutamic acid decarboxylase (GAD65) shows that 64k autoantibody positivity at onset predicts diabetes type. *J Clin Invest* 1993; **91**: 368–74.

22 Richter W, Endl J, Eiermann TH, Brandt M, Kientsch-Engel R, Thivolet C, Jungfer H, Scherbaum WA. Human monoclonal islet cell antibodies from a patient with insulin-dependent diabetes mellitus reveal glutamate decarboxylase as the target antigen. *Proc Natl Acad Sci* 1992; **89**: 8467–71.

23 Serjeantson SW, Court J, Mackay IR, Matheson B, Rowley MJ, Tuomi T, Wilson JD, Zimmet P. HLA-DQ genotypes are associated with autoimmunity to glutamic acid decarboxylase in insulin-dependent diabetes mellitus patients. *Human Immunol* 1993; **38**: 97–104.

24 Christie MR, Tun RYM, Lo SSS, Cassidy D, Brown TJ, Hollands J, Shattock M, Bottazzo GF, Leslie RDG. Antibodies to glutamic acid decarboxylase and tryptic fragments of islet 64kD antigen as distinct markers for the development of insulin-dependent diabetes. Studies with identical twins. *Diabetes* 1992; **41**: 782–7.

25 Bingley PJ, Christie MR, Bonifacio E, Bonfanti R, Shattock M, Fonte M, Bottazzo GF, Gale EAM. Combined analysis of autoantibodies improves prediction in islet cell antibody positive relatives. *Diabetes* 1994; **43**: 1304–10.

26 Velloso LA, Winqvist O, Gustafsson J, Kampe O, Karlsson FA. Autoantibodies against a novel 51kDa islet antigen and glutamate decarboxylase isoforms in autoimmune polyendocrine syndrome type 1. *Diabetologia* 1994; **37**: 61–9.

27 Christie MR, Genovese S, Cassidy D, Bosi E, Brown TJ, Lai M, Bonifacio E, Bottazzo GF. Antibodies to islet 37k-antigen, but not to glutamate decarboxylase, discriminate rapid progression to insulin-dependent diabetes mellitus in endocrine autoimmunity. *Diabetes* 1994; **43**: 1254–9.

28 Tuomilehto J, Zimmet P, Mackay IR, Koskela P, Vidgren G, Toivanen L, Tuomilehto-Wolf E, Kohtamaki K, Stengard J, Rowley MJ. Antibodies to glutamic acid decarboxylase as predictors of insulin-dependent diabetes mellitus before clinical onset of disease. *Lancet* 1994; **343**: 1383–5.

29 Richter W, Shi Y, Baekkeskov S. Autoreactive epitopes defined by diabetes-associated human monoclonal antibodies are localized in the middle and C-terminal domains of glutamate decarboxylase. *Proc Natl Acad Sci* 1993; **90**: 2832–6.

30 Mauch L, Abney CC, Berg H, Scherbaum WA, Liedvogel B, Northemann W. Characterization of a linear epitope within the human pancreatic 64-kDa glutamic acid decarboxylase and its autoimmune recognition by sera from insulin-dependent diabetes mellitus patients. *Eur J Biochem* 1993; **212**: 597–603.

31 Butler MH, Solimena M, Dirkx R, Hayday A, De Camilli P. Identification of a dominant epitope of glutamic acid decarboxylase (GAD-65) recognized by autoantibodies in stiff-man syndrome. *J Exp Med* 1993; **178**: 2097–106.

32 Kaufman DL, Clare-Salzer M, Tian J, Forsthuber T, Ting GSP, Robinson P, Atkinson MA, Sercarz EE, Tobin AJ, Lehmann PV. Spontaneous loss of T-cell tolerance to glutamic acid decarboxylase in murine insulin-dependent diabetes. *Nature* 1993; **366**: 69–72.

33 Tisch R, Yang X-D, Singer SM, Liblau RS, Fugger L, McDevitt HO. Immune response to glutamic acid decarboxylase correlates with insulitis in non-obese diabetic mice. *Nature* 1993; **366**: 72–5.

7

Humoral Immune Markers: Additional Islet Cell Antigens—Important Clues To Pathogenesis or Red Herrings?

ROBERT C. McEVOY[1], NANCY M. THOMAS[1], and JANICE NESS[2]
[1]Department of Pediatrics, Mount Sinai School of Medicine, New York, USA and
[2]Department of Pediatrics, University of Washington School of Medicine and
Children's Hospital & Medical Center, Seattle, Washington, USA

"Red Herring"—something used to confuse, or to divert attention from something else. (*Webster's New World Dictionary*)

INTRODUCTION

There is no question that sera from individuals with diabetes contain immunoglobulins which bind more or less specifically to islet cells on tissue sections, so-called islet cell antibodies or ICAs. At least two of the specific antigens of ICAs have been unequivocally identified as insulin and glutamic acid decarboxylase (GAD). These antigens and the data supporting the presence of autoimmune processes against them during the pathogenesis of insulin-dependent diabetes mellitus (IDDM) in humans are reviewed elsewhere in this volume. The continuing search for additional antigens has led to the subsequent identification of a myriad of islet cell components to which antibodies in the sera of newly diagnosed diabetic patients bind. The present review will attempt to organize the extensive data, accumulated largely over

Prediction, Prevention and Genetic Counseling in IDDM. Edited by Jerry P. Palmer.
© 1996 John Wiley & Sons Ltd.

the last five years, suggesting that autoimmune responses can be detected against many other antigens which are more or less unique to the islet beta cells. This area has been reviewed elsewhere in detail[1-5]. The data have been gathered using samples from individuals at the diagnosis of IDDM and from family members and others who have been followed prospectively and who eventually develop hyperglycemia and are diagnosed with IDDM. The discussion here will be limited to data obtained from human diabetes and to the humoral autoimmune response to the individual islet cell constituents, although in some cases the data from experimental animals are more complete. It must be recognized, however, that the presence of a high titer autoantibody response implies the involvement of at least the helper arm (CD4+) of the T-cell immune response. The presence of a cellular immune response in human diabetes will be discussed elsewhere in the volume.

The impetus for the examination of alternative islet cell antigens came from the original experiments which used sera from humans with diabetes to immunoprecipitate protein antigens from extracts of radio-labeled human islet cells (see Figure 7.1). Those antigens that were precipitated by sera from individuals with diabetes and not from non-diabetic controls were believed to have some role in the development of IDDM. The first antigen to be identified by this technique was the so-called 64K-antigen[6] which was eventually identified as GAD[7]. Over the last several years, a number of other antigens have been identified by this and similar techniques. Some of these antigens have been found to be identical to previously known substances, but the identities of many have not been unequivocally established as yet. Many, if not most, are present in minute amounts in the islets, limiting the usefulness of even the exquisitely sensitive techniques of molecular biology to aid in their identification. Since the molecular nature of many of these antigens remains elusive, they have frequently been identified by their molecular weights. Therefore, the antigens will be presented here in order of increasing size after first presenting the limited data on autoantigens that do not appear to be protein in nature.

NON-PROTEIN ANTIGENS

Fixation of pancreatic sections and extraction in organic solvents resulted in a different pattern of immunoreactivity from that seen using frozen sections, suggesting that at least some of the antigens were lipids or glycolipids. Importantly, neuraminidase treatment of islet sections markedly decreased binding of antibodies in ICA positive sera. Subsequently, at least two specific antigens have been identified. Initially, an islet sialoglycolipid was implicated as a autoantigen and detailed purifications by thin layer chromatography suggested that GM2-1 was a likely target as antibodies from 13 of 21 ICA

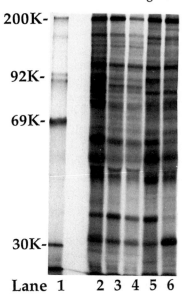

Lane 1   2 3 4 5 6

Figure 7.1. Autoradiograph of metabolically labeled ([³⁵S]methionine) human islet proteins immunoprecipitated and separated by polyacrylamide gel electrophoresis. Lane 1 contains molecular weight standards as labeled on the left side in kiloDaltons (K). Lanes 2–4 represent proteins immunoprecipitated by sera taken from three human patients at diagnosis of IDDM. These can be compared to lanes 5 and 6 which represent proteins immunoprecipitated by polyclonal antisera from two different rabbits immunized with human islets. (Autoradiograph kindly provided by Dr William Hagopian, Department of Medicine, University of Washington School of Medicine)

positive first degree relatives bound to this antigen[2,8]. While the rat islet ganglioside, GT3, has been shown to bind ICA, there is probably no relevance of this phenomenon in human diabetes as human islets lack this ganglioside. Sulfatides have also been shown to bind ICA. One study demonstrated binding of sulfatide by serum antibodies from 50 of 57 newly diagnosed patients[9]. Unfortunately, there have not as yet been prospective studies to demonstrate a temporal relationship between the appearance of the antibodies to these lipid components of the islet and those to the protein antigens. Also, the subcellular localization of the glycolipid antigens has not been attempted. Immune phenomena have been implicated in the development of neuropathy in diabetic patients and it is tempting to speculate as to the possible immunological cross-reactivity between glycolipid antigens in the islet and in the nervous system.

PROTEIN ANTIGENS

As would be expected from the myriad of bands seen after electrophoresis of immunoprecipitated metabolically labeled islet cell antigens (Figure 7.1), a number of islet proteins have been implicated as autoantigens in diabetes (Table 7.1). There has been substantial evidence gathered from many different laboratories and patient populations to establish that specific autoimmunity to human insulin and human glutamic acid decarboxylase is a frequent finding at the diagnosis of diabetes and that the presence of antibodies to these antigens identifies non-diabetic individuals as being at increased risk for developing the disease. These same criteria have not yet been as rigorously applied to most of the other protein antigens. Whether antibodies to any of these other antigens will increase the specificity and sensitivity of the prediction of diabetes as defined by the non-specific identification of ICAs and the specific identification of antibodies to insulin and GAD remains to be proven. Some of these antigens have been identified as specific proteins with known functions, others have yet to be completely characterized and can only be identified at present by their molecular weights.

GLUT 2—BETA CELL GLUCOSE TRANSPORTER

Immunoglobulins from the sera of patients at the diagnosis of IDDM were found to decrease glucose uptake into rat islet cells in vitro[10]. Subsequently, the same investigators were able to demonstrate that the inhibition was due to the presence of antibodies in the diabetic sera against GLUT-2, the specific

Table 7.1. Islet protein antigens detected by autoantibodies in human sera

Antigen	Identity	Reference
—	GLUT-2	11
30K	Chymotrypsin-like	12
37K	Tryptic fragment of 65K	25
38K	Unknown	6
38K	Carboxypeptidase-H	13
38K	Unknown cell-mediated assay	14
52K	Rubella-like antigen	16
60–65K	HSP 60/62/65	22
65K	Non-GAD/37K tryptic fragment	24
69K	Unknown	27
69L	ABBOS	28
120K	Unknown	31
155K (118K)	Unknown	32

glucose transporter of the beta cells[11]. Using fluorescence-activated cell sorting, sera from 24 of 30 patients had antibodies which bound to this cell surface protein. These assays are technically difficult and because the sensitivity is no greater than the standard ICA assay, it is unlikely that these antibodies will be routinely measured.

30K (CHYMOTRYPSINOGEN)

Antibodies in newly diagnosed patient sera (4 of 16) have been found which bound to a novel human pancreatic islet protein of approximately 30K[12]. This antigen was identified by microsequencing as identical at least in the N-terminal amino acid sequence to human chymotrypsinogen. This observation has not yet been confirmed by other laboratories and it is not yet known whether detection of antibodies to this acinar antigen will add either sensitivity or specificity for the prediction of IDDM.

37K PROTEIN

This protein is a proteolytic fragment of an islet antigen of 64K that is not GAD. This antigen is discussed in detail under the 64K antigen.

38K PROTEINS

At least two proteins with a molecular weight of 38K are precipitated with sera from IDDM patients. One of these proteins has been identified as a beta cell granule membrane enzyme, carboxypeptidase H, responsible for processing proinsulin to insulin[13]. The protein was immunoprecipitated by sera from IDDM patients at diagnosis and from 5 of 20 first degree relatives.

Perhaps another protein with a similar molecular weight had previously been identified by immunoprecipitation by about 25% of sera from IDDM patients at diagnosis[6] and a similar or identical protein by proliferation of a T-cell clone raised from peripheral blood lymphocytes from a patient at the diagnosis of IDDM[14]. Humoral and T-cell responses against a 38K protein have also been reported by another laboratory[15]. Whether these different methods and different laboratories have detected the same or different proteins remains to be determined, but the T-cell clone[14] did not recognize carboxypeptidase H. At the present time, the non-carboxypeptidase 38K protein has not been further identified or characterized.

52K PROTEIN

Sera from 58% of newly diagnosed IDDM patients have been shown to bind to a protein antigen of approximately 52K on Western blots of islet and rat insulinoma cell extracts[16]. The antigen is not found in other organs and is found in the secretory granule fraction from both insulinoma cells and human islets. Although the antigen has not yet been cloned, the *N*-terminal sequence is now known. A polyclonal antibody to a peptide synthesized from the *N*-terminal sequence data recognizes islet secretory granules by electron microscopic immunocytochemistry. Further characterization of this antigen appears to support the hypothesis of molecular mimicry in that the antigen is also recognized by a monoclonal antibody to rubella virus antigen[17]. Rubella virus is the only known human pathogen that has been definitely linked to an increased risk for IDDM, at least when the individual is infected prenatally resulting in congenital rubella syndrome (reviewed in reference 18)[18].

60–62K (HEAT SHOCK PROTEINS)

Before the 64K antigen had been shown to be GAD, one of the candidates for the identity of this protein was the human heat shock protein (hsp) with a molecular weight of about 60–65K. This was a particularly attractive hypothesis because of the postulated roles for heat shock proteins in the immune response and in a variety of autoimmune diseases including arthritis and systemic lupus erythematosus[19,20]. The hypothesis was strengthened by the demonstration that immunization of pre-diabetic NOD mice with the human heat shock protein prevented diabetes[21] and by the demonstration that an islet cell secretory granule antigen was chemically similar to hsp 62[22]. In contrast, specific autoantibodies to human hsp 65 could not be demonstrated in the sera of newly diagnosed human diabetics[23]. This remains an area of controversy, but at the time of writing there is no strong evidence of a direct role for heat shock proteins or an autoimmune response against this family of proteins in the pathogenesis of human IDDM.

NON-GAD 64–65K PROTEIN

In addition to GAD, the attempts to characterize the 64K protein also resulted in the elucidation of another islet antigen of approximately the same molecular mass which was also precipitated by sera from newly diagnosed patients with IDDM[24]. Proteolysis with trypsin resulted in fragments of different molecular weights than did treatment of GAD[25]. Of interest was the observation that antibodies to a 37K trypsin fragment were more closely associated with IDDM than those to the original protein[26].

69K, ABBOS, BOVINE SERUM ALBUMIN

Part of the considerable controversy over the identity of the 64K protein was due to possible cross-reactivity in the assay with bovine serum albumin

(BSA). There was increasing evidence that many individuals had serum antibodies against BSA, but there has been great controversy as to whether there was any association between the presence of these antibodies and IDDM. When solid tumors of rat insulinoma cells were used as a target for ICAs in IDDM serum, the staining of the cells appeared in a polar distribution, unlike the uniform labeling of the classic ICAs. This polar antigen has been identified and cloned[27]. It is a 69K protein and contains a region of sequence homology with a portion of BSA. This homologous sequence has been termed the ABBOS peptide. There is a positive correlation between cow's milk consumption and the prevalence of diabetes among the countries of the world, with the highest rates of both in Scandinavia and particularly Finland. Further, nutrition studies in the animal models of IDDM revealed that cow's milk protein is the principal protein source in rat chow and when BB rats were fed a diet from which milk protein had been removed, the rate of diabetes fell to very low levels[28]. Also, the expression of the 69K antigen is increased in islet cells after exposure in vitro to interferon-γ. Thus, it is possible that early exposure to BSA from cow's milk sensitizes genetically susceptible individuals to this protein. A viral infection in the pancreas could increase interferon-γ production locally, secondarily increasing expression of the 69K antigen containing the ABBOS peptide on the beta cells. Expression of this novel peptide could elicit a secondary immune response by the T cells already sensitized to BSA and thus destroy the beta cells. While this is an extremely attractive hypothesis, several investigators have found no relati onship between anti-BSA immunity and IDDM[29]. In addition, autoantibodies to the 69K antigen do not increase the sensitivity or specificity of the prediction of diabetes beyond that demonstrated by classic ICA and anti-GAD[30].

120K PROTEIN

Monoclonal antibodies have been used to define novel islet cell surface antigens. One such monoclonal antibody, designated 4F2, stained human islet cells by histochemical detection methods and identified a glycoprotein of approximately 120K[31]. Since this first observation in 1987, no further information has been reported as to the possible identity of this protein or its role in the beta cell.

155K (138K) PROTEIN

Using a monoclonal antibody raised against rat insulinoma cells (RIN m5F) a novel antigen of the pancreatic beta cells has been detected[32]. The antigen is a glycoprotein found in the pancreas of rat, dog, pig, monkey and human[33]. The antigen has an apparent molecular weight of 155K and 160K in rat pancreas and islets by Western blotting and immunoprecipitation, but only about 138K in human material[34]. The epitope detected by the monoclonal antibody is thus highly tissue specific, but highly conserved among species. That this epitope is relevant to IDDM is demonstrated by the observation that 87–94% of over 300 children with IDDM have antibodies in their sera against this epitope at or soon after diagnosis versus about 4% of over 1600 control children[32,35]. Unlike ICA but similar to antibodies to GAD, these antibodies persist in many patients for as long as 20 years after diagnosis. The 155K rat antigen has been purified to homogeneity by electrophoresis and high performance liquid chromatography. The expression of the antigen is increased by dexamethasone treatment in vivo[36] but not in vitro[37], suggesting that its expression is linked to stimulation of the beta cells. Of particular interest is the recent observation that a human T-cell clone, isolated from cells taken at the onset of IDDM, proliferates specifically in response to this rat antigen[38], again suggesting a cross-reactivity between the rat and human antigens. While these observations are provocative, the antigen has not yet been identified and the high prevalence of autoantibodies to this antigen in first degree family members[35] limits its utility in screening studies.

SUMMARY AND CONCLUSIONS

As the subtitle of this chapter implies, there is no agreement as yet as to the meaning of the autoimmune response to this myriad of different cell- and/or organ-specific antigens. Without exception, the humoral immune response, generating antibodies to these antigens, is clearly associated with diabetes as individuals with IDDM have been found to express antibodies against these antigens far more frequently than do individuals from control populations. Relative to the significance of these antibodies to the pathogenesis of IDDM, at least two possibilities must be considered. First, in genetically susceptible individuals, an autoimmune response to a specific antigen (not necessarily the same antigen in every subject) triggers a series of immunological processes which eventually accumulate to destroy sufficient beta cell mass to produce insulin deficiency leading to hyperglycemia, and the clinical diagnosis of IDDM. In this scenario, the broad spectrum humoral immune response to this wide variety of antigens could be seen as "antigen spreading", that is recruitment of clones responding to additional antigens as a consequence of the original, inappropriate autoimmune attack against a "primary" antigen. If there is a single primary antigen, knowledge of the identity of this first antigen which triggers the cascade of immune responses may be critical to prevention of the ultimate destruction of the islets. Intervention strategies would therefore need to be aimed at the response to the primary antigen as any specific intervention against the secondary immune responses would be less effective.

The second view of the autoimmune nature of diabetes implicates a failure of normal control mechanisms to contain or block inappropriate autoimmune attacks on the islets. As long as these autoreactive phenomena would be limited by regulated control mechanisms, they would never produce enough beta cell loss to result in IDDM. This view places a defect in the regulation of the immune response as fundamental, with the specificity of the autoimmune detected against the islet antigens having a secondary role.

There is evidence from the experimental animal models of IDDM to support each of these views. Certainly, additional investigation will be necessary before either of these mechanisms can be given a pathogenetic role in the development of IDDM in humans. However, the rapid expansion of knowledge in this field, largely accumulated in this decade, should soon clarify the merits of each of these potential mechanisms or perhaps suggest new ones.

REFERENCES

1 Bärmeier H, Christie M, Herold B, Herold K, Lernmark Å. The humoral anti-islet response: biochemical characterization. In Ginsberg-Fellner F, McEvoy RC (eds), *Autoimmunity and the Pathogenesis of Diabetes* New York: Springer-Verlag, 1990, pp 87–105.

2 Karounos DG, Nell, LJ, Thomas JW. Autoantibodies present at onset of type 1 diabetes recognize multiple islet cell antigens. *Autoimmunity* 1990; 6: 79–91.

3 Thai A-C, Eisenbarth GS. Natural history of IDDM. *Diabetes Revs* 1993; 1: 1–14.

4 Atkinson MA, MacLaren NK. Islet cell autoantigens of IDDM. *Diabetes Revs* 1993; 1: 191–203.

5 Bosi E, Bonifacio E, Bottazzo GF. Autoantigens in IDDM. *Diabetes Revs* 1933; 1: 204–14.

6 Baekkeskov S, Nielson JH, Marner B, Bilde T, Ludvigsson J, Lernmark Å. Antibodies in newly diagnosed diabetic children immunoprecipitate human pancreatic islet cell proteins. *Nature* 1982; 298: 167–9.

7 Baekkeskov S, Aanstoot HJ, Christgau S, Reetz A, Solimena M, Cascalho M, Folli F, Richter-Olesen H, De Camili P. Identification of the 64K autoantigen in insulin dependent diabetes as the GABA-synthesizing enzyme glutamic acid decarboxylase. *Nature* 1990; 347: 151–6.

8 Dotta F, Dionisi S, Gianini R, Lollobridgida L, Perviti M, Lenti L, Eisenbarth GS, Di Mario U. Expression of antibodies to the GM-2 islet ganglioside precedes the onset of type 1 in high risk subjects. *Diabetologia* 1933; 36: A24 (Abstract).

9 Buschard K, Josefsen K, Rygaard J, Spitalnik S. Pancreatic islet cell epitope recognized by an anti-sulfatide monoclonal antibody. *APMIS* 1991; 99: 1151–6.

10 Johnson JH, Crider BP, McCorkle K, Alford M, Unger RH. Inhibition of glucose transport into rat islet cells by immunoglobulins from patients with new onset insulin dependent diabetes mellitus. *New Engl J Med* 1990; 322: 653–9.

11 Inman L, McAllister C, Chen L, Hughes S, Newgard C, Kettman J, Unger R, Johnson J. Autoantibodies to the GLUT-2 glucose transporter of beta cells in insulin dependent diabetes of recent onset. *Proc Natl Acad Sci (USA)* 1993; 90 1281–4.

12 Kim YJ, Zhou Z, Hurtado J, Wood DL, Choi AS, Pescovitz MD, Warfel KA,

Vandagriff J, Davis JK, Kwon BS. IDDM patients' sera recognize a novel 30 Kd pancreatic autoantigen related to chymotrypsinogen. *Immunol Invest* 1993; **22**: 219–27.

13 Castano L, Russo E, Zhou L, Lipes M, Eisenbarth GS. Identification and cloning of a granule autoantigen (carboxypeptidase H) associated with type 1 diabetes. *J Clin Endocr Metab* 1991; **73**: 1197–201.

14 Roep BO, Kallen AA, Hazenbos WLW, Bruining GJ, Bailyes EM, Arden SD, Hutton JC, DeVries RRP. T-cell reactivity to 38kD insulin secretory granule protein in patients with recent onset of type 1 diabetes. *Lancet* 1991; **337**: 1439–45.

15 DeAizpurua HJ, Honeyman MC, Harrison LC. A 64 kDa antigen/glutamic acid decarboxylase (GAD) in fetal pig pro-islets: co-precipitation with a 38 kDa protein and recognition by T cells in humans at risk for insulin dependent diabetes. *J Autoimmun* 1992; **5**: 759–70.

16 Karounos D, Thomas JW. Recognition of a common antigen by autoantibodies from NOD mice and humans with IDDM. *Diabetes* 1990; **39**: 1085–90.

17 Karounos D, Wolinsky J, Thomas J. Monoclonal antibody to rubella virus capsid protein recognizes a beta cell antigen. *J Immunol* 1993; **150**: 3080–5.

18 Yoon J-W. Role of viruses in the pathogenesis of IDDM. *Ann Med* 1991; **23**: 437–45.

19 Bahr GM, Rook GA, AlSaftar M, VanEmbden J, Stanford JL, Behbehani K. Antibody levels to mycobacteria in relation to HLA type: evidence for non-HLA-linked high levels of antibody to the 65kD heat shock protein of M. bovis in rheumatoid arthritis. *Clin Exp Immunol* 1988; **74**: 211–15.

20 Tsoulfa G, Rook GA, Van Embden JD, Young DB, Mehlert A, Isenberg DA, Hay PC, Lydyard PM. Raised serum IgC and IgA antibodies to mycobacterial antigens in rheumatoid arthritis. *Ann Rheum Dis* 1989; **48**: 118–23.

21 Elias D, Reshef T, Birk O, van der Zee R, Walker M, Cohen I. Vaccination against autoimmune mouse diabetes with a T-cell epitope of human 65kDa heat shock protein. *Proc Natl Acad Sci (USA)* 1991; **88**: 3088–91.

22 Brudzynski K, Martinez V, Gupta RS. Secretory granule antoantigen in insulin dependent diabetes mellitus is related to 62 kDa heat-shock protein (hsp60). *J Autoimmun* 1992; **5**: 453–63.

23 Atkinson M, Holmes L, Scharp D, Lacy P, MacLaren N. No evidence for serological autoimmunity to islet cell heat shock proteins in insulin dependent diabetes. *J Clin Invest* 1991; **87**: 721–4.

24 Christie MR, Vohra G, Champagne P, Daneman D, Delovitch TL. Distinct antibody specifies to a 64-kD islet antigen in type 1 diabetes as revealed by trypsin treatment. *J Exp Med* 1990; **172**: 789–94.

25 Christie MR, Tun RY, Lo SS, Cassidy D, Brown TJ, Hollands J, Shattock M, Bottazzo GF, Leslie RD. Antibodies to GAD and tryptic fragments of islet 64K antigen as distinct markers for development of IDDM. Studies with identical twins. *Diabetes* 1992; **41**: 782–7.

26 Christie MR, Hollands JA, Brown TJ, Michelsen BK, Delovitch TL. Detection of pancreatic islet 64,000 M(r) autoantigens in insulin dependent diabetes distinct from glutamate decarboxylase. *J Clin Invest* 1993; **92**: 240–8.

27 Pietropaolo M, Castano L, Babu S, Buelow R, Kuo Y-L, Martin S, Martin A, Powers AC, Prochazka M, Naggert J, Leiter EH, Eisenbarth GS. Islet cell autoantigen 69 kD (ICA 69): molecular cloning and characterization of a novel diabetes associated autoantigen. *J Clin Invest* 1993; **92**: 359–71.

28 Karjalainen J, Matin JM, Knip M, Ilonen J, Robinson BH, Savilahti E, Åkerblom H, Dosch HM. A bovine albumin peptide as a possible trigger of insulin dependent diabetes melitus. *N Engl J Med* 1992; **327**: 302–7.

29 Atkinson MA, Bowman MA, Kao K-J, Campbell L, Dush PJ, Shah SC, Simell O,

MacLaren NK. Lack of immune responsiveness to bovine serum albumin in insulin dependent diabetes. *New Engl J Med* 1993; **329**: 1853–8..

30 Pietropaolo M, Eisenbarth GS. Biochemical determination of antibodies to three recombinant autoantigens: high predictive value and stability of patterns. *Diabetes* 1994; **43**: 153A.

31 Srikanta S, Telen M, Posillico JT, Dlinar R, Krisch K, Haynes BF, Eisenbarth GS. Monoconal antibodies to a human islet cell glycoprotein: 4F2 and LC7-2. *Endocrinology* 1987; **120**: 2240–4.

32 Thomas NM, Ginsberg-Fellner F, McEvoy RC. Strong association between diabetes and displacement of a mouse anti-rat insulinoma cell monoclonal antibody by human serum *in vitro*. *Diabetes* 1990; **39**: 1203–11.

33 Felix I, Vargas-Rodriguez I, Pan Y-X, Thomas NM, McEvoy RC. Identification of rat islet cell surface antigens by monoclonal antibodies, PAGE, and Western blotting. *Anat Rec* 1992; **232**: 32A–33A.

34 McEvoy RC, Pan Y-X, Thomas NM. Purification and initial characterization of a novel beta cell antigen. *Autoimmunity* 1993; **15**: 77.

35 McEvoy RC, Thomas NM, Ginsberg-Fellner F. Displacement of MAB 1A2 by islet cell antibodies (ICA) in sera from diabetic patients persists after diagnosis, is increased in families with diabetic children, and precedes the development of insulin dependent diabetes (IDDM). *Ped Res* 1991; **29**: 196A.

36 Vargas-Rodriguez I, Felix, I, Ginsberg-Fellner F, Pan Y-X, Thomas NM, McEvoy RC. Dexamethasone induces increased expression of the diabetes associated β cell plasma membrane antigen detected by monoclonal antibody (MAb) 1A2. *Diabetes* 1992; **43**: 95A.

37 McEvoy RC, Thomas NM. Dexamethasone (DEX) fails to induce increased expression of a 155 kD beta cell antigen on rat insulinoma cells *in vitro*. *Ped Res* 1994; **35**: 205A.

38 McEvoy RC, Kallen AA, Thomas NM, Roep BO, De Vries RRP. Recognition of purified 155 kD and 160 kD β cell antigens by a T cell clone from an IDDM patient. *Diabetes* 1994; **43**: 154A.

8

T-Cell Markers

MARK A. ATKINSON and MARK A. BOWMAN
Department of Pathology, University of Florida College of Medicine, USA

INTRODUCTION

WHY USE T-CELL MARKERS FOR IDD?

As is evident from various chapters throughout this book, insulin-dependent diabetes (IDD) is a chronic disorder which results from an autoimmune destruction of the insulin-producing pancreatic β cells. Much has been learned during the past decade of the underlying genetics, natural history and pathogenesis of IDD. It is now well understood that the disease has a long prodromal period prior to the onset of symptoms. Recently, important advances in the use of markers to identify individuals during this pre-diabetic period have allowed large clinical intervention trials to be started with the ultimate goal of preventing the development of insulin dependence. A vast majority of studies utilize autoantibodies (e.g. islet cell (ICA), insulin (IAA), glutamate decarboxylase (anti-GAD), etc.) as the predominant markers for identifying those at increased risk for IDD, and many studies include genetic and/or metabolic (i.e. intravenous glucose tolerance testing) markers to more precisely define the predicted risk. Despite the usefulness of autoantibodies as markers for the disease, abundant evidence suggests that IDD results from a cell-mediated destruction of islet β cells. This evidence includes the demonstration of β-cell antigen-specific T-cell responses in IDD patients and in those at increased risk for the disease, the mononuclear cell infiltrate of the pancreatic islets, observations of animal models which suggest that T cells are required for and actively involved in β-cell destruction (e.g. adoptive transfer, lymphocyte depletion, etc.), and the beneficial response of humans with IDD to immunospecific therapy aimed at cellular immune activity. This

Prediction, Prevention and Genetic Counseling in IDDM. Edited by Jerry P. Palmer.
© 1996 John Wiley & Sons Ltd.

preponderance of evidence, arguing that IDD results from a cell-mediated immune destruction of the β cells, makes it reasonable to hypothesize that markers of cellular immunity will ultimately prove superior to the aforementioned autoantibody markers in terms of their ability to delineate the natural history of IDD, as well as to determine an individual's risk for the disease. This chapter describes the current status of T-cell markers for IDD, and illustrates how this information might be used in the future to enhance our ability to predict IDD and determine the pathogenesis of this disorder.

THE INSULITIS LESION

When examining the role of cellular immunity in IDD, one of the most intriguing places to initiate the investigation is at the site of the destructive lesion, the pancreatic islet. Unfortunately, these descriptions are rare due to the extended natural history and chronic nature of the disease. The most striking histological feature of the pancreas from patients with long-standing IDD is the near total lack of insulin-secreting β cells[1]. By contrast, islet cells secreting glucagon, somatostatin, or pancreatic polypeptide (i.e. the α, δ, or PP cells, respectively) are remarkably preserved. Since β cells constitute approximately 70% of the islet population, most islets in these patients are abnormally small[1]. Aside from mild interstitial fibrosis and exocrine atrophy, there are no other obvious histological abnormalities.

By the time of IDD onset, most islets are deficient in β cells similar to those observed in patients with long-standing disease[2]. Many of the remaining islets contain cells with enlarged nuclei, variable numbers of degranulated β cells, and a chronic inflammatory infiltrate commonly referred to as insulitis. This infiltrate consists mostly of CD8 T cells, plus variable numbers of CD4 T cells, B lymphocytes, macrophages, and natural killer cells[3,4]. The expression of both human leukocyte antigen (HLA) class I and class II molecules within the islets is increased, but whether the abundance of class II molecules is accounted for by an over-expression of this antigen on the β cells, or by its occurrence on endothelium or infiltrating leukocytes is controversial[3,5,6]. In addition, the expression of intercellular adhesion molecule-1 (ICAM-1) on the vascular endothelium of the islets is increased, a feature consistent with leukocytic infiltration[4].

The distribution of islets with insulitis within the pancreas of newly diagnosed patients can be strikingly uneven. The islets within one pancreatic lobule may appear normal, while those in adjacent lobules may contain insulitic islets[2]. This variability may reflect differing insulin secretory activities of the β cells, with the most metabolically active ones being preferentially destroyed. Histologic evidence of islet regeneration is modest, but has been reported in the pancreata of some young patients with IDD[6].

WHAT FACTORS REGULATE THE DESTRUCTIVE ACTIVITIES OF T CELLS INVOLVED IN IDD?

A key issue with respect to analysis of autoreactive T cells involves the identification of potentially pathogenic cells, a population which constitutes only a small fraction of the entire pool of autoantigen reactive T cells (reviewed in references 7 and 8)[7,8]. Indeed, naive (i.e. inactive) T cells have no pathogenic quality, and those that are specific for self-antigens can persist indefinitely within an individual without mediating pathology. However, if naive T cells become primed by antigen recognition and make the transition to an activated/memory state, they can function as effector cells, mediate self-cell destruction, and subsequently induce autoimmune disease.

With respect to experimental models of IDD, when naive T cells transgenically express a β-cell antigen-specific T-cell receptor, they can persist indefinitely in the host while neglecting the β-cell antigen in the target organ[9]. However, these same cells become pathogenic if primed (i.e. activated) by immunization. From these and other data, it appears that pathogenic T cells include only those which first encounter antigen under the appropriate priming conditions[10]. Recent studies have also highlighted the importance of cell adhesion molecules (e.g. VLA-4, a cell activation marker) for pathogenicity of T cells[11]. Unfortunately, we do not know in human IDD the agent(s) which transform naive T cells into primed pathogenic cells.

In cell-mediated immunological diseases such as experimental allergic encephalomyelitis (EAE), of the primed autoantigen-specific CD4 T-cell pool, primary cells of the T helper 1 (Th1) subtype are pathogenic[12,13]. By contrast, T helper 2 (Th2) cells, which among other activities promote antibody formation, are known to suppress the activities of Th1 lymphocytes by secreting lymphokines such as interleukin-4 and -10[14,15]. The immune response can also work in the opposite direction, in that production of lymphokines by Th1 cells (e.g. interferon-γ, interleukin-2) can inhibit Th2 cells as well. If both cell types are present in the target organ and both are triggered by autoantigen recognition, one population may downregulate the other via its lymphokines. The potential for IDD to result from a Th1/Th2 disorder has been described elsewhere[16] with a schematic interpretation of that model shown in Figures 8.1 and 8.2. There is evidence of Th1 cell involvement in IDD in that interferon-γ, production correlates with the development of IDD in NOD mice, and that anti-interferon-γ antibodies prevent the disease[17]. It is therefore possible that for a Th-1-mediated disease such as IDD, the generation of Th2 cells may be able to derail the autoimmune pathology. Evidence for this process in human IDD will be discussed later in this chapter.

Finally, the clonal size (i.e. precursor frequency) of pathogenic T cells may also be critical for disease development. In most systems studied to date where passive autoimmune disease is induced by injection of T cells, there

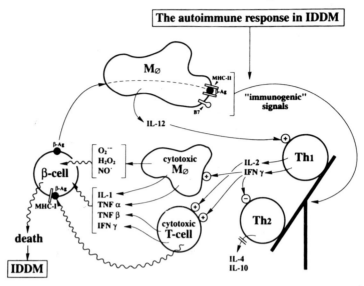

Figure 8.1. A scheme illustrating the immune system cells that may be involved in the autoimmune response leading to destruction of pancreatic islet β cells and IDDM. The concept illustrated posits that certain β-cell protein(s) act as autoantigens (β-Ag) after being processed by macrophages (Mϕ) or other antigen-presenting cells and presented in a complex with MHC class II molecules on the surface of the Mϕ. The β-Ag–MHC class II complex, accessory molecules on the Mϕ (e.g. the B7 molecule), and perhaps other signals together may comprise immunogenic signals that activate T cells, predominantly of the Th1 subset. Also, Mϕ-derived IL-12 activates Th1 cells. The antigen-activated Th1 cells produce IL-2 and IFN-γ, which inhibit Th2 cell production of IL-4 and IL-10. Also, Il-2 and IFN-γ activate Mϕ and cytotoxic T cells to kill islet β cells by a variety of mechanisms, including oxygen free radicals (O_2^- and H_2O_2)), NO, cytokines (IL-1, TNF-α, TNF-β, IFN-γ), and cytotoxic T cells that interact with a β-cell autoantigen–MHC class I complex on the β cell. Figure is taken from reference 16 and is reproduced by permission of the American Diabetes Association

exists a strict dose dependency for the passive transfer of disease. For example, in studies of graft versus host disease utilizing injection of anti-host reactive CD4 T-cell clones, a dose of 5×10^6 cells induced 100% lethality in recipient mice, while a dose of 1×10^6 cells failed to elicit even mild signs of the disease[18]. Therefore, in addition to the necessity for recent activation of an autoreactive Th1 subtype, a minimum clonal size of effector cells is required to induce disease. A recent hypothesis that incorporates these observations posits that high clonal sizes of recently activated Th1 cells could allow a spreading of the autoimmune T-cell receptor repertoire which may underlie the observed response to several β-cell antigens most often seen prior to symptomatic IDD[19]. Thus, the clonal sizes of recently activated Th1 cells may correlate with disease progression. Alternatively, given their antagonistic

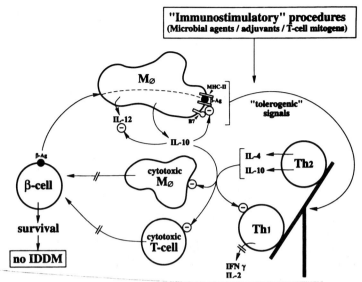

Figure 8.2. A scheme illustrating possible mechanisms by which different immunostimulatory procedures (microbial agents, adjuvants, T-cell mitogens) may provide "tolerogenic" signals that would substitute for the "immunogenic" signals mediating the autoimmune response in IDDM (Figure 8.1). Thus, islet β-cell autoantigen (β-Ag) processing and presentation by macrophages (Mφ) would deliver "tolerogenic" signals that activate a Th2 subset of T cells producing IL-4 and IL-10 that down-regulate Th1 cells and IFN-γ and IL-2 production. Also, IL-10 production by Mφ may be up-regulated by these immunostimulatory procedures, with consequent down-regulation of β-Ag presentation and reinforcement of a "tolerogenic signal" for recognition of β-Ag as self by the immune system. In addition, IL-10 inhibits production of IL-12, a Th1-cell activator. The combination of up-regulated IL-4 and IL-10 production and down-regulated IFN-γ and IL-2 production would inhibit cytotoxic Mφ and T-cell functions and thereby prevent β-cell damage and IDDM. Figure is taken from reference 16 and is reproduced by permission of the American Diabetes Association

relationship to Th1 cells, the clonal size of autoantigen reactive Th2 cells may inversely correlate with progression to β-cell destruction and insulin dependency. In summary, activation, cytokine production, and precursor frequency all may influence the destructive activity of T cells.

T-CELL ACTIVITIES AS MARKERS OF CELLULAR IMMUNITY IN IDD

The literature is marked with considerable controversy regarding the functional characteristics of peripheral blood mononuclear cells (PBMCs) obtained from individuals with or at increased risk for IDD. Analyses of functional activity range from crude studies to those which are highly technical in nature. Unfortunately, many promising observations have not shown a high degree of reproducibility. Furthermore, since many methodological aspects are not in standardized formats, comparative analysis between laboratories is often difficult.

One novel assay for measurement of functional cellular immune activity in persons with IDD involved the transfer of insulitis into mice utilizing PBMCs from new-onset patients[20]. Specifically, when athymic CD1/nu/nu mice were injected intraperitoneally with PBMCs from 10 new-onset IDD patients and 10 control subjects, no mice developed overt hyperglycemia. However, PBMCs from six of the new-onset patients and none of the controls induced significant pancreatic mononuclear cell infiltration. The infiltrate was specific for islets, with control tissues devoid of cellular infiltrate. The authors contend that human cellular immunity to islet cells can be detected utilizing this model[20], however the practical application of the technique is questionable.

Another proposed model for the detection of cellular immunity in IDD involves measurement of cytoadherence of or cytolysis by lymphocytes from IDD subjects to rodent insulinoma cells or erythrocytes coated with islet cells. In one such study, lymphocytes from recent-onset IDD subjects displayed an enhanced ability to form rosettes with RINm5f cells compared with lymphocytes from health control subjects or non-insulin-dependent diabetes (NIDD) subjects[21]. Further analysis characterized these cells as predominantly T cells, with smaller numbers of natural killer cells. In later investigations of 63 new-onset patients and 153 healthy controls, cellular specificity was observed as cytoadherence to transformed hamster insulinoma cells (i.e. HIT) but not towards a panel of seven non-β-cell lines[22]. The cytoadherence could be blocked by the addition of anti-CD3 or anti-CD4 antibodies, but not by anti-CD8 antibodies. One technique for monitoring cell-mediated cytolysis activity involves the coating of ^{51}CR-labeled chicken erythrocytes with human or mouse pancreatic islet homogenate, and subsequently incubating the erythrocytes with T cells obtained from IDD patients or normal control subjects[23]. Utilizing this methodology, T cells from IDD patients (in comparison to those from controls) showed a significantly increased degree of cytotoxicity towards the labeled erythrocytes. When erythrocytes were coated with homogenates of other cell types, the same effect was not observed. However, the practicality, reproducibility, and interassay variation of these cytoadherence techniques are not yet resolved.

PHENOTYPIC MARKERS OF CELLULAR IMMUNITY IN IDD

Cytometric analysis of cell-mediated immunity in patients with IDD may provide a practical basis for the investigation of the natural history of this disease and may contribute to a better definition of patients at risk of IDD. As the aforementioned functional studies have raised the question of laboratory practicality, many researchers have sought phenotypic markers of cellular immune activity. Significant abnormalities of lymphocyte populations reported in persons with or at increased risk for the disease include a reduced percentage of CD4 (helper/inducer) and CD8 (cytoxic/suppressor) lymphocytes as well as enrichment of lymphocytes possessing HLA class II molecules and interleukin-2 receptors, both of which indicate cellular activation[24-29].

To determine whether IDD represented a generalized immunological disorder, the phenotypes of PBMCs of pre-diabetic (i.e. ICA positive first degree relatives), new-onset, and long-standing IDD patients have been measured with a series of monoclonal antibodies for CD45R (anti-2H4) and CD29 (anti-4B4) which mark cells as suppressors/inducers or helpers/inducers respectively[26]. In these studies, pre-diabetic patients showed elevated numbers of suppressor/inducer cells and depressed helper/inducer cells compared to healthy controls, an observation also observed in both diabetic and non-diabetic twins with IDD[24]. Also, the mean CD4/CD8 ratio in the pre-diabetic subjects of this study[26] was decreased compared to controls, an observation confirmed by others[27]. Interestingly, new-onset IDD patients did not differ from controls, suggesting that the imbalances observable in the prodromal state resolve by the time of disease onset[26]. A persistent reduction of the CD4/CD8 T-cell ratio and cell activation before the onset of IDD has also been reported[27]. In a prospective analysis of 56 first degree relatives of IDD probands in which six individuals later developed IDD, five of these showed a persistent reduction of the CD4/CD8 lymphocyte ratio before the clinical onset of disease as compared to relatives who remained diabetes free. The authors contended that the imbalance of immunoregulatory subsets may mark a process leading towards β-cell destruction and IDD, and that this persistently reduced ratio may identify relatives at increased risk for IDD. In contrast, others[28] have observed similar lymphocyte percentages (i.e. CD4 and CD8 T-cell subset numbers and ratios) between ICA positive individuals and controls, thereby leaving the issue at this time in a controversial state.

More accepted is the observation of differences in the subpopulations of CD4 subsets (i.e. decreased CD29+ helper/inducer T cells)[26,28]. To determine the role of CD4 regulatory abnormalities in the pathogenesis of IDD, a series of studies measuring the function of CD4 helper/inducer and suppressor/ inducer T-cell populations in ICA positive non-diabetic subjects were performed[28]. Helper/inducer T-cell function, as measured in a mitogen-induced T lymphocyte/B lymphocyte co-culture system, was decreased in the ICA positive subjects as compared to controls. Furthermore, individuals with the highest titers of ICA displayed the most significant disturbances in function. Similarly, a separate group has reported rising IAA levels correlate with rising elevations in the CD4 CD45R+/CD29+ ratio[29]. Both studies contend that the functional defect in the CD4 helper/inducer population may contribute to the pathogenesis of IDD and may provide a marker for identifying persons at increased risk for the disease.

T-CELL ANTIGENS

A plethora of islet cell autoantigens have been associated with IDD[30]. These antigens may be involved in the pathogenesis of IDD, or (alternatively) may merely be the targets of autoantibodies that serve as markers of anti-β-cell immunity. Co-culture of islet cells or insulinomas with PBMC has provided one means to demonstrate cellular responses to autoantigens, and co-culture with T cells or T-cell clones (supplemented with antigen presenting cells) has provided another. The biochemical identification and recombinant production of putative β-cell autoantigens has allowed for recent investigations measuring the T-cell activity against these compounds.

ISLET/INSULINOMA CELLS

The utilization of islet cells in assays of cellular proliferation or generation of T-cell lines theoretically provides all potential sources of β-cell autoantigen. However, the scarcity of human islet cells has made the performance of such assays difficult. Therefore, most studies have utilized rodent islet cell tumor lines (e.g. RIN, HIT, NIT, etc.) for these purposes. For example, with insulinoma (i.e. rat RINm5F cell) membranes as an antigenic source, T-cell lines have been generated from PBMC of recent-onset IDD patients[31]. Utilizing this technique, a series of HLA-DR restricted clones specifically responsive to insulinoma membrane antigens were developed including those reactive to a 38 kDa antigen (discussed later).

With the aim of directly measuring T-lymphocyte activity, one assay has been developed which measures PMBC proliferation in the presence of adult human islets and fetal pig proislets. In those studies[32], the proliferative response to islets in 6 out of 6 subjects at increased risk for IDD (i.e. ICA positive) and 7 of 11 (64%) new-onset IDD patients exceeded the reference range of 12 control subjects. In addition, granulocyte macrophage colony-stimulating factor secretion was monitored, and paralleled the stimulation observations. The authors contend that this assay was at least as sensitive as the GAD autoantibody for marking preclinical IDD.

In follow-up studies[33] by those same investigators, sonicated fetal pig proislets were observed to stimulate the PBMC of 15 out of 22 (68%) increased risk subjects, 12 of 29 (41%) new-onset IDD patients, and 1 of 6 (17%) Graves disease patients to a proliferative response greater than the reference range of

14 control subjects. In terms of disease prediction, the majority (15 of 22, 68%) of increased risk (i.e. ICA or 64 kDa autoantibody positive) subjects had significant T-cell reactivity to the proislets. Indeed, the authors suggest that the presence of T-cell reactivity to proislets was as predictive as a high titer ICA (i.e. > 40 JDF units), a widely regarded prognostic indicator for IDD.

INSULIN

Although insulin would appear to be an obvious candidate antigen for investigation, there are surprisingly few reports analyzing cellular immunity against insulin in non-insulin treated subjects. In one study, PBMC responses to insulin were observed in 8 of 9 (89%) ICA positive first degree relatives of IDD subjects and 4 of 12 (33%) healthy controls[34]. Furthermore, in the ICA positive subjects, no relationship was observed between the cellular and humoral (i.e. insulin autoantibodies) response to this antigen. This study, however, utilized a low definition of positive (i.e. a stimulation index of greater than 1.5) which influences both the sensitivity and the specificity of the assay for discriminating between individuals at risk of developing IDD and individuals not so predisposed. In another study[32], PBMC responses to insulin as compared to those against fetal pig proislets (mentioned above) were fewer in frequency and magnitude (i.e. 4 of 6 increased risk, 3 of 11 new onset, 0 of 12 controls). These data are similar to those observed by others[35] wherein insulin reactive PBMC were identified more often in patients with new-onset or established IDD than ICA negative relatives of IDD patients or healthy control subjects. In summary, under a strict definition of a positive response, insulin specific T-cell responses appear to occur at a lower frequency than responses reported for other autoantigens. The reasons for this observation are as yet unclear, and their value as a predictive marker may therefore be limited.

GLUTAMIC ACID DECARBOXYLASE

Autoantibodies in new-onset IDD patients reactive to a 64 kDa islet cell protein were initially described in 1982[36]. The biochemical identification of this antigen occurred as a result of the observation that autoantibodies to the enzyme GAD were present in IDD-prone patients with Stiff-man syndrome, and that 64 kDa-reactive autoantibodies from patients with IDD reacted with GAD[37,38]. As indicated in other chapters of this text, GAD autoantibodies have now been shown in multiple studies to be valuable as markers in predicting the disease. Two molecular weight forms of GAD (M_r 65 000 and 67 000) exist; GAD 65 is the primary isoform expressed by human β cells.

GAD is also a target of cellular immunity in human IDD. In analysis[39] of PBMC proliferative responses to recombinant GAD 65 in newly diagnosed

IDD patients, ICA-positive and ICA-negative relatives of IDD patients, and healthy controls, the likelihood of a positive response was higher among the diabetic patients (12 of 18, 67%) and ICA-positive relatives (5 of 8, 63%) than among subjects at low risk for IDD (i.e. controls (0 of 14) and ICA-negative relatives (2 of 19, 11%)). This finding points strongly towards measurement of GAD 65 immunity as a potential marker for IDD. Cellular immunity to GAD 67 also exists in IDD. In studies analyzing cellular immunity to the middle portion (i.e. amino acids 208–404) of GAD 67, PBMC activity was significantly higher in both at-risk relatives (12 of 29, 41%) and recent-onset IDD subjects (11 of 29, 38%) than in other autoimmune disease subjects (1 of 7, 14%) and healthy controls (1 of 23, 4%)[40]. The authors of this report contend that GAD 67 reactivity may delineate asymptomatic subjects at increased risk for IDD.

One study[41] simultaneously investigated both humoral (i..e. autoantibodies) and cellular (i.e. PBMC responses) anti-GAD immunity in 31 relatives of IDD patients at increased risk for the disease due to the presence of ICA. Subjects with high PBMC activity towards GAD were more reactive to tetanus toxoid than low GAD PMBC responders, perhaps indicating an overall heightened state of T-cell activity. Interestingly, these authors reported an inverse relationship between GAD antibody titer and PBMC reactivity to GAD. Specifically, high concentrations of autoantibodies capable of precipitating native pig brain GAD were observed in subjects with low PBMC reactivity to GAD. Conversely, low GAD autoantibody concentrations were observed in subjects with increased GAD PBMC activity. These studies may also explain the paradoxical findings that GAD autoantibodies are highly predictive of IDD, yet when in extremely high titer they mark individuals with a low risk of progression to disease[42,43]. The question as to whether this differential display of anti-GAD immunity is representative of the aforementioned Th1/Th2 paradigm is extremely controversial, and attempts to confirm these findings are actively being pursued as this information (if true) would be very valuable in terms of prioritizing markers for IDD. An analysis of the epitopic recognition of GAD during the prodromal phase of human IDD may better illuminate the natural history of the disease. Furthermore, the predictive power of cellular immunity to GAD may lie in the epitopic recognition of GAD. Specifically, PMBC reactive with certain GAD epitopes may mark individuals destined for IDD, whereas PBMC reactive with other GAD epitopes may not mark impending IDD—rather they may mark proneness towards Stiff-man syndrome, polyendocrine autoimmunity, or relatives of IDD patients with little likelihood of developing IDD. In order to find the dominant epitopes of GAD, PBMC reactivity to GAD 65 and GAD 67 peptides was measured in both recent-onset IDD and control subjects[44]. Interestingly, PBMC reactivity to GAD peptides was observed in 9 of the 10 control and 13 of the 15 recent-onset IDD patients tested, findings markedly different from previous reports analyzing the responses to whole GAD[39–41]. In addition, control subjects most often reacted to peptides of residues 161–243 of GAD 65 while IDD subjects responded to amino acids 473–555[44]. Responses to GAD 67 peptides were similar in IDD patients and controls. Other studies[45] varied dramatically from those in that while responses to GAD peptides were also observed in controls, the primary region of cellular immunity to GAD resided within residues 247 to 266, a region with extensive sequence homology to the P2-C protein of coxsackievirus[46], an environmental agent long associated via epidemiological studies with IDD. Clearly a longitudinal analysis of cellular immune activities to GAD and its component peptides is required to answer questions related to both disease specificity and the pathogenic role (if any) of anti-GAD immunity.

38 kDa

To identify the autoantigenic targets of cellular immunity in IDD, a series of T-cell lines were generated against RIN cell membranes[31] from the PBMC of a new-onset IDD patient. A majority of the T-cell lines were reactive against the cellular sub-fraction enriched in insulin-secretory granules, and more specifically against a 38 kDa fraction of those granules[47]. To assess the specificity of cellular immunity to the 38 kDa fraction, both new-onset and healthy controls have been tested for anti-38 kDa reactivity, and 14 (74%) of 19 new-onset and only 2 of 16 (13%) controls were positive in one published study[48].

Utilizing IDD sera with high titer activity against a 38 kDa islet cell protein, other investigators immunoscreened a human islet cell cDNA library and identified the nuclear transcription factor jun-B[49] as a target autoantigen. This protein, with an M_r of 38 000, stimulated the PBMC of 12 out of 17 (71%) new-onset patients, 8 of 16 (50%) ICA-positive relatives of IDD patients, and 0 of 10 healthy controls[49]. The authors contend that the cellular immune response to jun-B identifies subjects at risk for the development of IDD. The identification of jun-B as the 38 kDa autoantigen is controversial, and further attempts to identify this antigen biochemically are actively being pursued.

OTHER AUTOANTIGENS

Newly diagnosed patients with IDD may have antibodies to bovine serum albumin (BSA) and a 17 amino acid BSA peptide termed ABBOS[50]. It has been hypothesized that ingestion of cow's milk in early life can initiate β-cell destruction through molecular mimicry between the ABBOS sequence common to both BSA and a 69 kDa β-cell protein. However, the 69 kDa β-cell protein has limited amino acid sequence homology with BSA[51], the specificity of anti-BSA immunity for IDD has not been confirmed[52], and evidence of active cellular immunity against BSA in IDD patients is limited[52].

Heat shock protein immunity (i.e. hsp 60, hsp 65) has formed the basis for exciting yet controversial findings in IDD research. While reports exist both for[53] and against[54,55] the role of autoantibodies to hsp as being markers for IDD, studies utilizing therapeutic regimens which actively involve cellular immunity to hsp have shown dramatic results in terms of inducing a remission of IDD in humans and NOD mice[56,57]. Given the need to identify potential environmental agents which may initiate IDD, and the necessity to understand the role of cellular immunity in therapeutic interventions, cellular immunity to BSA and hsp will undoubtedly form the basis for further investigations.

WHAT DO T-CELL MARKERS REVEAL TO US?

DO CELLULAR IMMUNE RESPONSES RISE OR FALL NEAR THE ONSET OF IDD?

Unfortunately, little longitudinal information is available regarding the patterns of cellular immune responsiveness to specific β-cell antigens in subjects prior to the onset of IDD. However, the implications of the study regarding cellular and humoral immune responses against GAD[41], if true, would be dramatic. If GAD is an antigen of pathogenic significance, then GAD-reactive T cells could serve as better predictive markers of IDD than GAD autoantibodies. Specifically, a potent anti-GAD Th1 response might be correlated with a strong cytotoxic T-lymphocyte response against β cells. In contrast, high-GAD autoantibody titers may mark an active Th2 response against GAD which would diminish the cytotoxic T-cell response against β cells. Furthermore, as this is the first autoimmune condition for which a dichotomy in the cellular and humoral immune responsiveness to an autoantigen has been reported, these findings may help unravel the role of specific Th subsets in the pathogenesis of autoimmune disease. Future studies will expand on these questions by analyzing the level of activity (both cellular and humoral) not only against GAD, but also against other islet cell autoantigens associated with IDD in the period prior to the onset of IDD.

HOW DO T-CELL MARKERS COMPARE TO AUTOANTIBODY AND METABOLIC MARKERS?

The identification of islet cell reactive autoantibodies in 1975 not only served to bolster the hypothesis that IDD resulted from an autoimmune process, but also set the stage for a series of studies aimed at determining the natural history of events prior to the onset of symptomatic IDD. In nearly all natural history studies, islet cell autoantibodies have served as powerful markers of β-cell autoimmunity in non-diabetic individuals as they are able to identify those at increased risk for IDD. Specifically, they can occur years before the onset of hyperglycemia, show high specificity for disease (i.e. 0.1 to 2% of normal subjects and approximately 3% of non-diabetic relatives of patients with IDD, versus 70 to 80% of patients with newly diagnosed IDD), show an age- and titer-dependent risk for IDD, and when observed in combination with each other in a single person confer a much greater risk for the development of IDD than does a single autoantibody alone.

As the disease progresses towards clinical onset, there is a loss in the normal early (i.e. first-phase) response of insulin to intravenous glucose administration. However, the metabolic profiles of subjects in the period before the onset of IDD differ greatly (i.e. slow versus rapid loss of first-phase insulin release to intravenous glucose administration). Therefore, although they can provide a valuable tool to supplement autoantibody analysis, variability in metabolic markers has hampered the design of methods for utilizing them to predict accurately the time of disease onset.

Given the arguments for the cellular immune basis for IDD, and the promising preliminary studies regarding T-cell markers for IDD, the future of utilizing T-cell markers looks promising. However, the number of subjects analyzed for T-cell markers during the period prior to the onset of IDD represents only a fraction of those studied utilizing either autoantibody and/or metabolic markers. Therefore, comparing the predictive value of antibodies with T-cell responses would be premature at this point in time.

FUTURE QUESTIONS AND DIRECTIONS

DOES CELLULAR IMMUNE ACTIVITY AS MEASURED IN THE PERIPHERY MIRROR THE EVENTS ASSOCIATED WITH PANCREATIC β-CELL DESTRUCTION?

Because the pancreas is not safely accessible for biopsy, immune effector mechanisms in humans have largely been studied using peripheral blood cells. Such studies might not adequately represent the immune activities occurring within the cellular infiltrate of islets during the prodromal phase of IDD. Currently, PBMC proliferation in vitro upon exposure to islet cells or other antigen sources is the most commonly used method to identify T-cell activities which may serve as markers for IDD. The use of PBMC, however, leaves unresolved the intra-islet events, which cannot be addressed at the level of the periphery.

It is unknown which immune system component ultimately destroys the majority of β cells. As previously indicated, CD8+T cells are the predominant lymphocytes in the insulitis lesion of patients dying at the time of IDD diagnosis[3,4]. In NOD mice, however, treatment with anti-CD4 antibodies is able to prevent IDD, suggesting that CD4+ cells are required for disease[58,59]. Furthermore, the elaboration of cytokines by cells within the insulitis lesion is thought to have an important pathogenic function. Interleukin-1 inhibits insulin secretion by β cells in vitro and is cytotoxic to β cells at high concentrations[60]. β cells themselves can produce IL-6, which powerfully stimulates the immune response and may therefore enhance insulitis and β-cell destruction[17]. Interferon-α has been consistently detected in the pancreas of patients dying of diabetic ketoacidosis[5], and transgenic mice expressing interferon-α in their β cells develop insulitis and diabetes unless given anti-interferon-α antibodies[61]. Both superoxide radicals and nitric oxide have been implicated as important mediators of β-cell damage in IDD[62,63]. These toxic chemical species may be produced in relatively high concentrations during inflammation often leading to tissue injury. β cells also produce nitric oxide in response to cytokine stimulation in vitro[63], and it has been suggested that cytokines released by inflammatory cells within the insulitis lesions may induce β-cell self-destruction through the expression of nitric oxide.

All of these aforementioned immunological features are localized to the site of tissue destruction, and it is unlikely that their ultimate relative contributions towards β-cell loss will be resolved in the near future, since only the cellular immune events of the peripheral compartment can be assessed at present.

IS THERE A SPECIFIC CASCADE OF ANTIGENIC RESPONSES IN IDD?

Two reports[19,64] have recently provided evidence that the anti-GAD immune response is one of the earliest events in a cascade of autoimmune reactions in the NOD mouse. Both studies report that T cells from four-week-old NOD mice proliferate in response to GAD-65, that this proliferation occurs concurrently with the onset of insulitis and that it occurs prior to proliferation in response to other antigens of interest, including carboxypeptidase H. In one of the studies, the intrathymic injection of GAD-65 in three-week-old mice significantly decreased the frequency of diabetes at 25 weeks of age as compared to peripherin-injected mice. These observations suggest that cellular immunity to GAD is a primary event in the natural history of IDD in these mice. One of the two reports included data showing that the T-cell response in NOD mice is initially confined to a small linear region of GAD-65 (between amino acids 509 and 543) and later spreads to other determinants[64], an observation consistent with earlier reports concerning immune responses in mice with EAE.

The two aforementioned studies demonstrated that spreading of cellular immune responses to various cellular determinants/peptides within the GAD molecule (i.e. intramolecular spreading) and to other target cell autoantigens (i.e. intermolecular spreading) exists in the NOD model of IDD.

It remains to be resolved whether the autoimmune phenomena associated with the etiology of human IDD are indicative of a primary T-cell-mediated autoimmune process against β cells, or whether these events arise as secondary autoimmune phenomena via intermolecular antigenic spreading of autoimmune responsiveness following a primarily T-cell response against a virus or other environmental agent. Furthermore, given the heterogenic nature of human IDD and the extensive known repertoire of β-cell autoantigens, if a similar cascade of antigen recognition underlies the natural history of human IDD, it is likely to be much more problematic to dissect.

Based on the previously described observations of a dynamic autoimmune T-cell repertoire, the following model for the pathogenesis of cell-mediated autoimmune disease in general, and of IDD in particular, has been proposed[65]. A first generation of effector T cells is triggered either by a self-antigen or by an environmentally derived determinant able to mimic self. At this point, the autoimmune T-cell repertoire is limited and therefore amenable to selective therapeutic immuno-interventions. This initial response has a pro-inflammatory, Th1 bias characterized by the release of lymphokines in the target organ that up-regulate antigen presentation, resulting in a second wave of priming of autoimmune T cells with distinct specificities for autoantigens. The second wave of activated T cells is more diverse with respect to antigen recognition (which manifests as intramolecular as well as intermolecular spreading of target antigenic determinants), and the pathology progresses. In the absence of antigenic determinant spreading (in this model) autoimmunity will not progress. Likewise, if at this or a later point, the autoimmune T-cell pool becomes skewed towards a Th2 cell predominance the disease process will be slowed or halted (Figures 8.1 and 8.2)[16]. Only an unrestricted, Th1-dominated response will progress to total β-cell destruction and fulminant disease.

The data supporting this model argue for a prospective study in which individuals at high risk of developing IDD are frequently tested for their cellular responses to various candidate auto- and alloantigens during the period prior to the onset of IDD. These investigations will establish parameters of the T-cell response to β cells that are fundamental for the interpretation of T-cell autoimmunity in IDD.

DOES CELLULAR PROLIFERATION PROVIDE THE BEST MEASURE OF T CELL RESPONSES LEADING TO IDD?

The evaluation of T-cell reactivity, based solely on proliferation, is hampered by several factors. First, the apparent precursor frequency of autoreactive T cells within the periphery in most autoimmune diseases is low (i.e. most pathogenic T cells are theoretically at or near the site of tissue destruction). Furthermore, the measurement of proliferation does not take into account the fact that regulatory T cells may be modulating the activity of destructive T cells at the local level. Therefore, proliferation (reported as stimulation index towards an antigen) may not relate to the status of or proneness towards disease. In addition, new-onset IDD patients, a key population group to these studies, are hyperglycemic and occasionally lymphopenic, characteristics which could conceivably confound comparison of their lymphocyte proliferations to those of normal control volunteers.

As previously indicated, autoantigen-specific T cells represent a minor fraction of the total lymphocyte pool even during autoimmune disease. For example, in testing the blood of multiple sclerosis patients for myelin basic protein (MBP) reactive T cells, frequencies of 1 in 30 000 were reported using an interferon-γ ELISA spot assay. This frequency was 10–100-fold higher than in normal controls[66,67]. Importantly, when patients with clear reactivity to MBP in the ELISA spot system were tested for proliferative T-cell responses, either no responses or only weak responses with marginally significant proliferation were detected. The ELISA spot assay, therefore, appears to be more sensitive than proliferation as a marker for disease. Furthermore, these two assay systems measure unrelated T-cell functions. The proliferation assay ultimately measures IL-2-induced bystander proliferation rather than direct blastogenesis by antigen-specific cells, as is frequently assumed. The ELISA spot assay can be used to measure the production of a lymphokine of interest (e.g. Th1 function with interleukin-2 and interferon-γ release, and interleukin-4, -5, or -10 secretion for Th2 cells).

The most commonly used strategies to overcome the low frequency of autoantigen-specific T cells involve restimulating T cells in vitro before testing them (e.g. establishing T-cell lines or clones) and although widely practiced they are clearly unsuited for unbiased determination of T-cell markers in IDD. These approaches fail to discriminate between T cells actively engaged in the autoimmune process (i.e. primed/memory cells), and passive (i.e. naive) autoreactive T cells. Indeed, autoreactive T-cell lines can be readily isolated from healthy controls[68] and HIV-reactive T-cell lines can be generated from individuals who have never encountered the virus[69] using T-cell restimulation systems. A clear advantage of defining cytokine production as the end-point is that it measures T-cell function in freshly isolated PBMCs, which better represent the in vivo state. Unfortunately, studies monitoring cytokine production as well as precursor frequency of autoreactive cells in persons either with IDD or at increased risk for the disease have not been performed, but will form the basis for future investigations. In summary, critical parameters to monitor future investigations involve defining the antigenic specificity of the autoimmune repertoire, as well as its clonal size, state of activation, and functional bias (Th1 versus Th2).

REFERENCES

1 Gepts W. Pathologic anatomy of the pancreas in juvenile diabetes mellitus. *Diabetes* 1965; **14**: 619–33.

2 Foulis AK, Lidde CN, Farqharson MA, Richmond JA, Weir RS. The histopathology of the pancreas in type 1 (insulin-dependent) diabetes mellitus: A 25 year review of death in patients under 20 years of age in the the United Kingdom. *Diabetologia* 1986; **29**: 267–74.

3 Bottazzo GF, Dean BM, McNally JM, Mackay EH, Swift PGF, Gamble DR. In situ characterization of autoimmune phenomena and expression of HLA molecules in the pancreas in diabetic insulitis. *N Engl J Med* 1985; **313**: 353–60.

4 Hanninen A, Jalkanen S, Salmi M, Toikkanen S, Nikolakaros G, Simell O. Macrophages, T cell receptor usage, and endothelial cell activation in the pancreas at the onset of insulin-dependent diabetes mellitus. *J Clin Invest* 1992; **90**: 1901–10.

5 Foulis AK, McGill M, Farquaharson MA. Insulitis in type 1 (insulin-dependent) diabetes mellitus in man-macrophages, lymphocytes, and interferon-gamma containing cells. *J Pathol* 1991; **165**: 97–103.

6 Gepts W, LeCompte PM. The pathology of type 1 (juvenile) diabetes. In Volk BW, Arguilla ER (eds), *The Diabetic Pancreas*, 2nd edn. New York: Plenum, 1992, pp 337–65.

7 Powrie F, Coffman RL. Cytokine regulation of T cell function: potential for therapeutic intervention. *Immunol Today* 1993; **14**: 270–4.

8 Seder RA, Paul WE. Acquisition of lymphokine-producing phenotype by CD4+T cells. *Ann Rev Immunol* 1994; **12**: 635–73.

9 Ohashi PS, Oehen S, Boerki K, Pirchner H, Ohashi CT, Odermatt B et al. Ablation of "tolerance" and induction of diabetes by virus infection in viral antigen transgenic mice. *Cell* 1991; **65**: 305–17.

10 Brocke S, Gaur A, Piercy C, Gautam A, Gijbels K, Fathman CG et al. Induction of relapsing paralysis in experimental autoimmune encephalomyelitis by bacterial superantigen. *Nature* 1993; **365**: 642–4.

11 Baron JL, Madri JA, Ruddle NJ, Hashim G, Janeway CA. Surface expression of alpha 4 integrin by CD4 T cells is required for their entry into brain parencyma. *J Exp Med* 1993; **177**: 57–68.

12 Sedgwick JD, Macphee IA, Puklavec M. Isolation of encephalitogen CD4+T cell clones in the rat. Cloning methodology and interferon-gamme secretion. *J Immunol Methods* 1989; **121**: 185–96.

13 Ando DG, Clayton J, Kono D, Urban JL, Sercarz EE. Encephalitogenic T cells in the B10.PL model of experimental allergic encephalomyelitis (EAE) are of the Th-1 lymphokine subtype. *Cell Immunol* 1989; **124**: 132–43.

14 Khoury SJ, Hancock WW, Weiner HL. Oral tolerance to myelin basic protein and natural recovery from experimental autoimmune encephalomyelitis are associated with downregulation of inflammatory cytokines and differential upregulation of transforming growth factor beta, interleukin 4, and prostaglandin E expression in the brain. *J Exp Med* 1992; **176**: 1355–64.

15 Mosmann TR, Moore KW. The role of IL-10 in cross regulation of TH1 and TH2 responses. *Immunol. Today* 1993; **12**: 49–53.

16 Rabinovitch A. Immunoregulatory and cytokine imbalances in the pathogenesis of IDDM. Therapeutic intervention by immunostimulation? *Diabetes* 1994; **43**: 613–21.

17 Campbell I, Kay TWH, Oxbrow L, Harrison LC. Essential role for interferon-gamma and interleukin-6 in autoimmune insulin-dependent diabetes in NOD/Wehi mice. *J Clin Invest* 1991; **87**: 739–42.

18 Lehmann PV, Schumm G, Moon D, Hurthenbach U, Falcioni F, Muller S et al. Acute

lethal graft-versus-host reaction induced by major histocompatibility complex class II-reactive T helper cell clones. *J Exp Med* 1990; **171**: 1485–96.

19 Tisch R, Yang XD, Singer SM, Liblay RS, Fugger L, McDevitt HO. Immune response to glutamic acid decarboxylase correlates with insulitis in non-obese diabetic mice. *Nature* 1993; **366**: 72–5.

20 Calcinaro F, Hao L, Chase HP, Klingensmith G, Lafferty KJ. Detection of cell mediated immunity in type 1 diabetes mellitus. *J Autoimmun* 1992: **5**: 137–47.

21 Lang F, Maugendre D, Houssaint E, Charbonnele B, Sai P. Cytoadherence of lymphocytes from type 1 diabetic subjects to insulin secreting cells. *Diabetes* 1987; **36**: 1356–64.

22 Segain JP, Valentin A, Bardet S, Feve B, Sevestre H, Houssainte E *et al*. In vitro relationship of CD4 cells from type 1 diabetic patients and xenogenic β-cell membranes. *Diabetes* 1989; **38**: 634–40.

23 Horvath M, Schroder D, Varsanyi M, Balazsi I. Human pancreatic extract and rat pancreatic islet homogenate-coated chicken erythrocytes as targets of lymphocyte mediated cytotoxicity in Type I diabetic patients. *Exp Clin Endocrinol* 1989; **93**: 151–6.

24 Johnston C, Alviggi L, Millward BA, Leslie RDG, Pyke DA, Vergani D. Alterations in T-lymphocyte subpopulations in type 1 diabetes. *Diabetes* 1988; **37**: 1484–8.

25 De-Berandinis PD, Londei M, Kahan M, Balsano F, Kontianen S, Gale EA *et al*. The majority of the activated T cells in the blood of insulin-dependent diabetes mellitus (IDDM) patients are CD4+. *Clin Exp Immunol* 1988; **73**: 255–9.

26 Faustman D, Eisenbarth G, Daley J, Breitmeyer J. Abnormal T-lymphocyte subsets in type 1 diabetes. *Diabetes* 1989; **38**: 1462–8.

27 Al-Sakkaf L, Pozzilli P, Tarn AC, Schwarz G, Gale EAM, Bottazzo GF. Persistent reduction of CD4/CD8 lymphocyte ratio and cell activation before the onset of Type I (insulin-dependent). *Diabetologia* 1989; **32**: 322–5.

28 Schatz DA, Riley WJ, Maclaren NK, Barrett DJ. Defective inducer T-cell function before the onset of insulin dependent diabetes mellitus. *J Autoimmun* 1991; **4**: 125–36.

29 Faustman D, Schoenfeld D, Ziegler R. T-lymphocyte changes linked to autoantibodies. *Diabetes* 1992; **40**: 590–7.

30 Atkinson MA, Maclaren NK. The islet cell autoantigens of insulin-dependent diabetes. *J Clin Invest* 1993; **92**: 1608–16.

31 Van Vliet E, Roep B, Meulenbroek L, Bruining GJ, Devries RRP. Human T cell clones with specificity for insulinoma cell antigens. *Eur J Immunol* 1989; **19**: 213–16.

32 Harrison LC, Deaizpurua H, Loudovaris T, Campbell IL, Cebon JS, Tait BD *et al*. Reactivity to human islets and fetal pig proislets by peripheral blood mononuclear cells from subjects with preclinical and clinical insulin-dependent diabetes. *Diabetes* 1991; **40**: 1128–33.

33 Harrison LC, Chu SX, Deaizpurua HJ, Graham M, Honeyman MC, Colman PG. Islet-reactive T cells are a marker of preclinical insulin-dependent diabetes. *J Clin Invest* 1992; **89**: 1161–5.

34 Keller RJ. Cellular immunity to human insulin in individuals at high risk for the development of type 1 diabetes mellitus. *J Autoimmun* 1990; **3**: 321–7.

35 Atkinson MA, Bowman MA, Kao JK, Campbell L, Dush PD, Shah SC *et al*. Absence of peripheral blood mononuclear cell responses to bovine albumin or ABBOS peptide in insulin dependent diabetes. *N Engl J Med* 1993; **329**: 1853–8.

36 Baekkesov S, Neilsen JH, Marner B, Bilde T, Ludvigsson J, Lernmark A. Autoantibodies in newly diagnosed diabetic children immunoprecipitate human pancreatic islet cell proteins. *Nature* 1982; **298**: 167–9.

37 Solimena M, Folli F, Aparisi R, Pozza G, De Camilli P. Antoantibodies to GABA-ERGIC neurons and pancreatic beta cells in stiff-man syndrome. *N Engl J*

Med 1990; **322**: 1555–60.

38 Baekkesov S, Aanstoot HJ, Christgau S, Reetz A, Solimena M, Cascalho M, Folli F, Richter-Olesen H, DeCamilli P. The 64kD autoantigen in insulin-dependent diabetes is the GABA synthesizing enzyme glutamic decarboxylase. *Nature* 1990; **347**: 151–6.

39 Atkinson MA, Kaufman DL, Campbell L, Gibbs KA, Shah SC, Bu DF *et al*. Response of peripheral blood mononuclear cells to glutamate decarboxylase in insulin dependent diabetes. *Lancet* 1992; **339**: 458–9.

40 Honeymoon MC, Cram DS, Harrison LC. Glutamic acid decarboxylase 67-reactive T-cells: a marker of insulin dependent diabetes. *J Exp Med*; **177**: 535–40.

41 Harrison LC, Honeyman MC, Deaizpurua HJ, Schmidi RS, Colman PG, Tair BD *et al*. Inverse relation between humoral and cellular immunity to glutamic acid decarboxylase in subjects at risk of insulin-dependent diabetes. *Lancet* 1993; **341**: 1365–9.

42 Gianani RA, Pugliese A, Bonner-Weir S, Shiffrin AJ, Soeldner JS, Elrich H *et al*. Prognostically significant heterogeneity of cytoplasmic islet cells antibodies of patients with type 1 diabetes. *Diabetes* 1992; **41**: 347–53.

43 Atkinson MA, Kaufman DL, Newman D, Tobin AJ, MacLaren NK. Islet cell cytoplasmic autoantibody reactivity to glutamate decarboxylase in insulin-dependent diabetes. *J Clin Invest* 1993; **91**: 350–6.

44 Lohmann T, Leslie RDG, Hawa M, Geysen M, Rodda S, Londei M. Immunodominant epitopes of glutamic acid decarboxylase 65 and 67 in insulin dependent diabetes-mellitus. *Lancet* 1994; **343**: 1607–8.

45 Atkinson MA, Bowman MA, Campbell L, Darrow BL, Kaufman DL, Maclaren NK. Cellular immunity to an epitope common to glutamate decarboxylase and Coxsackie virus in insulin-dependent diabetes. *J Clin Invest* (in press).

46 Kaufman DL, Erlander MG, Clare-Salzler M, Atkinson MA, Maclaren NK, Tobin AJ. Autoimmunity to two forms of glutamate decarboxylase in insulin dependent diabetes. *J Clin Invest* 1992; **83**: 283–92.

47 Roep BO, Arden SD, Devries RR, Hutton JC. T-cell clones from a Type I diabetes patient respond to insulin secretory granule proteins. *Nature* 1990; **345**: 632–4.

48 Roep BO, Kallan AA, Hapenbos WLW, Bruining J, Bailyes EM, Arden SD *et al*. T-cell reactivity to 38kD insulin-secretory-granule protein in patients with recent-onset type I diabetes. *Lancet* 1991; **337**: 1439–41.

49 Honeymoon MG, Cram D, Harrison LC. Transcription factor jun-B is target of autoreactive T-cells in IDDM. *Diabetes* 1993; **42**: 626–30.

50 Karjalainen J, Martin JM, Knip M, Ilonen J, Robinson B, Savilahti E, Akerblom HK, Dosch H-M. A bovine albumin peptide as a possible trigger of insulin-dependent diabetes mellitus. *N Engl J Med* 1992; **327**(5): 302–27.

51 Pietropaolo M, Castano L, Babu S, Roland B, Kuo YLS, Martin S *et al*. Islet cell autoantigen 69kD (ICA69). *J Clin Invest* 1993; **92**: 359–71.

52 Atkinson MA, Bowman MA, Kao KJ, Campbell L, Dush PJ, Shah SC *et al*. Lack of immune responsiveness to bovine serum albumin in insulin dependent diabetes. *N Engl J Med* 1993; **329**: 1853–8.

53 Jones DB, Hunter NR, Duff GW. Heat shock protein 65 as a beta cell antigen of insulin-dependent diabetes. *Lancet* 1990; **335**: 583–5.

54 Atkinson M, Holmes LH, Scharp DW, Lacy PE, Maclaren NK. No evidence for serological autoimmunity to islet cell heat shock proteins in insulin dependent diabetes. *J Clin Invest* 1991; **87**: 721–4.

55 Christie MR, Hollands JA, Brown TJ, Michelsen BK, Delovitch TL. Detection of pancreatic islet 64,000 M_r autoantigens in insulin-dependent diabetes distinct from

glutamate decarboxylase. *J Clin Invest* 1993; **92**: 240–8.
56 Shehadeh N, Calcinaro F, Bradley BJ, Bruchlim I, Vardi P, Lafferty KJ. Effect of adjuvant therapy on development of diabetes in mouse and man. *Lancet* 1994; **343**: 706–7.
57 Elias D, Cohen IR. Peptide therapy for diabetes in NOD mice. *Lancet* 1994; **343**: 704–6.
58 Shizuru JA, Taylor-Edwards C, Banks B, Gregory AK, Fathman CA. Immunotherapy of the nonobese diabetic mouse: Treatment with antibody to T-helper lymphocytes. *Science* 1988; **241**: 659–61.
59 Wang Y, Hao L, Gill RG, Lafferty KJ. Autoimmune diabetes in NOD mouse is L3T4 T-lymphocyte dependent. *Diabetes* 1987; **36**: 535–8.
60 Rabinovitch A, Sumoski W, Rajotte RV, Warnock GL. Cytotoxic effects of cytokines on human pancreatic islet cells in monolayer culture. *J Clin Endocrinol Metab* 1990; **71**: 151–6.
61 Stewart TA, Hultgren B, Huang X, Pitts-Meek S, Hully J, MacLachlan NJ. Induction of Type I diabetes by interferon alpha in transgenic mice. *Science* 1993; **260**(5116): 1942–6.
62 Corbett JA, Mikhael A, Shimizu J, Frederick K, Misko TP, McDaniel ML *et al*. Nitric oxide production in islets of nonobese diabetic mice: aminoguanidine-sensitive and -resistant stages in the immunological diabetic process. *Proc Natl Acad Sci USA* 1993; **90**: 8992–5.
63 Corbett JA, Sweetland MA, Hang JL, Lancaster JR, McDaniel ML. Nitric oxide mediates cytokine-induced inhibition of insulin secretion by human Islets of Langerhans. *Proc Natl Acad Sci USA* 1993; **90**: 1731–5
64 Kaufman DL, Clare-Salzler M, Tian J *et al*. Spontaneous loss of T cell self tolerance to glutamate decarboxylase is a key event in the pathogenesis of murine insulin-dependent diabetes. *Nature* 1993; **366**: 69–71.
65 Atkinson MA, Maclaren NK. The pathogenesis of insulin dependent diabetes. *N Engl J Med* (in press).
66 Olsson T, Sun J, Hillert J, Hojeberg B, Ekre HP, Andersson G *et al*. Increased numbers of T cells recognizing multiple myelin basic protein epitopes in multiple sclerosis. *Eur J Immunol* 1992; **22**: 1083–7.
67 Soderstrum M, Link H, Sun JB, Fredrikson S, Kostulas V, Hojeberg B *et al*. T cells recognizing multiple peptides of myelin basic protein are found in blood and enriched in cerebrospinal fluid in optic neuritis and multiple sclerosis. *Scand J Immunol* 1993; **37L**: 355–68.
68 Utz U, Biddison WE, McFarland HF, McFarlin DE, Flerlage M, Martin R, Skewed T-cell receptor repertoire in genetically identical twins correlates with multiple sclerosis. *Nature* 1993; **364**: 243–7.
69 Manca F, Habeshaw J, Dalgleish A. The naive repitoire of human T helper cells specific for gp120, the envelope glycoprotein of HIV. *J Immunol* 1991; **146**: 1964–71.

9

Metabolic Assessment in the Pre-clinical Period of Type 1 IDDM

DAVID K. McCULLOCH
Diabetes Clinical Research Unit, Virginia Mason Research Center, Seattle, Washington, USA

INTRODUCTION

From a clinical point of view, autoimmune diseases (like rheumatoid disease or autoimmune thyroid disease) have several features in common, most notably that there is a wide spectrum of clinical presentation. This is readily apparent in a disease like rheumatoid arthritis. Patients can be found who appear similar genetically (at least with respect to relevant HLA genes) and immunologically (from the presence of relevant autoantibodies) and yet have very different disease courses. At one end of the spectrum are those who have mild grumbling arthralgias, where the diagnosis of rheumatoid arthritis may be in doubt for many months or years. At the other end are unfortunate individuals who undergo a fulminant and rapidly progressive course, leading to crippling destructive disease. In all cases, however, it is clinically apparent that some organic disease affecting the joints is underway. With Type 1 diabetes, however, this spectrum of disease activity has not been appreciated until recently, because the only people who present clinically are those who are at one extreme of the spectrum, having "end-stage" pancreatic β-cell dysfunction, and who are frankly hyperglycemic and symptomatic. For those with any lesser degree of autoimmune damage, there would be nothing in the person's history, or on physical examination, to suggest that any active

Prediction, Prevention and Genetic Counseling in IDDM. Edited by Jerry P. Palmer.
© 1996 John Wiley & Sons Ltd.

disease is occurring in the pancreas, or to know whether the disease is progressing. The importance of metabolic assessment during this pre-clinical period is that it is the only method currently available to evaluate the target end-organ. Ideally, metabolic assessment should allow us to demonstrate that the β cells are malfunctioning, to quantify the damage, to document and follow changes in β-cell function, to distinguish those with progressive disease, from those who may be in remission, with stable non-progressive β-cell dysfunction, and to demonstrate improvement in β-cell function in response to therapeutic intervention. In this review, I will discuss how close we are to achieving these ideals with currently available tests, review areas where controversy has arisen, and suggest how metabolic testing can be applied in a practical way, singly or in combination, to help predict which subjects are suitable for preventive treatment.

EVALUATION OF GLUCOSE TOLERANCE

Since the most important function of the pancreatic β cells is to maintain normal glucose homeostasis, it is tempting to use glucose tolerance as an overall assessment of β-cell function. In this, we can learn a lot from strategies used to detect the development of non-insulin-dependent diabetes (NIDDM). Although technically simple, the use of random or fasting blood glucose values has been shown to be inadequate as a screening test for diabetes[1]. The oral glucose tolerance test (OGTT) gives considerably more information and has been widely used in epidemiologic studies. In 1979, the National Diabetes Data Group (NDDG), in concert with the World Health Organization (WHO), proposed that the term "impaired glucose tolerance" (IGT) be introduced to describe individuals who met criteria during the OGTT which was between a normal and diabetic response[2]. There is a spectrum from normal through IGT, ending with overt diabetes, and the proportion of the population in the latter two categories increases with age. The Second National Health and Nutrition Examination Survey (NHANES II) has estimated that about 11% of Americans aged between 20 and 74 have IGT, and a further 6% have NIDDM[2]. At all ages the proportion of the population with IGT or NIDDM increases with obesity. The results of an OGTT can therefore be used as a metabolic marker which predicts the likelihood for developing NIDDM in the future. In studies of pre-clinical IDDM where OGTTs have been performed prospectively on islet cell antibody positive (ICA+) non-diabetic relatives from family studies, or on cohorts of patients with polyendocrine disease, results often remain normal until just before the clinical onset of IDDM[3], although subsets of patients can show impaired glucose tolerance for many months or years before IDDM develops[4].

Glycated hemoglobin has received much less favor in the prospective evaluation of pre-clinical IDDM, for reasons that deserve discussion. Glycated hemoglobin (HbA1) has been widely used for almost twenty years as a reliable indicator of metabolic control in diabetic patients. It reflects average blood glucose levels over a six–eight-week period and correlation between HbA1 and several measures of diabetic control are well known. It is less clear, however, how valuable HbA1 measurements are in the diagnosis of diabetes or impaired glucose tolerance. Studies have attempted to evaluate this by comparing HbA1, and particularly its sub-fraction HbA1c, to OGTT results. Although some correlation between them has been found, significant discrepancies and disparities were apparent[5]. This may reflect problems in the inter- and intra-subject reliability and reproducibility of both the early HbA1 assays and also the OGTT.

Much recent improvement in the HbA1c assays has taken place and interassay Cvs of 2–3% can now be achieved[6]. Recent prospective studies on 381 non-diabetic individuals from the Pima Indian population (who are at high risk for developing NIDDM) have suggested that the measurement of glycated hemoglobin (HbA1c) is not only a simpler and more reproducible test than the OGTT, but may be a better predictor of which subjects are likely to develop NIDDM in future[6]. After being followed for up to six years, 38% of those with IGT at baseline developed diabetes, compared with 50% of those who had an elevated HbA1c, and 69% of those with both IGT and elevated HbA1c[6]. Although there were some false negatives in this study (about 10% of those who had a normal HbA1c at baseline developed NIDDM up to six years later) these predictions were based on a single HbA1c estimation at baseline. It is likely that if HbA1c were measured annually, at the same time every year, the predictive power would increase significantly.

There is evidence that small changes in glucose tolerance such as that seen in pregnancy, seasonally or as a result of a change in diet can be reflected in significant changes in HbA1c, even within the normal reference range. There are obvious advantages to the use of the HbA1c assays rather than the OGTT in the detection of diabetes or changes in glucose tolerance. The OGTT is a time-consuming test, difficult to standardize and requiring a great deal of patient preparation and cooperation. HbA1c is a single blood test requiring 1–2 ml of blood and demanding no special dietary measures prior to the test for its reproducibility. It therefore has much more potential as a practical screening test.

In the past few years we have begun a prospective screening program of healthy school children (aged 12–18 years) in Washington State to evaluate their risk for developing IDDM[7]. As part of this study we have drawn blood on the same children at the same time every year (April/May) for measurement of HbA1c (using the same assay as that used in the DCCT, with an interassay CV of <3%). Several interesting findings have already emerged. Although the normal range for this assay is 3.5–6.05%, healthy individuals maintain their own HbA1c within a much narrower range. Figure 9.1 shows data from four representative children in the study who are persistently negative for islet cell autoantibodies (represented by the open circles), and whose initial HbA1c, at entry to the study, were at different levels within the normal range. The figure shows that, if a healthy individual has a HbA1c of around 3.8% one year, it will be around 3.8% at the same time the next year, whereas someone whose normal set point is around 5.3% will remain at that level. Among 216 subjects measured 12 months apart there was a strong correlation ($r = 0.69$, $p < 0.005$) with the mean intrasubject CV of less than 5%. Among the 15 individuals who were at higher risk of developing IDDM (ICA+ > 20 JDF units, and/ or the presence of IAA in addition to ICA), HbA1c was $5.0 \pm 0.15\%$, significantly higher than those with low titer ICA ($4.7 \pm 0.04\%$, $n = 49$, $p < 0.008$) or those who were ICA negative controls ($4.6 \pm 0.03\%$, $n = 164$, $p < 0.002$). We postulate that a rise in HbA1c within the defined "normal" range, may be an early indicator of subclinical loss of pancreatic β-cell

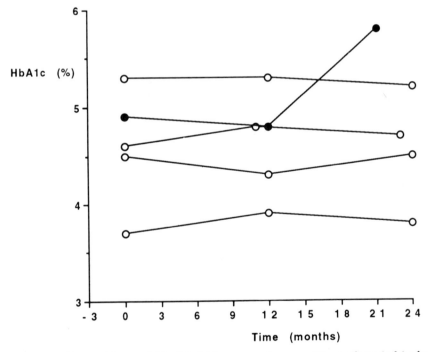

Figure 9.1. Glycated hemoglobin (HbA1c) measured over a 24 month period in four teenage school children who are autoantibody negative (open circles) and one who was strongly positive for both islet cell antibody and insulin autoantibody (solid circles)

function and are following subjects prospectively to evaluate HbA1c as a predictor of IDDM. Figure 9.1 shows data from one subject (a 15-year-old girl, subject number 10 in reference 7) who was strongly positive for ICA and IAA at entry to the study (represented by the solid circles). After 12 months of follow-up she had maintained her HbA1c at the same level as baseline, similar to the ICA negative subjects. The following year, however, her HbA1c had risen from 4.8 to 5.8%. Although this is still within the normal range, and was associated with a normal fasting blood glucose and no symptoms, it was a much larger rise than we had seen in other children in the study. Eleven months later she presented in mild ketoacidosis with a blood glucose of 510 mg dl^{-1} (28 mM) and was promptly started on insulin.

Direct comparisons between HbA1c and OGTT for prediction of progression to clinical IDDM, such as those being done in NIDDM[6] are not currently available, but would be very useful.

EVALUATION OF INSULIN SECRETION

Even when sensitive measures of glucose tolerance are used, abnormalities in glucose homeostasis will not be seen until a significant amount of islet damage has occurred. In order to detect damage to the pancreatic islets at an earlier stage, β-cell function must be measured directly. One of the simplest ways is to evaluate insulin secretion in response to standardized secretagogues[3]. Although a variety of secretagogues has been used over the past few decades (such as glucose, arginine, glucagon and isoproterenol), the most widely used is the acute insulin response to intravenous glucose (AIRg), also referred to as the first phase insulin response (FPIR), which measures the rise in insulin above baseline in the first 10 minutes after an intravenous glucose challenge. Although used by several research groups over the past 30 years[3], there has been no standardization of the dose or concentration of the glucose used, time over which the glucose should be infused, and which samples should be taken afterwards for insulin measurement to calculate the AIRg (or FPIR). The ICARUS (Islet Cell Antibody Register Users Study) group has evaluated some of the methodological details of the test[8], and has developed a consensus protocol, summarized in Table 9.1. An infusion time of 3 minutes ± 15 seconds is easy to achieve, even in subjects with small veins, using either an infusion pump or manual infusion. Shorter infusion times (30 seconds or less) require larger veins, a more concentrated glucose infusion, and may be associated with an unpleasant hot flushing feeling for the subject. A glucose dose of 35 grams seems to be above a maximally stimulating dose for any subject. It has been suggested that timing of samples begin at the end of the 3 minute infusion (4 minutes after the start of the glucose). This may cause a problem for those who wish to measure insulin sensitivity (Si) using

Table 9.1. Summary of the ICARUS protocol for the intravenous glucose tolerance test

Preparation	3 days of unrestricted diet, containing at least 150 grams carbohydrate. Avoid unusual physical exertion for previous 24 hours. Defer test if subject has intercurrent illness.
Fast	At least 10 but less than 16 hours. Plain water permitted but no smoking or caffeine.
Start time	0730–1000 hours.
Glucose dose	0.5 grams per kilogram up to 35 grams maximum of 25% glucose.
Infusion	Manual or pump driven infusion over 3 minutes±15 seconds, with time zero set at the end of the infusion.
Sample collection	A minimum of 2 baseline samples 5 minutes apart, taken immediately before the start of the glucose infusion, and 1, 3, 5, and 10 minutes after the end of the infusion.
Cannulae	Antegrade cannulation of the antecubital fossa is preferred. A single cannula may be used, although a separate cannula in each arm is helpful if multiple samples are taken during and after the glucose infusion for estimation of insulin sensitivity.

Bergman's minimal model, since this defines the beginning of the glucose infusion as time zero, and uses the 1, 2, and 3 minute insulin values in the model[9]. In my lab we have resolved this problem by having two IV lines inserted so that glucose can be infused in one arm over 3 minutes while, from the other arm, samples can be taken every minute during, as well as after, the end of the infusion.

After the end of the glucose infusion, how many time points for insulin measurement should be taken to calculate the AIRg (or FPIR)? The longest running and largest prospective clinical study in the world has been the Joslin family study (started by Soeldner and colleagues three decades ago). This group simply added the insulin values 1 minute and 3 minutes after the end of the infusion and used this to represent the FPIR. Others have felt that taking the average of 5–10 samples during the first 10 minutes, or calculating the areas above baseline for the insulin curve form 1 to 10 minutes would give a better representation of AIRg (or FPIR) and would yield less intrasubject variability[3]. When this was compared directly it was found that the correlation between the AIRg measured using the mean of seven samples versus two was extremely good, but that the intrasubject CV was slightly improved by taking more samples (11.6 ± 2.3% versus 14.9 ± 2.8%)[8]. For young children, however, the use of a 3 minute infusion in a small vein, and taking only two samples after the end of the infusion may make the difference between whether the test is possible to do or not. Clearly, getting some useful data is better than no data, although I believe that for those who can tolerate a longer study, with more samples taken, the additional information and more reliable measurement is worthwhile.

One major practical problem which remains with this test is that, despite efforts at standardization, the intrasubject coefficient of variation for the measurement is still 10–25%. Rayman *et al.* suggested that intrasubject CV could be reduced to under 5% if the blood samples were drawn from a retrogradely cannulated hand vein as opposed to the usually antegrade cannulation of a vein in the antecubital fossa[10]. If this were true, it would represent a dramatic improvement over any other published methodology and would give a very much more precise and reproducible measurement of β-cell function with which to follow individuals. However, in their study they did not simultaneously draw blood retrogradely and antegradely in the same subjects at the same time, but used historical data for AIRg for antegradely drawn samples, and so the validity of their findings has been in some doubt. We recently completed a study in nine healthy subjects where we performed three intravenous glucose tolerance tests over an eight week period and obtained simultaneous measurements (antegradely and retrogradely) in every subject[11]. We found no difference in intrasubject CV for the two methods (both being around 20%). However, the values for AIRg were significantly higher, when using retrograde sampling, since this blood is closer to arterial blood than that obtained during antegrade sampling. It would appear then that retrograde cannulation (which is technically more difficult, and has a higher failure rate in subjects with small veins) does not offer significant advantages, and that an intrasubject CV of around 20% is about as good as one can expect with the AIRg at the present time.

At least part of the intrasubject variability in the measurement of AIRg arises as a result of physiologic changes in insulin secretion that can occur because of changes in insulin sensitivity. There is a strong curvilinear inverse correlation between measures of insulin secretion (like AIRg) and how sensitive the person's body is to insulin (measured as an insulin sensitivity index, or Si)[12]. Insulin sensitivity seems to be a fairly labile physiological function which varies at different times during the day and during the menstrual cycle. It is markedly affected by obesity, exercise, intercurrent illness, and changes during puberty and as people age. We have argued that it would be sensible to measure both AIRg and Si simultaneously, if possible, so that the AIRg can be interpreted in relation to the person's Si at the time[12]. There are several problems with this approach, however. Measurement of Si using the euglycemic hyperinsulinemic clamp technique, or using the frequently sampled intravenous glucose tolerance test requires frequent blood sampling over several hours. This makes it a very impractical test to undertake on many of the high risk children who are being followed prospectively. Galvin *et al.* have recently demonstrated that a reasonable estimate of Si can be obtained more simply by doing a 40 minute intravenous glucose tolerance test and calculating the rate of glucose disposal (*Kg*) and dividing this by the area under the insulin response curve[13].

Despite the theoretical importance of evaluating AIRg in relation to Si, prospective studies have not yet shown that this improves the ability to predict which high risk subjects are more likely to develop IDDM. However, in studies where newly diagnosed IDDM subjects have been treated with cyclosporine, the measurement of Si uncovered some surprising findings[14]. In 16 patients who underwent clinical remission during cyclosporine treatment, both AIRg and Si improved at 3 and 6 months. Although the endogenous insulin secretion (as estimated by stimulated C-peptide levels) improved to 12 months, loss of remission occurred in several patients and was associated with a decrease in insulin sensitivity, rather than insulin secretion (Figure 9.2). The potential for any immunotherapeutic agents to affect Si as well as insulin secretion suggests that measurement of both is preferable during intervention trials. There has been recent concern about the use of nicotinamide in the prevention of IDDM, and whether this drug might induce insulin resistance and compensatory increases in AIRg. A closely related compound, nicotinic acid, is known to induce profound insulin resistance, sufficient to induce hyperglycemia in asymptomatic individuals with subclinical β-cell dysfunction[15]. However, no increase in fasting insulin, or decrease in insulin sensitivity has been found, when nicotinamide has been tested in normal volunteers[16], although data are not available for the effects of nicotinamide in ICA positive individuals who have impaired β-cell function.

What has the measurement of AIRg (with or without simultaneous measurement of Si) taught us about the natural history of pre-clinical IDDM? The most striking finding in most studies is that there is tremendous heterogeneity. Although some individuals show an inexorable decline in insulin secretion which culminates in clinical IDDM, the rate of decline is very variable, and many ICA positive first degree relatives have impaired insulin secretion which is stable and does not appear to change or decline over many years of follow-up[17]. An important focus of current research is to predict which individuals will progress towards clinical IDDM from those who will remain euglycemic. It has been shown that once the AIRg is very low (below the first percentile) then progression to clinical IDDM becomes much more likely, especially among IDDM relatives who have high titers of ICAs and insulin autoantibodies (IAAs)[18]. With AIRg values above the first percentile, however, prediction of IDDM is much less confident.

It is hoped that measurements of pancreatic β-cell function will give us information about the extent of islet destruction, during the pre-clinical period, and yet some misperceptions still exist in this area. It is often said that 90% of the β-cells need to be destroyed before clinical IDDM will develop, despite the fact that this dogma was based on some assumptions in pancreatectomized rats and humans which have been shown to be false. At the time of clinical onset of IDDM, considerably more than 10% of the β cells probably remain functional. In studies of streptozocin-treated baboons where

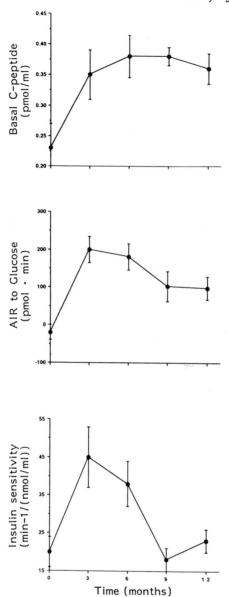

Figure 9.2. Insulin secretion and insulin sensitivity parameters over 12 months, in 16 patients with recently diagnosed IDDM, treated with cyclosporine (adapted from Hramiak *et al.*)[14]

correlations were made between the in vivo evaluation of β-cell function and in vitro estimates of β-cell mass, we found that 40–50% of β cells could be present and viable at a time when the AIRg is essentially zero[19]. In addition, histologic and in vitro physiologic data from the pancreas of a human patient who died soon after the onset of IDDM found that a substantial β-cell mass was still viable[20]. It is possible that, at the time of clinical presentation of IDDM, cytokines and other factors from the cells involved in the autoimmune insulitis may cause functional impairment of the remaining β cells, and that considerable recovery of function may be possible, if the autoimmune process could be stopped or suppressed[21]. Support for this has been obtained in studies on the non-obese diabetic (NOD) mouse[22]. When islets undergoing severe insulitis are removed from 12–13-week-old NOD mice and studied in culture, they show a profound impairment in insulin secretion on day zero. However, there is almost complete recovery of function by day 7 in culture (Figure 9.3). There are important implications of all these data for the interpretation of metabolic tests in pre-clinical IDDM. When the AIRg (or FPIR) is measured on a high risk non-diabetic and is found to be at the first percentile, this does *not* mean that 99% of the person's β cells have been destroyed. It is more likely that 50% or more of the pancreatic β cells are still potentially salvageable, but that they are suffering, functionally, because of the surrounding autoimmune milieu.

To detect β-cell dysfunction at an even earlier stage, the insulin response to a number of other secretagogues has been evaluated[3]. Glucose potentiates the ability of many non-glucose secretagogues to stimulate insulin release. The acute insulin response to a maximally stimulating dose of the amino acid arginine (AIRarg), for example, can be over five times greater when the plasma glucose is clamped at >450 mg dl^{-1} (>25 mM) than when tested at basal levels[23]. A decrease in the ability of glucose to potentiate AIRarg has been shown to be a more sensitive measure of β-cell dysfunction than AIRg in streptozocin-treated baboons, in women with former gestational diabetes, in pancreas and kidney transplant recipients, and in healthy human donors who have donated part of their pancreas. From a practical point of view, however, it is a more difficult, time-consuming and uncomfortable test for the patient. In our prospective family and population studies in pre-clinical IDDM, I have not found that this test is sufficiently more sensitive than AIRg to merit its use on a routine basis. Figure 9.4 shows data from 11 ICA positive non-diabetic teenagers from the Washington State Diabetes Prediction Study[7]; who had both AIRg and glucose potentiation slope to AIRarg measured within three weeks of each other, expressed in relation to insulin sensitivity, and compared to normal data[24]. There is a strong correlation between the two measurements ($r = 0.81$, $p < 0.05$), but the percentile for glucose potentiation is not consistently lower than for AIRg, as would be expected if this test were a more sensitive indicator of β-cell dysfunction.

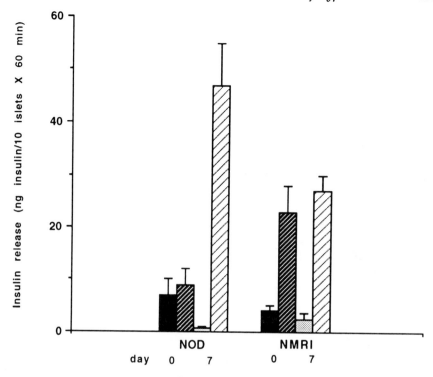

Figure 9.3. Insulin release from isolated pancreatic islets of 12-week-old female NOD mice and male NMRI mice. The islets were incubated in medium containing 1.67 Mm glucose, and after 60 min the medium was removed and the islets were incubated for another 60 min in medium containing 16.7 Mm glucose. The insulin release was examined immediately after isolation (day 0) (■, 1.67 Mm glucose; ▨ 16.7 Mm glucose) and after 1 week in culture (day 7) (▦, 1.67 Mm glucose; ▨ 16.7 Mm glucose) (adapted from Strandell *et al*.)[22]

EVALUATION OF OTHER ASPECTS OF β-CELL FUNCTION

Since C-peptide is secreted from the β cells in equimolar concentration with insulin, but is not extracted by the liver to any significant degree, it is attractive as a measure of β-cell function, although complexities in the kinetics and metabolism make interpretation of C-peptide measurements tricky in some situations. Because its measurement is unaffected by the presence of insulin antibodies, C-peptide levels, either fasting or stimulated by glucagon or a mixed meal, have been used extensively to follow the natural history of β-cell function in Type 1 diabetic patients after they have been started on insulin[25,26]. However, C-peptide measurements have not shown any advantage over insulin for the prediction of IDDM in the pre-clinical period.

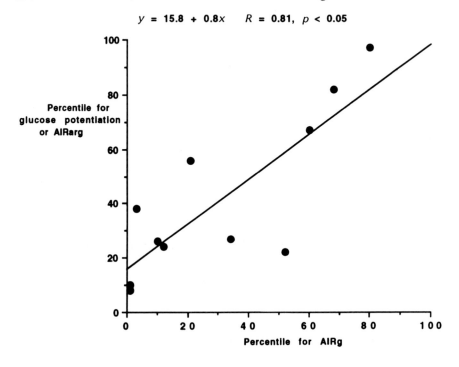

Figure 9.4. Correlation between the acute insulin response to intravenous glucose (AIRg) and the glucose potentiation slope of the acute insulin response to arginine (AIRarg), expressed as a percentile of normal (derived from reference 24), in 11 non-diabetic teenagers who were ICA positive

It has been found, in normal healthy subjects, that ~15% of circulating "immunoreactive insulin" is in fact proinsulin[27], and that the proportion of proinsulin increases in situations of impaired islet function. Studies in HLA identical siblings, and non-diabetic twins of IDDM patients showed elevated proinsulin levels, but failed to show differences among those at higher risk for developing IDDM (HLA identical siblings, or twins only recently discordant), from those at lesser risk (HLA non-identical siblings, or twins long discordant from the proband). Spinas *et al.* on the other hand, found that proinsulin levels were 3–4 times higher among ICA positive relatives of IDDM subjects compared with ICA negative relatives[28]. Some of these discrepancies may reflect differences in assay methodology. Improved understanding of how proinsulin is processed and cleared may increase the usefulness of this measurement[29]. However, no prospective studies to date have shown that proinsulin measurements offer any advantages over AIRg (or FPIR) in predicting the development of IDDM.

It has been shown that insulin is secreted in a series of rapid regular oscillations at intervals of 10 to 15 minutes and that this phenomenon is an intrinsic pancreatic function, occurring in the isolated pancreas[30]. This normal pattern is disturbed, with a significant reduction in pulse amplitude, following treatment with relatively small (non-diabetogenic) doses of streptozocin in baboons[31], suggesting that this might also be a useful measure of subclinical β-cell dysfunction. When nine ICA positive, non-diabetic first degree relatives were compared to normal controls, matched for age, sex and height, there was almost a complete absence of oscillatory activity in the ICA positive individuals, despite no significant differences in AIRg between the groups[32]. These findings suggest that oscillatory disturbances may be an even earlier indication of β-cell dysfunction than AIRg. Unfortunately the measurement of insulin cycling requires blood sampling at 1 minute intervals for up to 120 minutes followed by complex computerized time-series analyses, which make it unappealing as a clinical test. In addition, no prospective data are available to evaluate whether any disturbances in insulin cycling are different among ICA positive subjects who do not progress to clinical IDDM, compared to those who ultimately develop diabetes.

SUMMARY AND STRATEGIES FOR THE FUTURE

Careful measurement of glucose tolerance, insulin secretion and other aspects of pancreatic β-cell function has improved our understanding of the natural history of the pre-clinical period of Type 1 diabetes. Careful attention to methodological detail and standardization of protocols have allowed metabolic assessments to give useful information which can be followed prospectively and compared in laboratories around the world. Based on our current understanding, I would offer the following suggestions for the use of metabolic testing in ongoing and future studies:

1. After identification of potentially high risk non-diabetic individuals, based on immunologic and genetic testing, document the presence or absence of β-cell dysfunction by measuring AIRg (or FPIR), using the ICARUS protocol (Table 9.1). Where possible, do enough time points to document insulin sensitivity (Si). My preference is to use the tolbutamide or insulin modifications to the frequently samples IVGTT and Bergman's minimal model for this. By so doing, insulin sensitivity can be followed after therapeutic intervention has been started, and even after IDDM has developed and insulin treatment has been started.
2. Using a sensitive assay with a good interassay CV, measure HbA1c annually, at the same time every year (to avoid confusion from physiological rises in HbA1c in winter).

3. If and when intervention is contemplated, repeat AIRg, HbA1c and Si, and measure C-peptide in response to a standard mixed meal before and at intervals after treatment has been started.

ACKNOWLEDGMENTS

Many of the data from my own laboratory referred to here were supported by NIH grant DK-40627. My thanks also for the generous support of the families of Peter and Sharlee Eising, and Del and Mary Buse. I am grateful for the technical help, intellectual stimulation and support of numerous friends and colleagues over the past decade who have helped ask and answer many of the questions discussed in this chapter, particularly Jerry Palmer, Donna Koerker, Les Klaff, Åke Lernmark, Steve Kahn, Marli McCulloch, Jean Bucksa, Nicky Leech, Rachel Rowe, Jim Neifing and Niecey Meldrum.

REFERENCES

1 Harris MI, Modan M. Screening for NIDDM: Why is there no national program? *Diabetes Care* 1994; **17**: 440–4.
2 Harris MI. Impaired glucose tolerance in the US population. *Diabetes Care* 1989; **12**: 464–74.
3 McCulloch DK, Palmer JP, Benson EA. Beta cell function in the preclinical period of insulin-dependent diabetes. *Diabetes Metab Rev* 1987; **3**: 27–43.
4 Wagner R, Genovese S, Bosi E *et al.* Slow metabolic deterioration towards diabetes in islet cell antibody positive patients with autoimmune polyendocrine disease. *Diabetologia* 1994; **37**: 365–71.
5 Little RR, England JD, Wiedmeyer H-M *et al.* Relationship of glycosylated hemoglobin to oral glucose tolerance: implications for diabetes screening. *Diabetes* 1988; **37**: 60–4.
6 Little RR, England JD, Wiedmeyer HM *et al.* Glycated haemoglobin predicts progression to diabetes mellitus in Pima Indians with impaired glucose tolerance. *Diabetologia* 1994; **37**: 252–6.
7 Rowe RE, Leech NJ, Nepm GT, McCulloch DK. High genetic risk for IDDM in the Pacific Northwest: First report from the Washington State Diabetes Prediction Study. *Diabetes* 1994; **43**: 87–94.
8 McCulloch DK, Bingley PJ, Colman PG, Jackson R, Gale EAM, the ICARUS group. Comparison of bolus and infusion protocols for determining acute insulin response to intravenous glucose in normal humans. *Diabetes Care* 1993; **16**: 911–15.
9 Bergman RN, Ider YZ, Bowden CR, Cobelli C. Quantitative estimation of insulin sensitivity. *Am J Physiol* 1979; **236**: E667–E677,
10 Rayman G, Clark P, Schneider AE, Hales CN. The first phase insulin response to intravenous glucose is highly reproducible. *Diabetologia* 1990; **33**: 631–4.
11 Rowe RE, Leech NJ, Finegood DT, McCulloch DK. Retrograde versus antegrade cannulation in the intravenous glucose tolerance test. *Diabetes Res Clin Prac* 1994; **25**: 131–36.

12 Kahn SE, Prigeon RL, McCulloch DK *et al.* The contribution of insulin-dependent and insulin-independent glucose uptake to intravenous glucose tolerance in healthy human subjects. *Diabetes* 1994; **43**: 587–92.

13 Galvin P, Ward G, Walters J *et al.* A simple method for quantification of insulin sensitivity and insulin release from an intravenous glucose tolerance test. *Diabetic Med* 1992; **9**: 921–8.

14 Hramiak IM, Dupre JD, Finegood DT. Determinants of clinical remission in recent-onset IDDM. *Diabetes Care* 1993; **16**: 125–32.

15 Kahn SE, Beard JC, Schwartz MW *et al.* Increased β-cell secretory capacity as mechanism for islet adaptation to nicotinic acid-reduced insulin resistance. *Diabetes* 1989; **38**: 562–8.

16 Paul TL, Hramiak IM, Mahon JL *et al.* Nicotinamide and insulin sensitivity. *Diabetologia* 1993; **36**: 369.

17 Palmer JP, McCulloch DK. Prediction and prevention of IDDM—1991. *Diabetes* 1991; **40**: 943–7.

18 Thai A-C, Eisenbarth GS. Natural history of IDDM. *Diabetes Revs* 1993; **1**: 1–14.

19 McCulloch DK, Koerker DJ, Kahn SE, Bonner-Weir S, Palmer JP. Correlations of in vivo β-cell function tests with β-cell mass and pancreatic insulin content in streptozocin-administered baboons. *Diabetes* 1991; **40**: 673–9.

20 Conget I, Fernandez-Alvarez J, Ferrer J *et al.* Human pancreatic islet function at the onset of type 1 (insulin-dependent) diabetes mellitus. *Diabetologia* 1993; **36**: 358–60.

21 Eizirik DL, Sandler S, Palmer JP. Repair of pancreatic β-cells: a relevant phenomenon in early IDDM? *Diabetes* 1993; **42**: 1383–91.

22 Strandell E, Eizirik DL, Sandler S. Reversal of β-cell suppression in vitro in pancreatic islets isolated from nonobese diabetic mice during the phase preceding insulin-dependent diabetes mellitus. *J Clin Invest* 1990; **85**: 1944–50.

23 Ward WK, Bolgiano DL, McKnight B, Halter JB, Porte D, Jr. Diminished β-cell secretory capacity in patients with non-insulin dependent diabetes mellitus. *J Clin Invest* 1984; **74**: 1318–26.

24 Kahn SE, Prigeon RL, McCulloch DK *et al.* Quantification of the relationship between insulin sensitivity and β-cell function in human subjects: evidence for a hyperbolic function. *Diabetes* 1993; **42**: 1663–72.

25 Madsbad S. Prevalence of residual B cell function and its metabolic consequences in type 1 (insulin-dependent) diabetes. *Diabetologia* 1983; **24**: 141–7.

26 Landin-Olsson M, Nilsson KO, Lernmark Å, Sundkvist G. Islet cell antibodies and fasting C-peptide predict insulin requirement at diagnosis of diabetes mellitus. *Diabetologia* 1990; **33**: 561–8.

27 Ward WK, LaCava EC, Paquette TL, Beard JC, Wallum BJ, Porte D, Jr. Disproportionate elevation of immunoreactive proinsulin in type 2 (non-insulin-dependent) diabetes mellitus and in experimental insulin resistance. *Diabetologia* 1987; **30**: 698–702.

28 Spinas GA, Snorgaard O, Hartling SG, Oberholzer M, Berger W. Elevated proinsulin levels related to islet cell antibodies in first-degree relatives of IDDM patients. *Diabetes Care* 1992; **15**: 632–7.

29 Rhodes CJ, Alarcon C. What β-cell defect could lead to hyperproinsulinemia in NIDDM? Some clues from recent advances made in understanding the proinsulin-processing mechanism. *Diabetes* 1994; **43**: 511–17.

30 Weigle DS. Pulsatile secretion of fuel-regulatory hormones. *Diabetes* 1987; **36**: 764–75.

31 Goodner CJ, Koerker DJ, Weigle DS, McCulloch DK. Decreased insulin- and glucagon-pulse amplitude accompanying β-cell deficiency induced by streptozocin in baboons. *Diabetes* 1989; **38**: 925–31.

32 Bingley PJ, Matthews DR, Williams AJK, Bottazzo GF, Gale EAM. Loss of regular oscillatory insulin secretion in islet cell antibody positive non-diabetic subjects. *Diabetologia* 1992; **35**: 32–8.
33 Bingley PJ, Colman P, Eisenbarth GS *et al.* Standardization of IVGTT to predict IDDM. *Diabetes Care* 1992; **15**: 1313–16.

10

Environmental Factors: Viruses

JI-WON YOON
Laboratory of Viral and Immunopathogenesis of Diabetes, Julia McFarlane Diabetes
Research Centre, University of Calgary, Calgary, Alberta, Canada

INTRODUCTION

Type 1 diabetes, also known as insulin-dependent diabetes mellitus (IDDM), results from the destruction of insulin-producing pancreatic beta cells, which leads to the development of hypoinsulinemia and hyperglycemia[1]. There is considerable evidence that beta cell destruction in pre-diabetic patients is progressive and takes place over a lengthy asymptomatic period. During the past few decades, researchers have extensively studied genetic factors, environmental factors (viral infections, diet, toxins), and autoimmunity as possible causes of pancreatic beta cell destruction.

Viruses are suspected as causative factors in some cases of IDDM for several reasons. It was first noted almost 70 years ago, that there appears to be a seasonal incidence in the onset of acute IDDM with a peak in the autumn[2] and diseases with seasonal incidences are often caused by viral infections. There have also been many anecdotal reports of a viral infection preceding or coinciding with the onset of IDDM, as well as case reports of virus isolation from pancreata of acutely diabetic deceased patients[3]. Epidemiological studies examining newly diagnosed, recent-onset IDDM patients for the presence of virus-specific IgM antibodies have also suggested a role for viruses in the etiology of IDDM[4]. In animals, several viruses have been demonstrated to definitely cause diabetes, including encephalomyocarditis (EMC) virus[5], coxsackie B4 virus[6], Kilham's rat virus (KRV)[7], and rubella virus[8], while other viruses, such as retrovirus[9] and bovine viral diarrhea-mucosal disease virus[10] are suspected of causing diabetes in non-obese diabetic (NOD) mice and cattle respectively.

Prediction, Prevention and Genetic Counseling in IDDM. Edited by Jerry P. Palmer.
© 1996 John Wiley & Sons Ltd.

Viruses may be involved in the pathogenesis of IDDM in at least two distinct ways. First of all, viruses may directly infect and destroy insulin-producing pancreatic beta cells, resulting in clinical IDDM. Alternatively, since many cases of IDDM are known to involve a rather long pathologic process, it is also possible that viruses may in some way trigger or contribute to the autoimmune destruction of beta cells (Table 10.1). In this chapter, I will discuss the evidence for viral involvement in IDDM, the possible mechanisms by which viruses may act, and also the mechanisms whereby viruses may protect against the development of the disease (Figure 10.1).

Table 10.1. Viruses associated with the development of IDDM

Mechanism	Virus	Host	Remarks
	EMC	Mice	Genetically susceptible animals only
		APA strain of Syrian hamsters	
	Coxsackie B	Mice	Genetically susceptible animals only
Cytolytic Infection		Non-human primates	Genetically susceptible animals only
		Humans	
	Coxsackie A	Humans	Some epidemiological evidence
	Rubella	Humans	Especially congenital rubella syndrome
		Hamsters	
	Cytomegalovirus	Humans	Several case studies
	Mumps virus	Humans	
Triggering of autoimmunity	Epstein-Barr	Humans	
	Retrovirus	NOD mice	
	Reovirus	Mice	
	Kilham's rat virus	DRBB rats	No distinct infection of rat beta cells
	Bovine viral diarrhea-mucosal disease virus	Cattle	Suspected of triggering autoimmunity
	Coxsackie B	Humans?	Persistent infection and/or induction of cytokines?

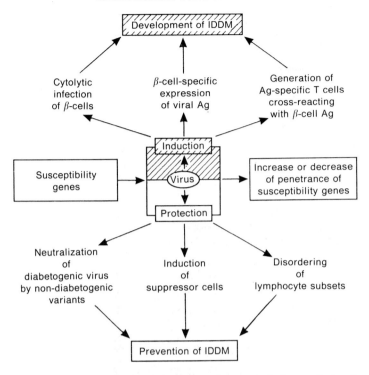

Figure 10.1. Role of viruses in the destruction of pancreatic beta cells leading to an increase or decrease in the penetrance of susceptibility genes. Genetic susceptibility appears to be a prerequisite for the development of IDDM, however, environmental factors such as viruses, may act as inductive or preventive agents. Some viruses may induce diabetes by directly infecting and destroying beta cells, while others may trigger beta cell-specific autoimmune IDDM. Regarding prevention, vaccination with viruses can neutralize infectious virus, while in some instances infection with viruses may induce suppressor T cells or may selectively deplete the CD4 positive T cell subset. In these ways, viruses as environmental factors, may affect the penetrance of susceptibility genes

DIRECT CYTOLYTIC INFECTION AND DESTRUCTION OF PANCREATIC BETA CELLS BY VIRUSES AND DEVELOPMENT OF IDDM

ENCEPHALOMYOCARDITIS VIRUS

Encephalomyocarditis (EMC) virus is a picornavirus, meaning that it is a small RNA virus with a capsid comprised of four polypeptides (VP1, 2, 3 and 4) and a genome that is a linear molecule of single-stranded RNA of positive polarity. EMC virus does not induce diabetes in humans, but in genetically susceptible strains of mice, the M variant of EMC (EMC-M) virus does induce a diabetes-like syndrome, characterized by hypoinsulinemia, hyperglycemia, glycosuria, polydipsia and polyphagia. EMC-M virus-infected mice do not however consistently develop these symptoms[11]. Two stable, antigenically indistinguishable variants, one of which produces diabetes in over 90% of infected animals (EMC-D), and the other completely non-diabetogenic (EMC-B), have been isolated by plaque purification[12]. After determination of the complete nucleotide sequences of the genomes of both variants, their comparison revealed a total of 14 nucleotide differences between the two variants[3]. Further investigation using several mutant viruses generated from stocks of both EMC-D and EMC-B variants revealed that a "G" base at nucleotide position 3155 (Ala [GCC]-776 on the VP1) is unique to all diabetogenic variants, while an "A" base at the same position (Thr[ACC]-776) is identical in all non-diabetogenic variants and that only one amino acid, alanine, is critical for the diabetogenicity of the EMC virus. The single point mutation ("G" to "A"; "Ala" to "Thr") results in the conversion of the diabetogenic variant to the non-diabetogenic variant of EMC virus. The 776th amino acid, alanine, lies in the highly conserved, strongly hydrophilic patch of the VP1. This site has been identified as the viral attachment to pancreatic beta cells and the amino acid change at this position from threonine of the EMC-B variant to alanine of the EMC-D variant reduces the hydrophilicity of the region by 37%. It appears that having alanine at this position in EMC-D, contributes to this variant's diabetogenicity by increasing the efficiency of viral attachment to pancreatic beta cells[3].

Only certain strains of inbred mice (SJL/J, SWR/J, DBA/1J and DBA/2J) develop diabetes after EMC-D viral infection, while other strains (C57BL/6J, CBA/J and AKR/J) do not, indicating that the genetic background of the host plays a role in the development of EMC-D virus-induced diabetes[12]. Results from studies using F1, F2, backcrosses, and hybrids of these animals, as well as in vitro viral attachment studies, indicate that susceptibility to EMC-D virus-induced diabetes is determined by a single autosomal recessive gene that is inherited in a Mendelian mode[3]. It is thought that the expression of viral receptors on beta cells may be modulated in genetically susceptible mice[3].

Initially it was thought that T lymphocytes might be involved in the destruction of beta cells in EMC-D virus-induced diabetes, but later studies showed that depletion of lymphocytes failed to alter the incidence of diabetes[3]. As well, EMC-D-infected athymic nude mice showed a diabetogenic response that was nearly identical to that of their heterozygous littermates[3], and treatment of EMC-infected mice with cyclosporin A did not prevent the disease, but rather enhanced both its incidence and severity[3]. Data showed that Mac-2 positive macrophages are predominant at an early stage of viral infection, while mixed immunocytes (other macrophages, helper/inducer T cells and cytotoxic/suppressor T cells) are present at intermediate and late stages of viral infection[3]. Depletion of macrophages resulted in the prevention of diabetes when mice were inoculated with a low dose of EMC virus. In contrast, activation of macrophages in mice prior to viral infection clearly enhanced the incidence of diabetes. A low dose of virus infection is not enough to destroy a sufficient number of beta cells for the development of overt clinical diabetes, but the involvement of activated macrophages at an early stage of viral infection clearly contributes to destruction of residual beta cells[3].

COXSACKIE VIRUSES

Coxsackie B viruses and human IDDM

In humans, there is a great deal of circumstantial evidence that coxsackie B viruses may be involved in the development of IDDM. Much of the evidence has come from epidemiological studies linking recent-onset IDDM with coxsackie B viral infections. Twenty-five years ago, Gamble *et al.*[13] conducted one of the first epidemiological studies to compare anti-coxsackie B antibody levels in patients with recent-onset diabetes and those in non-diabetic controls. They reported that patients with recent-onset IDDM (less than three months' duration) had higher titers of antibody to coxsackie virus, especially the B4 serotype. Since that time, researchers have continued to compare levels of anti-coxsackie B virus neutralizing antibodies in sera from diabetic and non-diabetic subjects. Many studies have found statistically significantly higher levels of coxsackie B virus-specific antibody in recent-onset diabetic patients compared to non-diabetic healthy controls[6]. These studies provide some evidence for coxsackie B viral involvement in the development of IDDM. However, there have been other epidemiological studies that have found no evidence of a correlation[6], while still others have found higher levels of anti-coxsackie B virus-specific antibodies in non-diabetic control subjects than in recent-onset IDDM patients[6]. The contrasting results from the above studies do not necessarily negate a relationship between coxsackie B viral infection and IDDM. There are different variants of the virus found within each serotype. For example, Prabhakar *et al.* (reviewed in reference 6) isolated 13 variants of coxsackie B4 virus. Of four coxsackie B4 variants tested in another study, only one proved to cause diabetes while the remaining three variants did not[6]. This is an indication of the possible rarity of diabetogenic variants of coxsackie B4 virus. As well, we are unable to distinguish between diabetogenic and non-diabetogenic variants using routine neutralizing antibody or ELISA testing, since the variants are cross-reactive. Therefore, if a person is exposed to a more common non-diabetogenic variant of coxsackie B4 virus prior to exposure to a more rare diabetogenic variant of the same serotype, the person will have already developed antibodies against the non-diabetogenic variant which will neutralize the diabetogenic variant during the subsequent infection and the person will not become diabetic, even if genetically predisposed to the disease. If this person is a subject in an epidemiological study, the results will not be meaningful as the lack of diabetes seen will not be a result of lack of exposure to a diabetogenic coxsackie B4 virus, and no correlation between coxsackie B4 virus infection and the incidence of diabetes would be found. In contrast, in certain areas, outbreaks of diabetogenic virus prior to outbreaks of non-diabetogenic virus would result in a high correlation between coxsackie B virus infection and the development of diabetes. In animal models, it has already been proven that prior infection with non-diabetogenic EMC-B virus results in no development of diabetes after subsequent infection by diabetogenic EMC-D virus[3]. Thus the correlation between coxsackie B virus infection and development of diabetes seen in some studies and the lack of correlation found in other studies may be dependent on the genetic make-up of the virus and genetic backgrounds of the individuals.

There have also been many anecdotal reports describing the development of IDDM in patients with a recent or concurrent coxsackie B viral infection[6]. One report in particular of a patient who died after a massive synchronous destruction of pancreatic islets, suggests that a viral infection must have been responsible, although unfortunately the serology was not studied in this case.

More direct supporting evidence of a role of coxsackie B viral infection in the onset of IDDM has come from research reporting the isolation of coxsackie B viruses from, or the presence of coxsackie B viral antigens in, pancreata of recent-onset IDDM patients. In 1976, Gladisch *et al.* reported the case of a five-year-old girl who developed myocarditis and diabetes two weeks after open heart surgery (reviewed in reference 6). At necropsy, her islets showed a lymphocytic infiltrate and beta cell necrosis. Coxsackie B4 antigens were detected in the islets by immunofluorescence and high levels of antibody against coxsackie B4 virus were present in the child's serum. Three years later a variant of coxsackie B4 virus isolated from the pancreas of a diabetic patient was found to induce diabetes in mice[6]. In this case, less than three days after the onset of a flu-like illness, a previously healthy ten-year-old boy was admitted to the hospital in diabetic ketoacidosis. Seven days after admission the child died when all attempts to ameliorate his deteriorating condition failed. At autopsy, lymphocytic infiltration of the islets and beta cell necrosis were observed. When several inbred strains of mice were inoculated with the coxsackie B4 variant isolated from the diabetic child, SJL/J male mice developed diabetes, while CBA/J, C57BL/6J and Balb/c mice did not.

Champsaur *et al.* reported an additional case of coxsackie B5 virus infection appearing to have triggered IDDM (reviewed in reference 6). A 16-month-old girl with a coxsackie B5 virus infection developed diabetic symptoms for a ten day period shortly after infection, went into remission for two months, then developed definite IDDM. In this case, the virus isolated from the girl's feces caused glucose intolerance in selected mouse strains. Islet cell antibodies were found in the child a week before the onset of diabetes, and immunogenetic analysis revealed that the child had markers indicating a high risk for the development of IDDM

Various studies of the capacity of coxsackie B3 and B4 viruses to infect beta cells have been conducted using human pancreatic cell cultures and clearly demonstrate that human beta cells can be infected by coxsackie B3 and B4 viruses[6]. Radioimmunoassays showed that intracellular insulin in infected beta cells decreased rapidly beginning at 24 hours after infection and that the decrease in insulin roughly paralleled the increase in viral titer. It is interesting to note from the results of these studies that coxsackie B4 viral infection can impair human islet cell metabolism in vitro without involvement of the immune system. These studies also demonstrate that human beta cells, at least under in vitro conditions, are not resistant to infection by coxsackie B viruses.

From results of the above research on humans and animals, it is speculated that coxsackie B viruses, especially the B4 serotype, may play a role in the development of IDDM either by directly initiating the development of the disease, or by operating as the final insult to beta cells in individuals where ongoing autoimmune beta cell destruction has already been taking place.

Coxsackie B viruses and animal IDDM

Mice   Naturally acquired coxsackie B viral infections of the pancreas normally produce a predominantly acinar cell pancreatitis and do not usually affect the endocrine pancreas. Coleman *et al.* infected CD1 mice, which are susceptible to diabetes, with a passaged coxsackie B4 isolate and 20–30% of the animals developed hyperglycemia[6]. In other strains of mice, unadapted coxsackie viruses did not infect pancreatic beta cells when inoculated, however, once repeatedly passaged in murine pancreatic cell-rich cultures, coxsackie B4 virus became much more beta cell tropic and was shown to be capable of producing hypoinsulinemia and hyperglycemia in several inbred strains of mice[6]. All six B serotypes of coxsackie virus, once repeatedly passaged in beta cells, have been shown to be capable of inducing diabetes in SJL/J mice. Studies on the influence of genetics on the response to coxsackie B virus infections in these mice have found that the "db" diabetic mutation on chromosome 4 exerted the most effect on susceptibility and host response to coxsackie B4 virus and was associated with an impaired humoral response to coxsackie B4 virus infection as these mice did not develop an adequate level of anti-coxsackie B4 IgM and IgG antibodies[6]. The animals were also found to be deficient in absolute and relative numbers of spleen lymphocyte subsets[6].

Several studies have found that preproinsulin mRNA levels in islet fractions prepared from mice after coxsackie B4 virus infection are reduced[6]. Investigation into long-term effects of coxsackie B4 virus infection on murine pancreatic islet function revealed that inoculation of mice with a pancreas-adapted coxsackie B4 virus caused a significant increase in insulin release in islets from inoculated mice at three and six months after inoculation[6]. Histological examination of the islets revealed no changes and islet cell antibodies were not detected. The abnormal insulin release occurred with minimum changes in blood glucose concentration. It would thus appear from these results that coxsackie B4 virus infection may lead to lasting changes in islet metabolism with only very slight changes in blood glucose levels. Another interesting study reported that chronic coxsackie B viral infection of the beta cells could result in the synthesis and result of interferon-α, which in turn induces MHC class I hyperexpression on adjacent endocrine cells[6].

Gerling *et al.*[14] monitored the expression of the 64 kDa autoantigen glutamic acid decarboxylase (GAD) in coxsackie B4 virus-infected SJL/J and CD1 mice. They found that the antigen's expression was increased two–three-fold before the onset of hyperglycemia indicating that coxsackie B4 virus infection may initiate or enhance an autoimmune reaction. This same group later found that 90% of coxsackie B4 virus-infected mice developed antibodies to GAD by 4–6 weeks after infection[6]. Consistent with other reports, infectious virus was not detected after 72 hous post infection. Since infection with Coxsackie B4 virus increased the expression of GAD, Hou *et al.*[15] analyzed immunoreactive GAD expression with a panel of antisera and polyclonal antisera against GAD and measured GAD activity in the brains, pancreata, and islets of coxsackie B4 virus-infected mice. GAD-65 and GAD-67 were detected in all these tissues in non-infected mice, and also in the brains of the infected mice. However, the pancreata from infected mice contained three times more GAD-65 than the pancreata of the non-infected mice. There was virtually no detectable GAD-67 in the pancreata from the infected mice. Coxsackie B4 infection therefore appeared to have an effect on GAD-65 and GAD-67 activity in pancreata, but not in the brains of infected mice.

Interestingly, it has been found that homology exists between GAD and coxsackie B4 non-capsid protein P2-C[16]. On the basis of this similarity, Kaufman and his co-workers initially proposed that molecular mimicry between the P2-C protein and GAD may be involved in viral induction of IDDM, whereby antibodies directed against the viral protein could cross-react with GAD on the beta cells A more recent study by Kaufman and his colleagues[17] has shown, through peptide mapping of GAD for the fine specificity of T-cell responses, that the region of sequence similarity of GAD with coxsackie B4 virus is not the region involved in the initial event in induction of autoimmune IDDM, but a region that subsequently reacts with T cells. This study and another[18] do suggest however that GAD plays a critical role in the initial development of IDDM in non-obese diabetic (NOD) mice. It may be that the part of the coxsackie B4 domain that has homology with GAD, the P2-C, may play a role later in the disease process in mice infected with coxsackie B4 virus rather than an initial role. The precise role that GAD or any of its peptides, including the P2-C, play in the initiation or process of autoimmune IDDM in NOD mice is not known.

Non-human primates　Coxsackie B4 virus was serially passaged in monkey beta cell cultures, then harvested and used to infect rhesus, cynomolgus, cebus and patas monkeys[6]. Glucose tolerance tests were performed before and after infection, and an elevation of the glucose tolerance curve and marked depression of the insulin secretion curve were seen only in the coxsackie B4 virus-infected patas monkey. The rhesus, cynomolgus and cebus monkeys did not show any changes in insulin or blood glucose levels after coxsackie B4 viral infection. As coxsackie B4 virus produced abnormalities in glucose tolerance tests and impaired insulin secretion in only the patas monkey, genetic factors therefore must be critical for the development of diabetes in monkeys infected with coxsackie B4 virus.

Studies in other animal cells　To investigate an alternative pathogenic mechanism for coxsackie B virus, Montgomery *et al.*[19] studied the effect of infection by coxsackie B4 virus isolated from a human pancreas on rat insulinoma (RINm5F) cells. Following acute infection, virus was detectable in cells for 10 days, then could not be detected. However, viral antigens could be detected using antibody and FACS within the cells or at the cell surface. The coxsackie B4-infected RINm5F (RIN CB4) cells were readily passaged and grown for over 6 months. In the RIN CB4 cells, insulin secretion and intracellular insulin content were decreased by 10–50% compared to control cells and had decreased numbers of insulin granules as seen by electron microscopy. It was also noted that MHC class I expression was increased by 50% on the RIN CB4 cells, compared to control cells. The investigators concluded that a normally lytic virus can persist in islet-derived tissue in a latent fashion and was associated with altered cell function. In this way, coxsackie B4 virus infection may possibly lead to IDDM without direct cytotoxicity.

　　Whatever the mechanism, evidence from studies on mice, non-human primates and humans, indicates that coxsackie B viruses affect glucose homeostasis. Research on coxsackie B4 virus has demonstrated that antigenic changes at the epitope level occur at a frequency greater than 1 in 10^6. This suggests that even within the same virus pool there may be many antigenic variants with different tissue tropisms and different physiologic properties, which could account for the wide spectrum of clinical disease produced by the coxsackie B viruses. Only rare variants may be diabetogenic, explaining why IDDM appears to be associated with coxsackie B virus infection in infrequent isolated cases[6].

COXSACKIE A VIRUS AND IDDM

There is some indirect evidence that coxsackie A virus may also be associated with IDDM[20]. In a recent study, Frisk *et al.* showed that of 108 recent-onset IDDM patients, 36 had IgM antibodies that reacted only with enteroviral procapsids, indicating a coxsackie A and/or echovirus infection.

VIRAL TRIGGERING OF AUTOIMMUNE TYPE I DIABETES

In certain cases of autoimmune IDDM, viruses such as retrovirus in NOD mice, and rubella virus in hamsters and humans, may have triggered the development of the disease. It is thought that some viruses may possibly induce beta-cell-specific autoimmunity by altering a normally existing beta cell antigen into an immunogenic form or by inducing a new antigen. Other viruses, such as Kilham's rat virus in DR-BB rats, may generate antigen-specific T effector cells which cross-react with a beta-cell-specific autoantigen, leading to autoimmune IDDM.

RUBELLA VIRUS

The fact that there is a high incidence of IDDM among patients with congenital rubella syndrome (CRS), provides some indication that viral infection may play a role in human diabetes[21]. Several reports, including a large prospective study of 242 patients, have shown that approximately 10–20% of individuals with CRS develop diabetes in 5 to 20 years[3]. A 50-year follow-up study of congenital rubella patients further supports these data[22]. There are indications that endocrine abnormalities in CRS might have an autoimmune basis. Islet cell and anti-insulin antibodies were found in 20% or more of non-diabetic patients with CRS and in 50–80% of diabetic patients with CRS. Patients with CRS and diabetes have a significantly increased frequency of HLA-DR3 and a significantly decreased frequently of HLA-DR2[20]. A majority of patients with CRS also have an abnormal carbohydrate metabolism.

An animal model that closely parallels the diabetes observed in humans with congenital rubella has been developed[8]. When neonatal golden Syrian hamsters are infected with beta-cell passaged rubella virus, they develop hyperglycemia and hypoinsulinemia at between seven and ten days of age. Islets from these animals reveal mononuclear cell infiltration and their beta cells show positive immunofluorescence for rubella virus antigen. In 40% of infected animals, cytoplasmic islet cell antibodies were detected and insulitis was observed in 34.5% of the hamster islets examined. These two phenomena are suggestive of an autoimmune process. As a togavirus, rubella virus might insert, expose or alter antigens in the plasma membrane of the host cell during infection, as it buds through the host cell membrane. Alternatively, the virus might induce an autoimmune syndrome by generation of viral antigen-specific cytotoxic T cells which recognize beta-cell-specific antigen(s) by molecular mimicry. This second mechanism is plausible as Karounos *et al.*[23] have examined a panel of monoclonal antibodies which recognize rubella virus capsid and envelope glycoproteins for reactivity with islet cell antigens and found that one monoclonal antibody which recognizes a domain within the rubella virus capsid protein reacts with extracts from rat, and human islets, as well as extracts from a rat insulinoma line. Through further testing the shared epitope was shown to be on a 52 Kda protein. Rubella virus exposure may therefore lead to a beta cell antigen response in susceptible individuals. There has been one case report of an adult simultaneously developing Still's disease and IDDM after a recent rubella infection[24]. The patient showed an isolated persistent increase of serum antibodies against rubella virus and the simultaneous onset of the two diseases does suggest that they were triggered by the same cause, possibly the rubella infection.

While rubella virus definitely appears to be involved in the development of IDDM in patients with CRS, more research is required to learn if the virus is unequivocally involved in other cases of IDDM.

RETROVIRUS

The retroviral genome is unique among mammalian viruses in that it is diploid, consisting of two identical molecules of single-stranded RNA of positive polarity which are linked together by hydrogen bonds at their 5' termini. The genome contains three genes: *gag*, which encodes the core proteins; *pol*, which encodes the enzyme reverse transcriptase; and *env*, which encodes the two envelope glycoproteins. Endogenous retroviruses exist as a provirus (viral DNA integrated into the genome of every cell of the host's body) and are transmitted vertically to the next generation via germ-line DNA. Endogenous retroviruses do not usually cause disease, but may be activated under certain conditions, as in some strains of inbred mice.

Beta-cell-specific expression of endogenous retroviruses has been associated with the development of insulitis and diabetes in NOD mice[9]. In these mice, cyclophosphamide significantly increases the incidence of diabetes either by inhibiting suppressor T cells or by activating cytotoxic T cells. The depletion of macrophages by silica treatment however results in the prevention of insulitis and diabetes in cyclophosphamide-treated NOD mice, suggesting that macrophages play an important role in the initiation of organ-specific autoimmunities in NOD mice and that the presentation by macrophages of autoantigens on specific target cells, such as beta cells, may result in initiation of the immune process[3].

An investigation in our laboratory was initiated to determine whether there are any specific changes on the beta cells of cyclophosphamide-treated male NOD mice that might lead to the attraction of macrophages for the initiation of beta-cell-specific autoimmune disease. Electron microscopic examination of thin sections of islets from male NOD mice, which had first received silica for the inhibition of insulitis, and then subsequently received cyclophosphamide, frequently found clusters of endogenous retrovirus particles in the beta cells[9]. In contrast, retrovirus particles were rarely found in the beta cells from male NOD mice which had received silica only. Virus particles were not contained in other endocrine cells, including alpha, delta, and polypeptide producing (ppp) cells, nor in exocrine acinar cells. Virus particles were also not found in the spleens, livers, or kidneys of either group of mice. A later study by Gaskins et al.[25] showed that beta cell expression of endogenous xenotropic retroviruses distinguished diabetes-susceptible NOD mice from diabetes-resistant NON mice, suggesting a potential pathogenic role for xenotropic retroviral gene expression in the development of diabetes in NOD mice.

Earlier studies had found C-type-like retrovirus particles in pancreatic beta cells from both C3H-db/db[26] and NOD mice[27]. As well, intracisternal A-type particles (IAP) had also been found earlier in beta cells from genetically diabetic mice including C57BL/KSJ (db/db), DBA/2J (db/db), and CheB/FeJ (db/db) mice[28]. There was a clear correlation between the presence of retrovirus particles in beta cells and insulitis lesions[3]. Studies from two separate laboratories, each using different methods, revealed that retroviral *gag* protein was present only in beta cells from diabetic NOD mice[3,29]. Cyclophosphamide treatment enhanced not only the expression of beta-cell-specific retrovirus particles, but also *gag* protein in the pancreatic islets of NOD mice.

It is not certain how retroviruses are involved in the pathogenesis of murine IDDM. The presentation of a retroviral antigen on the beta cells by antigen-presenting cells, such as macrophages, may be the initial step in the autoimmune destruction of beta cells. An immune response to a specific antigen on a target cell involves the activation of CD4 positive T cells, which are only activated when they interact with antigens presented on the surface of a macrophage or other antigen-presenting cell. Our previous experimental results support this possibility, since elimination of antigen-presenting macrophages resulted in the prevention of beta-cell-specific autoimmune processes in NOD mice[3]. Another possible mechanism whereby retroviruses could be involved in the initiation of autoimmune IDDM in NOD mice, is that retroviral genomes (e.g. IAP) in the beta cells may alter the expression of cellular genes possibly resulting in a beta-cell-specific altered antigen(s). An altered antigen might be recognized as foreign by immunocytes, leading to beta-cell-specific autoimmunity. In either situation, cytotoxic cross-reactive effector T lymphocytes that recognize specific determinants of "self-proteins" on beta cells may be generated, leading to the development of beta-cell-specific autoimmune IDDM in NOD mice.

As well as being associated with diabetes in animal models for human IDDM, such as the NOD mouse, retroviruses may be associated with the development of human IDDM. A recent report showed that insulin autoantibodies (IAAa) from human IDDM patients and non-diabetic first degree relatives cross-reacted with retroviral antigen p73[30]. 64% of sera from newly diagnosed patients which bound insulin by ELISA also bound retroviral protein p73 and sera from 75% of IAA-positive, non-diabetic first degree relatives also bound p73. In contrast, only 2.7% of sera from non-diabetic healthy controls bound p73. These results indicate that IAA-positive sera contain antibodies which recognize both insulin and p73. On the basis of studies on beta-cell-specific expression of retroviruses in NOD mice and the cross-reaction between human IAA and retroviral group specific antigen p73, it may be suggested that endogenous retroviruses may be involved in the pathogenesis of autoimmune IDDM in humans.

CYTOMEGALOVIRUS

Human cytomegalovirus (CMV) infection is ubiquitous and largely subclinical. As with many persistent viral infections, the initial infection takes place before birth, or very early in life, although disease may not appear until later. Once infected, an individual carries the virus for life. Infection can be passed through the sperm or ovum if CMV genomes are integrated into the host DNA. Viral infections can also be transmitted transplacentally, perinatally, or postnatally through close contact or breast milk. The immaturity of infant immune systems favors the establishment of persistent viral infections. CMV has also been implicated in IDDM as evidenced by a case report of a child with congenital cytomegalovirus infection that developed diabetes mellitus[31]. At 13 months of age, he presented with a two week history of polydipsia, vomiting and weight loss, and was found to be severely dehydrated and ketoacidotic, with a blood glucose level of 50 mmol l^{-1} (900 mg dl^{-1}). Another case report has described a 27-year-old woman infected with CMV[32]. In this instance, the infection resulted in rhabdomyolysis and renal failure, as well as triggering pancreatitis leading to diabetes. It has been suggested that in certain situations, pancreatitis in which whole islets and acini are destroyed can initiate IDDM. In other reports, characteristic inclusion bodies have been found in the beta cells of infants and children who died with disseminated CMV infections[33]. CMV is known to infect pancreatic islet cells, and in combination with more lethal betatropic agents may also be a causal factor in diabetes. In a study following 73 infants with a congenital CMV infection, one developed IDDM, compared to 38 of 19 483 non-infected control subjects[34]. The investigators believed that this indicated no statistical correlation between CMV infection and the development of IDDM. Using both dot and in situ hybridization techniques, Pak *et al.*[35] showed that 20% of IDDM patients appear to have cytomegaloviral genome in their pancreatic islets. Furthermore, 80% of patients who had both anti-CMV antibodies and cytomegaloviral genome also had islet cell autoantibodies[36]. Nicoletti *et al.*[37] found that there was a statistically significant association between high titers of anti-CMV IgG antibodies and islet cell autoantibodies in non-diabetic siblings of IDDM patients, but no correlation of CMV IgG with HLA-DR antigens. They felt these results suggested that a chronic CMV infection may be associated with islet cell autoantibody production, but that other factors may be needed for the development of clinical IDDM. Our recent study showed that human CMV can induce an islet cell antibody that reacts with a 38 kDa autoantigen isolated from human pancreatic islets[36]. This reaction probably arises from similar epitopes being shared by islet-cell-specific proteins and antigenic determinants of CMV, which may lead to islet-cell-specific autoimmunity.

The evidence that CMV infection is associated with IDDM remains circumstantial however and further studies are required to establish whether or not CMV infection is actually involved in the development of IDDM.

MUMPS VIRUS

Infection by mumps virus was one of the first viral infections recognized as being implicated in IDDM, when in 1899 Dr Harris noted the onset of diabetes after a case of mumps. Since that time there have been many cases where mumps infection appears to precede the onset of IDDM[3]. It has been hypothesized that an infection with mumps virus may also induce autoimmunity as some children appear to develop islet cell autoantibodies during parotiditis and human beta cells can be infected with mumps virus in vitro[3]. In an investigation into whether or not vaccination against mumps has had any impact on anti-mumps antibody activity in children with IDDM, or on the incidence of IDDM, Hyoty *et al.*[38] concluded that the elimination of natural mumps virus infection by vaccination may have been responsible for the decreased risk of developing IDDM observed. Cavallo *et al.* found that mumps infection of a human insulinoma cell line induced the release of interleukin-1 and interleukin-6 and also up-regulated the expression of HLA class I and II antigens[39]. From these data, the authors concluded that virally induced cytokine release and increased expression of HLA molecules by beta cells may somehow lead to an immune response against them. As with other viruses, however, further studies are required to determine whether or not mumps virus is definitely associated with the development of autoimmune IDDM.

EPSTEIN–BARR VIRUS

Epstein–Barr virus (EBV) has been implicated in the etiology of several autoimmune diseases and a temporal link between EBV infection and the onset of IDDM has been reported in a rare number of cases. In children with new-onset IDDM, EBV capsid antigen IgG antibody levels were significantly lower than in age-matched non-diabetic controls, suggesting that the diabetic children had abnormalities in their EBV-specific immune responses[40]. Recently, it was found that a five amino acid sequence, GPPAA, in the region of Asp-57 of the HLA-DQ β chain is successively repeated six times in the EBV BERF4-encoded epitope[41]. Two patients who produced antibodies against this epitope during acute EBV infections soon developed IDDM, while five individuals, also acutely infected but not producing antibodies against this epitope, did not develop IDDM[41]. This recent consideration of EBV as a candidate virus capable of possibly triggering autoimmune IDDM by molecular mimicry is interesting and worthy of further investigation.

REOVIRUS

When suckling SJL/J male mice were infected with the beta-cell-passaged reovirus type 3, some of the infected animals showed abnormal glucose tolerance tests within 10 days after infection, but these returned to normal after three weeks. Specific viral antigens were present in some beta cells as well as in acinar cells, and viral particles were detected by electron microscopy in the cytoplasm of some beta cells[42]. Similarly, mice infected with beta-cell-passaged reovirus type 1 also developed transient diabetes and a runting syndrome characterized by retarded growth, oily hair, alopecia and steatorrhea[43]. Sera from these mice contained autoantibodies which reacted with cytoplasmic antigens from the islets of Langerhans, anterior pituitary and the gastric mucosa of uninfected mice[43]. To rule out any role for these autoantibodies in the pathogenesis of reovirus-induced diabetes, infected SJL and NFS mice were treated with different immunosuppressive drugs. The administration of antilymphocyte serum, antithymocyte serum, or cyclophosphamide to infected mice reduced or prevented the development of reovirus-induced diabetes (reviewed in reference 3) and these animals gained weight at almost the same rate as uninfected controls. In addition, the mortality rate of infected mice was reduced by immunosuppression. Onodera *et al.*[43] therefore concluded that autoimmunity does play a role in reovirus-induced diabetes, though the precise mechanism is unclear.

KILHAM'S RAT VIRUS

Another virus that has been implicated in animal diabetes is Kilham's rat virus (KRV), which has been shown to cause autoimmune diabetes in diabetes-resistant BB (DRBB) rats, without distinct infection of beta cells[7]. Diabetes-prone (DP) BB rats, like NOD mice, spontaneously develop a diabetic syndrome that resembles human IDDM in many respects. DPBB rats are lymphopenic and about 70–80% of the animals become diabetic at about 120 days of age. In contrast to DPBB rats, DRBB rats, derived from DP-progenitors, have normal lymphocyte numbers and phenotypes and do not normally develop diabetes. When 21–25-day-old DRBB rats were infected with KRV, about 30% of the animals developed autoimmune diabetes within 2 to 4 weeks after infection[7]. An additional 48% showed evidence of lymphocytic insulitis without diabetes. Guberski *et al.* analyzed peripheral blood and lymph node cells of KRV-infected DRBB rats by flow cytometry for evidence of T-cell depletion[7]. When compared to vehicle controls, there were no significant changes in the percentages of peripheral blood CD4 positive and CD8 positive T cells or NK cells, 3, 6 or 10 days after infection, in the rats which eventually became diabetic. RT6.1 positive lymph node cells were also unchanged. One recent study suggested that widespread infection of peripancreatic and other lymphoid tissue but not pancreatic beta cells by KRV triggers autoimmune diabetes by perturbing the immune system of genetically predisposed DRBB/Wor rats[44], though exactly what role KRV plays in the induction of diabetes in DRBB rats is not known. It is speculated that KRV infection may generate antigen-specific cytotoxic T cells and the KRV-specific effector T cells may attack beta cells. Whether KRV-specific cytotoxic T cells cross-react with a beta cell surface antigen or recognize a viral peptide on KRV-infected beta cells remains to be determined.

PREVENTION OF IDDM BY VIRUSES

EMC-D virus-induced diabetes can be prevented in genetically susceptible mice by vaccination using the non-diabetogenic EMC-B variant[3]. Paradoxically, EMC-D virus infection of NOD mice has been shown to prevent the development of autoimmune diabetes or to specifically lessen the immune process in infected animals[45]. The development of diabetes in NOD mice can also be prevented by weekly immunization with retroviral proteins, such as the major envelope glycoprotein of C-type retrovirus (gp70) or group-specific antigen of A-type retrovirus (p73) from the age of 2 to 42 days[3]. Inoculation of newborn or 6-week-old NOD mice with lymphocytic choriomeningitis virus (LCMV) can also prevent or decrease the incidence of diabetes (0–6%)[46]. It is thought that LCMV may infect and deplete a subpopulation of CD4 positive T cells since selective suppression of some CD4 positive T cells has been observed during LCMV infection[47]. These findings have led Oldstone to suggest that LCMV by directly aborting autoimmune-producing T lymphocytes, may prevent insulitis and diabetes. In his model, LCMV-transgenic mice (expressing LCMV in beta cells) were able to generate a virus-specific cytotoxic T-lymphocyte response upon restimulation with the infecting virus[48]. This response, however, was retarded in its development in several sublines, suggesting a temporary state of T-cell hyporesponsiveness. In mice transgenic for both a LCMV-specific T-cell receptor and LCMV, self-reactive T cells remained functionally silent, apparently due to the inability of the beta cells to properly activate an immune response[49]. Mice transgenic for a LCMV glycoprotein developed CD8 positive T-cell-mediated diabetes within 8–14 days after LCMV infection, however if the mice were immunized with a synthetic peptide corresponding to the immunodominant LCMV glycoprotein before infection, autoimmune beta cell destruction and diabetes were prevented[50].

Inoculation of BB rats with LCMV (Armstrong strain, clone) also reduced their incidence of diabetes and prevented mononuclear cell infiltration into the islets, by somehow disordering particular lymphocyte subsets[51]. Viral antibody-free BB rats show an increased frequency and accelerated onset of diabetes, suggesting that infection may have a protective effect against the development of diabetes by these animals[3]. Thus we speculate that infection or immune stimulation in humans may also reduce the penetrance of susceptibility genes (Figure 10.1), which could account for the low concordance rate between identical twins of less than 40% for the development of diabetes.

CONCLUSIONS

While a genetic predisposition appears to be necessary for the development of IDDM, non-genetic environmental factors play an important role in the expression of the disease (Figure 10.1). Viruses, as one environmental factor, may directly infect and destroy pancreatic beta cells, or may trigger or contribute to beta-cell-specific autoimmunity. Certain viruses, such as retrovirus and rubella virus, may alter normally existing beta cell antigens into immunogenic forms or may induce new antigens leading to beta-cell-specific autoimmunity. In this situation, viral antigens or virus-induced autoantigens may be released from beta cells during normal cell turnover, then processed and presented by macrophages, in conjunction with MHC class II molecules to CD4 positive T helper cells, which then secrete interleukin-2. During this process, viral antigen-specific CD8 positive T effector cells might be generated which would in turn recognize the cross-reactive autoantigen expressed on unaffected beta cells, and then act to destroy the cells as final effectors, working synergistically with cytokines released from macrophages and other lymphocytes. Other viruses, such as KRV, may generate viral antigen-specific T effector cells. The viral antigen may have homology with proteins of the beta-cell-specific autoantigen and in this way the effector T cells may mistakenly recognize the beta-cell-specific autoantigen. Still other viruses, such as EMC-D and coxsackie B viruses, can induce IDDM by infecting and destroying beta cells in genetically susceptible animals. It is possible that coxsackie B viruses may also be associated with the development of autoimmunity by some undefined mechanism (the effects of persistent infection, molecular mimicry of a beta-cell-specific antigen such as GAD by a viral protein, or some other mechanism).

In this chapter, I have tried to produce a picture of how viruses are involved in the pathogenesis of IDDM, using the information currently available. However, the picture cannot be completed as many of the pieces of the puzzle are still missing. In order to find the missing pieces and fill in the picture, more research is needed on candidate viruses which appear capable of triggering or contributing to the initiation and/or process of autoimmune IDDM in humans. In animal models, more absolute, detailed information on the mechanisms of virus-induced IDDM is needed. Once the picture is complete, we will hopefully be able to develop methods to prevent that portion of IDDM which is caused by viruses.

ACKNOWLEDGMENTS

This work was supported by Grant MA9584 from the Medical Research Council of Canada to Ji-Won Yoon who is a Heritage Medical Scientist Awardee of the Alberta Heritage Foundation for Medical Research.

REFERENCES

1 Yoon, JW, Park YH, Santamaria PS. Autoimmunity of type I diabetes. In Flatt PR, Ionnides C (eds), *Drugs, Diet and Disease*. Volume 2: *Mechanistic Approaches to Diabetes*. London: Ellis Howard of Simon and Schuster International Group, 1994 (in press).

2 Adams SF. The seasonal variation in the onset of acute diabetes. *Arch Int Med* 1926; **27**: 861–2.

3 Yoon, JW. Viruses as triggering agents of insulin-dependent diabetes mellitus. In Leslie RDG (ed), *The Causes of diabetes*. London: John Wiley & Sons, 1993; pp. 83–103.

4 Szopa TM, Titchener PA, Portwood ND, Taylor KW. Diabetes mellitus due to viruses—some recent developments. *Diabetologia* 1993; **36**: 687–95.

5 Craighead JE, McLane MF. Diabetes mellitus: induction in mice by encephalomyocarditis virus. *Science* 1968; **162**: 913–15

6 Yoon JW, Kominek HI. Role of Coxsackie B viruses in the pathogenesis of diabetes mellitus. In Rose NR, Friedman H (eds). *Microbial Infections and Pathogenesis*. New York: Plenum Press 1994 (in press).

7 Guberski DL, Thomas VA, Shek WR, Like AA, Handler ES, Rossini AA, Wallace JE, Welsh RM. Induction of type I diabetes by Kilham's Rat Virus in diabetes-resistant

BB/Wor rats. *Science* 1991; **254**: 1010–13.

8   Rayfield E Kelly K, Yoon JW. Rubella virus-induced diabetes in hamsters. *Diabetes* 1986; **35**: 1276–81.

9   Suenaga K, Yoon JW. Association of beta cell-specific expression of endogenous retrovirus with the development of insulitis and diabetes in NOD mice. *Diabetes* 1988; **37**: 1722–6.

10 Tajima M, Yazawa T, Hagiwara K, Kurosawa T, Takahashi K. Diabetes mellitus in cattle infected with bovine viral diarrhea mucosal disease virus. *J Vet Med A* 1992; **39**: 616–20.

11 Ross ME, Onodera T, Brown KS, Notkins AL. Virus-induced diabetes mellitus IV. Genetic and environmental factors influencing the development of diabetes after infection with the M variant of encephalomyocarditis virus. *Diabetes* 1976; **25**: 190–7.

12 Yoon JW, McClintock PR, Onodera T, Notkins AL. Virus-induced diabetes mellitus. Inhibition by a non-diabetogenic variant of encephalomyocarditis virus. *J Exp Med* 1980; **152**: 878–92.

13 Gamble DR, Kinsley ML, Fitzgerald MG, Bolton R, Taylor KW. Viral antibodies in diabetes mellitus. *Br Med J* 1969; **3**: 627–30.

14 Gerling I, Nejman C, Chaterjee NK. Effect of coxsackievirus B4 infection in mice on expression of 64,000 Mr autoantigen and glucose sensitivity of islets before development of hyperglycemia. *Diabetes* 1988; **37**: 1419–25.

15 Hou J, Sheikh S, Martin DL, Chatterjee NK. Coxsackievirus B4 alters pancreatic glutamate decarboxylase expression in mice soon after infection. *J Autoimmun* 1993; **6**: 529–42.

16 Kaufman DL, Erlander MG, Clare-Salzler MJ, Atkinson MA, Maclaren NK, Tobin AJ. Autoimmunity to two forms of glutamate decarboxylase in insulin-dependent diabetes mellitus. *J Clin Invest* 1992; **89**: 283–92.

17 Kaufman DL, Clare-Salzler MG, Tian J, Forsthuber T, Ting G, Robinson P, Atkinson MA, Sercarz EE, Tobin AJ, Lehmann PV. Spontaneous loss of T-cell tolerance to glutamic acid decarboxylase in murine insulin-dependent diabetes. *Nature* 1993; **366**: 69–72.

18 Tisch R, Yang X, Singer S, Liblau R, Flugger L, McDevitt H. Immune response to glutamic acid decarboxylase correlates with insulitis in non-obese diabetic mice. *Nature* 1993; **366**: 72–5.

19 Montgomery L, Gordon D, George K, Maratos-Flier E. Coxsackie infection of insulinoma cells leads to viral latency and altered insulin and class I MHC expression. *Diabetes* 1991; **40**: 150A.

20 Frisk G, Nilsson E, Tuvemo T, Friman G, Diderholm H. The possible role of Coxsackie A and echo viruses in the pathogenesis of type I diabetes mellitus studied by IgM analysis. *J Infect* 1992; **24**: 13–22.

21 Ginsberg-Fellner F, Fedun B, Cooper, LZ, Witt ME, Franklin BH, Roman SH, Rubenstein P, McEvoy RC. Interrelationships of congenital rubella and type 1 insulin-dependent diabetes mellitus. In Jaworski MA, Molnar GD, Rajotte RV, Singh B (Eds), *The Immunology of Diabetes Mellitus*. Amsterdam: Elsevier Science Publishers, 1986; pp. 279–86.

22 McIntosh EDG, Menser MA. A fifty-year follow-up of congenital rubella. *Lancet* 1992; **340**: 414–5.

23 Karounos DG, Wolinsky JS, Thomas JW. Monoclonal antibody to rubella virus capsid protein recognizes a beta-cell antigen. *J Immunol* 1993; **150**: 3080–5.

24 Sibley JT. Concurrent onset of adult onset Still's disease and insulin dependent diabetes mellitus. *Ann Rheum Dis* 1990; **49**: 547–8.

25 Gaskins H, Prochazka M, Hamaguchi K, Serreze D, Leiter E. Beta cell expression of

endogenous xenotropic retrovirus distinguishes diabetes-susceptible NOD/Lt from resistant NON/Lt mice. *J Clin Invest* 1992; **90**: 2220–7.

26 Leiter EH. Type C retrovirus production by pancreatic beta cells: association with accelerated pathogenesis in C3H-db/db ("diabetes") mice. *Am J Pathol* 1985; **119**: 22–32.

27 Fukino-Kurihara H, Fujita H, Hakura A, Nonaka K, Tarui S. Morphological aspects on pancreatic islets of non-obese diabetic (NOD) mice. *Virchows Arch* 1985; **49**: 107–20.

28 Leiter EH, Kuff EL. Intracisternal type A particles in murine pancreatic β cells: immunocytochemical demonstration of increased antigen (p73) in genetically diabetic mice. *Am J Pathol* 1984; **114**: 46–55.

29 Nakagawa C, Hanafusa T, Miyagawa J, Yutsudo M, Nakajima H, Yakamoto K, Tomita K, Kono N. Retrovirus gag protein p30 in the islets of nonobese diabetic mice: relevance for pathogenesis of diabetes melitus. *Diabetologia* 1992; **35**: 614–18.

30 Hao W, Serreze DV, McCulloch DK, Neifing JL, Palmer JP. Insulin (auto) antibodies from human IDDM cross-react with retroviral antigen p73. *J Autoimmun* 1993; **6**: 787–98.

31 Ward KP, Galloway WH, Auchterlonie IA. Congenital cytomegalovirus infection and diabetes. *Lancet* 1929; **1**: 497.

32 Yasumoto N, Hara M, Kitamoto YU, Nakayama M, Sato T. Cytomegalovirus infection associated with acute pancreatitis, rhabdomyolysis and renal failure. *Intern Med* 1992; **31**: 426–30.

33 Jenson AB, Rosenberg HS, Notkins AL. Pancreatic islet cell damage in children with fatal viral infections. *Lancet* 1980; **2**: 354–8.

34 Ivarsson SA, Lindberg B, Nilsson KO, Ahlfors K, Svanberg L. The prevalence of type 1 diabetes mellitus at follow-up of Swedish infants congenitally infected with cytomegalovirus. *Diabetic Med* 1993; **10**: 521–3.

35 Pak CY, Eun HM, McArthur RG, Yoon JW. Association of cytomegalovirus infection with autoimmune type I diabetes. *Lancet* 1988; **2**: 1–4.

36 Pak CY, Cha CY, Rajotte RV, McArthur RG, Yoon, JW. Human pancreatic islet cell-specific 38kda autoantigen identified by cytomegalovirus-induced monoclonal islet cell autoantibody. *Diabetologia* 1990; **33**: 569–72.

37 Nicoletti F, Scalia G, Lunetta M, Condorellia F, DiMauro M, Barcellini W, Stracuzzi S, Pagano M, Meroni PL. Correlation between islet cell antibodies and anti-cytomegalovirus IgM and IgG antibodies in healthy first-degree relatives of type 1 (insulin-dependent) diabetic patient. *Clin Immunol Immunopathol* 1990; **55**: 139–47.

38 Hyoty H, Hiltunen M, Reunanen A, Leinikki P, Vesikari T, Lounamaa R, Tuomilehto J, Akerblom HK. Decline of mumps antibodies i type 1 (insulin-dependent) diabetic children and a plateau in the rising incidence of type 1 diabetes after introduction of the mumps-measles-rubella vaccine in Finland. Childhood Diabetes in Finland Study Group. *Diabetologia* 1993; **36**: 1303–8.

39 Cavallo MG, Baroni MG, Toto A, Gearing AJ, Forsey T, Andreani D, Thorpe R, Pozzilli P. Viral infection induces cytokine release by beta islet cells. *Immunology* 1992; **75**: 664–8.

40 Hyoty H, Rasanen L, Hiltunen M, Lehtinen M, Huupponen T, Leinikki P. Decreased antibody reactivity to Epstein-Barr virus capsid antigen in type 1 (insulin dependent) diabetes melitus. *APMIS* 1991; **99**: 359–63.

41 Parkkonen P, Hyoty H, Ilonen J, Reijonen H, Yla-Herttuala S, Leinikki P. Antibody reactivity to an Epstein-Barr virus BERF4-encoded epitope occurring also in Asp-57 region of HLA-DQ8 β chain. *Clin Exp Immunol* 1994; **95**: 287–93.

42 Onodera T, Jenson AB, Yoon JW, Notkins AL. 1981, Virus-induced diabetes mellitus: reovirus infection of pancreatic beta cells in mice. *Science* 1978; **301**: 529–31.

42a Onodera T, Toniolo A, Ray UR, Jenson AB, Knazek RA, Notkins AL. 1981, Virus-induced diabetes mellitus. *J Exp Med* 1981; **153**: 1457–65.

43 Brown DW, Welsh RM, Like AA. Infection of peripancreatic lymph nodes but not islets precedes Kilham's Rat Virus-induced diabetes in BB/Wor Rats. *J Virol* 1993; **67**: 5873–8.

44 Hermitte L, Vialettes B, Naquet P, Atlan C, Payan MJ, Vague P. Paradoxical lessening of autoimmune processes in non-obese diabetic mice after infection with the diabetogenic variant of encephalomyocarditis virus. *Eur J Immunol* 1990; **20** 1297–303.

45 Oldstone MBA. Prevention of type 1 diabetes in nonobese diabetic mice by virus infection. *Science* 1988; **239**: 500–2.

46 Oldstone MBA. Viruses as therapeutic agents: I. treatment of nonobese insulin-dependent diabetes mice with virus prevents insulin-dependent diabetes mellitus while maintaining general immune competence. *J Exp Med* 1990; **11**: 2077–89.

47 Oldstone MBA, Nerenberg M, Southern P, Price J, Lewicki H. Virus infection triggers insulin-dependent diabetes mellitus in a transgenic model: role of anti-self (virus) immune response. *Cell* 1991; **65**: 19–31.

48 Ohashi P, Oehen S, Buerki K, Pircher H, Ohashi C, Odermatt B, Malissen B, Zinkernagel RM, Hengartner H. Ablation of tolerance and induction of diabetes by virus infection in viral antigen transgenic mice. *Cell* 1991; **65**: 305–17.

49 Aichele P, Kyburz D, Ohashi PS, Odermatt B, Zinkernagel RM, Hengartner H, Pircher H. Peptide-induced T-cell tolerance to prevent autoimmune diabetes in a transgenic mouse model. *Proc Natl Acad Sci USA* 1944; **91**: 444–8.

50 Dryberg T, Schwimmbeck PL, Oldstone MBA. Inhibition of diabetes in BB rats by viral infection. *J Clin Invest* 1988; **81**: 928–31.

11

Environmental Factors: Milk and Others

WOLFRAM J. P. KARGES and H.-MICHAEL DOSCH
Research Institute, The Hospital For Sick Children, University of Toronto, Toronto, Canada

The involvement of genetic factors in the etiology and pathogenesis of insulin-dependent diabetes mellitus (IDDM) is well acknowledged. In addition, several clinical observations have long suggested that non-genetic factors may be critically involved in the development and even the course of IDDM (reviewed in reference 1)[1]. Among these observations are the incomplete concordance rate (30–50%) for IDDM in identical twins and the different IDDM incidence rates observed in genetically similar populations. A significant increase in IDDM incidence has been reported in different ethnic groups after geographical migration to new environments with different nutritional habits. Finally, the secular trend of increasing IDDM incidence rates, probably worldwide over the last 40 years and a shift towards younger age at time of diagnosis cannot be explained by hereditary factors.

There has been considerable debate on the nature of environmental causes of IDDM. Infectious agents, mainly viruses, have been long suspected as candidate triggers (see chapter 10). A protective rather than offensive role has recently been suggested for specific viral and bacterial antigen[2]. In the last decade, growing interest has focused on non-infectious, mostly nutritional factors in the etiology of IDDM; based on clinical and experimental data new concepts of diabetic autoimmunity have been developed with an implication for new approaches towards prediction and prevention of the disease.

Prediction, Prevention and Genetic Counseling in IDDM. Edited by Jerry P. Palmer.
© 1996 John Wiley & Sons Ltd.

NUTRITIONAL FACTORS AND IDDM: AN OVERVIEW

The involvement of numerous dietary and non-infectious environmental components has been considered in the etiology of insulin-dependent diabetes, either as primary triggers of the disease or as co-factors modifying the ongoing disease process (Table 11.1). Despite considerable indirect evidence for some (but not for all), no single nutritional factor has definitely been proven to trigger autoimmune diabetes.

Table 11.1. Dietary and other non-infectious factors implicated in the etiology of human IDDM

Offensive	Protective
Cow's milk protein[9–12,15,17–19,35,50,51,] bovine serum albumin[33,37,40,42,48,49] beta-lactoglobulin[21,36]	Breast feeding[13,15,16,20,52] Nicotinamide (pharmacological doses)[7]
Beta-cell toxic drugs[6] alloxan streptozotocin rodenticides	
Dietary toxins N-nitroso compounds[3]	
Others coffee[4] sugar[5]	

Food additives (N-nitroso compounds) to certain meat products have been suspected to contribute to the increased seasonal diabetes incidence in children from Iceland[3], possibly mediated through direct toxicity on fetal beta cells. Curiously, coffee[4] and sugar[5] have been added to the list of potential diabetes triggers, based on a moderate correlation between the per capita consumption of these nutrients and national diabetes incidence rates.

Streptozotocin, alloxan and other cytotoxic drugs as well as some rodenticides are known causes of insulinopenic diabetes in humans and rodents[6]. Although leading to beta cell destruction and eventually to insulin dependence, these forms of chemically induced diabetes lack typical immunological characteristics of IDDM. They may therefore be regarded as different disease entities clearly distinct from autoimmune diabetes.

Nicotinamide may antagonize toxic beta cell damage[7] through mechanisms that are not well defined. However, supra-physiological doses (X 1000 more than the natural dietary intake) are required to achieve beta cell protection in vivo whose extent and duration in humans is the subject of current clinical trials.

The increased incidence of IDDM after stressful life events is thought to reflect an unspecific decline in immune surveillance against self-reactive immune cells as has been suggested for other autoimmune diseases (e.g. of the thyroid or bowel). Similarly, malnutrition, zinc deficiency or frequent blood loss delay the diabetes onset in animal models by unspecifically down-regulating immune responsiveness.

The most consistent experimental and clinical evidence indicates that exposure to certain dietary antigens, in particular cow's milk protein, very early in life might specifically initiate immune mechanisms leading to autoimmune beta cell destruction and IDDM. This was recently acknowledged by the American Academy of Pediatrics by recommending the avoidance of cow's milk protein during the first year of life in children with a family history of autoimmune diabetes[8]. In this chapter we will mainly focus on current evidence for the role of cow's milk (and breast feeding) in IDDM development and discuss the concept of diabetic autoimmunity driven by molecular mimicry between a pancreatic self- and an environmental non-self-antigen.

COW'S MILK PROTEIN AND IDDM: CLINICAL EVIDENCE

A link of exposure to cow's milk, breast feeding and IDDM has been reported in more than a dozen epidemiological and case-control studies over the past decade. Only three early studies failed to detect a positive association between short or absent breast feeding and heightened IDDM risk (reviewed in reference 9)[9].

Two surveys of different countries delineated a strong positive correlation between the per capita cow's milk consumption and the national incidence rates of IDDM in children < 14 yr ($r = 0.96$)[10] or in all age groups ($r = 0.86$)[11]. More recently this correlation was confirmed for regional differences in diabetes incidence within a single country[12].

One of these studies also reported that the highest IDDM incidences are found in those countries with the lowest rate of breast feeding at 3 months of age ($r = -0.54$)[11]. Changes in breast feeding practices and the incidence of childhood IDDM (< 14 yr) were analyzed over the period from 1940 to 1982 in Norway and Sweden[13]. An inverse relation was found with an increasing diabetes incidence until the late 1960s as the percentage of children breast-fed ≥ 2 months (Sweden) or ≥ 3 months (Norway) dropped from 90% to 20%.

Several retrospective case-control studies have compared the dietary history of juvenile IDDM patients with that of random chosen age- and sex-matched controls, siblings, or the general population. In a recent meta-analysis[9] of 13 peer-reviewed reports, the adjusted overall odds ratio for IDDM in patients exposed to ≤ 3 months of breast feeding was 1.37 (95% confidence interval (CI) 1.22–1.53). Similarly, the overall odds ratio for exposure to cow's-milk-based baby formula before 3–4 months of age in patients was 1.57 (95% CI 1.19–2.07).

When studies most stringently designed to eliminate selection and recall bias were analyzed separately, the odds ratio for IDDM in patients with a breast feeding episode shorter than 3 months was 1.43 (95% CI 1.15–1.77); and 1.63 (95% CI 1.22–2.17) in patients with cow's milk exposure during the first 3 months of life[9].

In most of these studies control children were not matched for HLA genotype or other IDDM susceptibility markers, resulting in a low genetic risk in the control group to develop IDDM even if exposed to a critical trigger molecule of diabetic autoimmunity. The relatively low observed odds ratio of ~1.5 is therefore likely to underestimate the true contribution of cow's milk exposure to IDDM risk. In a detailed analysis of a small group of children at high genetic IDDM risk as defined by non-Asp57 alleles in the DQ β-chain, cow's milk exposure before 3 months of age was indeed associated with a much higher odds ratio of 3.7[14].

The protective effect of exclusive breast feeding and denial of cow's milk-based baby formula seems more pronounced in younger patients (Figure 11.1): the odds ratio was 3.81 (95% CI 1.10–13.29) for children developing diabetes before the age of 4 years[15], 2.78 (95% CI 1.08–7.14) for patients developing the disease before age 7[16,17], 2.12 for patients <9.2 years old[18] and the odds ratio declined to 1.06 (95% CI 0.66–1.70) and 1.40 (95% CI 1.00–1.95) for patients younger than 14[15] or 18 years[19]. This phenomenon could indicate that cow's milk protein would act as an accelerator of diabetes development, with later disease onset in breast fed children[20]. Alternatively, short breast feeding duration in the general population at the period when older patients were born (1970s) may have masked differences between patients and controls.

Breast feeding has been well known to protect against bacterial and viral infections in early infancy, mainly through the passive transfer of maternal antibodies in human milk. Indeed it has been speculated that insufficient breast feeding might predispose to beta cell infection and IDDM[13], although little clinical or experimental evidence is available to support that view.

Cow's-milk-based baby formulas are the most common substitute for mother's milk in infant nutrition in the western world. Overall breast-feeding duration is highly and inversely related to the introduction of cow's-milk-based formula before 4 months of age[21]. It has therefore been difficult to assess how much both factors independently contribute to diabetes risk, especially in breast-fed children receiving supplemental formula.

Statistical analysis has suggested that cow's-milk-based formulas confer increased IDDM risk independent of other nutrients, i.e. when used as supplemental food source during sustained (non-exclusive) breast feeding or after introduction of solid food[14]. The fact that cow's milk protein may be detectable in human breast milk in amounts sufficient to elicit immune responses in the child adds to the complexity of the issue[22,23].

As yet, no prospective clinical data are available on cow's milk exposure,

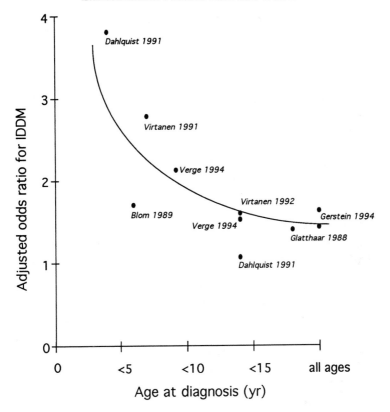

Figure 11.1. Adjusted odds ratios for IDDM in patients with early cow's milk exposure or short duration of breast feeding as a function of age at diagnosis

exclusive and non-exclusive breast feeding and IDDM risk. The development of such a prospective, randomized trial through international collaboration was recommended by the American Academy of Pediatrics[8]. A dietary intervention trial whose pilot phase is now under way, will provide important new information[24], in this blind, prospective trial, genetically susceptible newborns are randomized to receive formula with or without intact cow's milk protein and followed for the development of diabetes. In a just completed study in NOD mice, we confirmed near complete (>90%) protection with trial formula.

SUPPORT FROM MICE AND RATS

Since the early observation by Elliott and Martin[25], that chow free of cow's milk protein protected spontaneously diabetic BB rats[26], the diabetogenic or protective potential of a variety of natural ingredient or semi-synthetic diets has been tested in the BB rat and NOD mouse, both animal models of spontaneous autoimmune diabetes. The complex composition of diets and individual characteristics of animal colonies and experimental protocols have contributed to some controversy about the importance of single dietary components. However, several common findings have clearly emerged.

In all studies, hydrolyzed casein[27–29] or single amino acids[25,26] instead of intact protein reduced the diabetes incidence by 3- to 12-fold, and a casein hydrolysate even prevented destructive insulitis and hyperglycemia in NOD mice with a high spontaneous diabetes incidence (0% versus 74% incidence at 30 weeks of age)[30]. This effect could not be explained by malnutrition or specific nutrient deficiency.

It has been suggested that intact dietary protein, in particular cow's milk protein[31] is required to trigger or promote diabetic autoimmunity. Addition of cow's milk[25] or milk protein[27] to protective diets has been reported to restore a high diabetes incidence, although not in all studies[30]. When semi-purified lactalbumin was added to protective diets the diabetes incidence did not increase[27]. Of non-dairy proteins studied, gluten or corn did not abolish dietary protection[27], and neither hydrolyzed nor intact soy protein provided full protection in diabetes-prone rodents[28]. Efforts to characterize the diabetogenic potential of wheat have been inconclusive[29].

As in human IDDM, susceptibility to dietary factors (whether offensive or protective) seems to be limited to the early phase of life in rodents[26]. Only when introduced early after weaning did casein hydrolysate protect NOD mice from diabetes[27,28]; dietary protection was however not reversed by switching to non-purified diets at day 70 or 90 or at 30 weeks[30]. The narrow window of IDDM susceptibility suggests that dynamic host factors like post-natal immune maturation, gut epithelium closure or the development of mucosal immunity determine whether or not dietary antigen may elicit an autoreactive immune response that leads to diabetes.

Finally, breast feeding per se does not seem to be a major protective factor in diabetes-prone rodents. In all studies animals were naturally fed on breast milk from birth to weaning, usually at three weeks of age; however, the differential effects of diabetogenic or protective diets introduced a weaning were fully maintained in these animals.

The involvement of milk protein in diabetic autoimmunity has been mirrored by the presence of specific antibodies to these proteins in diabetic rodents. In NOD mice significantly increased levels of antibodies to bovine serum albumin (BSA) were found in diabetic animals as compared to non-diabetic controls and these antibodies became demonstrable already early in the pre-diabetic animal[32].

We observed that serum IgG antibodies to BSA were five times higher in diabetic BB rats than in non-diabetic BB or Wistar rats, with a gradual increase of antibody titers during the pre-diabetic phase and a peak at time of diagnosis at 90–120 days[31]. Levels were already significantly elevated in 40-day-old rats, providing an attractive marker of impending IDDM. Antibodies to β-lactoglobulin failed to demonstrate a correlation with disease expression[31,33]. Thus, in diabetes-prone rodents, anti-BSA antibodies are associated with the expression of the disease[32].

IMMUNE MARKERS TO MILK PROTEIN IN HUMANS

Antibodies against cow's milk protein and other dietary components are detectable in most healthy children and adults. The role of these antibodies to dietary protein is unclear, but they reflect an immunogenic contact with nutritional antigen that per se does not lead to allergy or other disorders.

Levels of cow's milk antibodies were not found to be different in children with and without atopy[23], excluding specific cow's milk allergies. Healthy infants with early introduction of cow's-milk-based formula develop much higher IgG cow's milk antibody levels than those where exposure occurred at ≥ 5 months of age[23]. However, differences disappear within 2 years. IgA and IgM cow's milk antibody levels are not modified by early infant nutrition in non-diabetic children[23].

Using ELISA techniques, antibody levels to cow's milk (IgA) and β-lactoglobulin (IgA and IgG) were found significantly higher in newly diag-nosed IDDM patients (mean age 9.1 yr) than in age-matched healthy children, but not in children with long lasting (>5 yr) diabetes (mean age 11.6 yr)[34]. Dietary cow's milk may increase antibody levels to milk protein, but daily milk consumption at time of diagnosis was not different in healthy and diabetic Finnish children[35], whereas significantly higher milk consumption was deli-neated in Australian children during the year before diagnosis of overt diabetes[18].

These observations have been confirmed in large population-based studies from Sweden[21] and Finland[36]. Recent-onset diabetic children (mean age 8.7 and 8.5 yr, respectively) had higher IgA and IgG antibodies to cow's milk and β- lactoglobulin than age-matched unrelated controls or non-diabetic siblings, with differences most prominent in patients younger than 3[36] or 5 years[21]. In a multiple regression analysis, IgA antibodies to cow's milk (odds ratio 8.83) and β-lactoglobulin (odds ratio 1.88) were significantly related to the risk of IDDM independently of islet cell antibodies[21].

BOVINE SERUM ALBUMIN: A TRIGGER OF DIABETIC AUTOIMMUNITY?

High levels of antibodies to BSA have been detected in both animal models of spontaneous autoimmune diabetes[31,32]. These antibodies were found to precipitate a novel islet cell protein, ICAp69, initially isolated from rat insulinoma cell lines and later identified in human, mouse and rat islets[37]. Using anti-BSA antibodies or human diabetic patient sera to screen islet cell CDNA libraries, the human ICAp69 gene was subsequently cloned and characterized independently by two groups[38,39]. ICAp69 and BSA share three conserved protein sequence homologies, one of which is located in the ABBOS region of the BSA molecule (pre-BSA position 152–169) where the bovine albumin sequence differs from human, rat, and mouse albumin[38].

Anti-BSA antibodies were analyzed in 142 children with newly diagnosed IDDM (mean age 8.4 ± 4.3 yr) and compared to age- and sex-matched healthy children[40]. At the time of diagnosis, all diabetic children had elevated IgG anti-BSA antibody levels (mean 8.5 kFU), but only ~3% of healthy children (mean 1.3 KFU). Anti-BSA levels were unchanged after three to four months but showed a sharp decline one to two years after diagnosis.

Blocking experiments revealed that at time of diagnosis on average more than half of total antibody reactivity to BSA (26–82%) was specific for the ABBOS peptide region, falling to 6% after one or two years. These results indicated that many of the BSA antibodies in diabetic children recognize an epitope in the ABBOS region and that these antibodies disappear in the first few years after diagnosis. ABBOS-specific antibodies are rarely found in healthy control children[40,41].

A large population-based study analyzed BSA antibodies and other disease markers for IDDM in French school children[42]—74.4% of children with recent-onset IDDM (mean age 8.4 yr) were found with elevated IgG anti-BSA antibody levels, two standard deviations above the mean value observed in age-matched healthy children. Of these controls 5.5% had elevated anti-BSA levels. Anti-BSA had a slightly lower sensitivity than ICA (74.4% versus 84%); 58% of patients were double positive (ICA+ and anti-BSA+), and none was negative for both markers. Elevated BSA antibody levels were found in 20% of ICA positive, healthy children[42] that had been recruited through screening a cohort of more than 13 000 French school children. Follow-up of these children will determine the predictive value of BSA serology in that subgroup.

An ongoing study of new cases from Finland confirmed the association of anti-BSA and childhood IDDM (Karjalainen, unpublished), with 60 out of 71 (84%) recent-onset IDDM patients having elevated IgG anti-BSA antibody levels as compared to 4.7% of healthy control children of the same age and sex (Figure 11.2).

The disease association of BSA antibodies with IDDM has been confirmed in other populations[43–45] but it was challenged in one US study[46]. The latter compared adult and adolescent IDDM patients with healthy adult controls, relatives or other autoimmune patients and found no significant differences in anti-BSA antibody levels. Immune parameters at time of diagnosis differ significantly in childhood and adult IDDM patients and the high mean age of

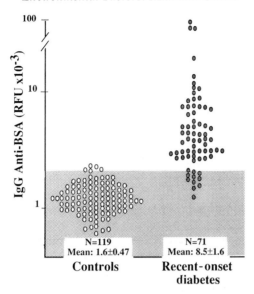

Figure 11.2. Anti-BSA antibody levels in a new series of Finnish children with recent-onset IDDM. Controls were age, sex and region matched. The shaded area includes 95% of all controls (mean±2SD), $p < 0.0001$

individuals in this study make comparison with earlier reports from pediatric patients difficult[47].

Technical aspects might contribute to the observed discrepancies[41], and other variables may in addition interfere with the detection of these antibodies. For example, drinking as little as one glass (180 ml) of cow's milk prior to blood sampling decreased IgG anti-BSA levels by 54% in diabetic children, with a nadir 2–3 hours after ingestion and recovery of pre-test levels over 12 hours. Total IgG, tetanus antibodies or serum osmolality were unchanged, suggesting a specific effect on circulating BSA antibodies, possibly through complex formation with absorbed BSA fragments (Dosch, unpublished). It is unclear why after milk ingestion BSA antibody levels decreased much less (14–26%) in healthy individuals with high or low baseline anti-BSA. Standardized assay and sampling conditions are thus mandatory: serum samples from the above French and Finnish studies had been obtained after overnight fasting.

Combining the discussed epidemiological and patient studies as well as animal experimentation, we have proposed that among all dietary proteins BSA stands out most as a candidate mimicry molecule in diabetic autoimmunity[1]. In a genetically IDDM susceptible host < 4 months old, dietary BSA would recruit a T-cell repertoire in which ABBOS-specific T cells cross-react with the ICAp69 self-antigen. Exposure later in life, after gut closure and more complete immune maturation, would not recruit such T cells, perhaps even generate oral tolerance. Large self-reactive T-cell pools would become the basis for pathogenic islet cell autoimmunity.

When peripheral blood mononuclear cells from newly diagnosed diabetic and age-matched control children were analyzed, a significant T-cell proliferative response to BSA (mean response 4834 cpm, stimulation index 4.84 ± 0.42), was observed in 28 of 31 patients, but not in 23 control children (mean response 1074 cpm, stimulation index 1.07 ± 0.12) (Figure 11.3). The fine specificity of these T cells was mapped to the ABBOS epitope[48]. These T cells also recognize recombinant ICAp69[38], their specificity mapping to the ABBOS-homologous region, called T-cell epitope 69 (Tep69)[49].

(Auto-) antigen-specific T-cell activation is regarded as a hallmark of the pre-diabetic phase of IDDM, and should therefore not only be detectable in animal models of the disease, but also in human IDDM. There is currently, however, no information available on BSA/ABBOS-specific cellular immune responsiveness in healthy individuals at increased diabetes risk. High cost and technical demands as well as the need for fresh blood samples are presently limiting the widespread use of T-cell assays in clinical settings. In addition to their scientific value, they may however become a useful tool to predict diabetes in selected, high risk populations.

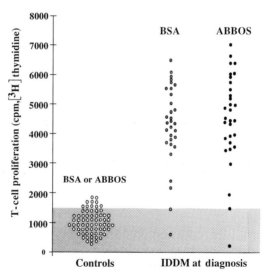

Figure 11.3. T-cell proliferative responses to BSA or ABBOS peptide in 31 newly diabetic children and 23 healthy control children. The shaded area indicates the range of responses in unstimulated cultures, $p < 0.0001$

CONCLUSIONS

Early introduction of cow's-milk-based formula to infant diet is associated with a moderate, but significant increase of IDDM risk in the general population (odds ratio ~1.5), especially in young children (odds ratio >3). This effect seems to be independent of the duration of breast feeding. The accumulated evidence provided the base for new recommendations by the American Academy of Pediatrics to avoid cow's milk exposure in young infants at risk to develop IDDM[8]. A prospective feeding trial will ultimately define the contribution of single dietary factors to IDDM risk in genetically susceptible individuals.

Elevated antibody levels to cow's milk protein may reflect an abnormal immune response to cow's-milk-derived dietary antigens in IDDM patients. It is far from clear whether, and in the positive case which, milk protein is involved in the etiology of IDDM. The presence in newly diagnosed diabetic children of antibodies to BSA and its ABBOS epitope as well as the sequence homology between BSA and the islet cell protein ICAp69 are compatible with a specific role of this antigen in diabetic autoimmunity. However, current antibody assays to BSA and other milk proteins do not substantially contribute to the prediction and diagnosis of IDDM.

REFERENCES

1 Karges WJP, Ilonen J, Robinson BH, Dosch H-M. Self and non-self antigen in diabetic autoimmunity: molecules and mechanisms. In Azzi A (ed), *Moleculer Aspects of Medicine*. Oxford, UK: Elsevier Science, 1995, pp 79–213.
2 Singh B, Rabinovitch A. Influence of microbial agents on the development and prevention of autoimmune diabetes. *Autoimmunity* 1993; **15**: 209–13.
3 Helgason T, Jonasson MR. Evidence for a food additive as a cause of ketosis-prone diabetes. *Lancet* 1981; **ii**: 716–20.
4 Tuomilehto J, Tuomilehto-Wolf E, Virtala E, LaPorte R. Coffee consumption as trigger for insulin-dependent diabetes in childhood. *Br Med J* 1990; **300**: 642–3.
5 Pozzilli P, Bottazzo GF. Coffee or sugar—which is to blame in IDDM? *Diabetes Care* 1991; **14**: 114–15.
6 Wilson GL, Patton NJ, McCord JM, Mullins DW, Mossman BT. Mechanisms of streptozotocin- and alloxan-induced damage in rat B-cells. *Diabetologia* 1984; **27**: 587–91.
7 Elliott RB, Chase HP. Prevention or delay of type 1 (insulin-dependent) diabetes mellitus in children using nicotinamide. *Diabetologia* 1991; **34**: 362–5.
8 American Academy of Pediatrics, Work Group on Cow's Milk Protein and Diabetes. Infant feeding practices and their possible relationship to the etiology of diabetes mellitus. *Pediatrics* 1994; **94**: 752–4.
9 Gerstein H. Cow's milk exposure and type 1 diabetes mellitus. *Diabetes Care* 1994; **17**: 13–19.
10 Dahl-Jørgensen K, Joner G, Hanssen KF. Relationship between cow milk consumption

178   Prediction, Prevention and Genetic Counseling in IDDM

and incidence of IDDM in childhood. *Diabetes Care* 1991; **14**: 1081–3.
11 Scott FW. Cow milk and insulin-dependent diabetes mellitus: is there a relationship. *Am. J. Nutrition* 1990; **51**: 489–91.
12 Di Fava D, Leslie RDG, Pozzilli P. Relationship between dairy product consumption and incidence of IDDM in childhood in Italy. *Diabetes Care* 1994; **17**: 1488–90.
13 Borch-Johnsen K, Mandrup-Poulsen T, Zachau-Christiansen B, Joner G, Christy M, Kastrup K, Nerup J. Relation between breast-feeding and incidence rates of insulin-dependent diabetes mellitus. *Lancet* 1984; **2**: 1083–6.
14 Kostraba JN, Cruickshanks KJ, Lawler-Heavner J, Jobim LF, Rewers MJ, Gay EC, Chase HP, Klingensmith G, Hamman RF. Early exposure to cow's milk, and solid foods in infancy, genetic predisposition and risk of IDDM. *Diabetes* 1993; **42**: 288–94.
15 Dahlquist G, Blom L, Lönnberg G. The Swedish childhood diabetes study—a multivariate analysis of risk determinants for diabetes in different age groups. *Diabetologia* 1991; **34**: 757–62.
16 Virtanen SM, Räsänen L, Aro A, Lindström J, Sippola H, Lounamaa R, Toivanen L, Tuomilehto J, Åkerblom HK, and the Childhood Diabetes in Finland Study Group. Infant feeding in Finnish children less than 7 yr of age with newly diagnosed IDDM. *Diabetes Care* 1991; **14**: 415–17.
17 Virtanen SM, Räsänen L, Ylönen K, Aro A, Clayton D, Langholz B, Pitkäniemi J, Savilahti E, Lounamaa R, Tuomilehto J, Åkerblom, HK, and the Childhood Diabetes in Finland Study Group. Early introduction of dairy products associated with increased risk of IDDM in Finnish children. *Diabetes* 1993; **42**: 1786–90.
18 Verge CF, Howard NJ, Irwig L, Simpson JM, Mackerras D, Silink M. Environmental factors in childhood IDDM. *Diabetes Care* 1994; **17**: 1381–9.
19 Glatthaar C, Whittall DE, Welborn TA, Gibson MJ, Brooks BH, Ryan MMP, Byrne GC. Diabetes in Western Australian children: descriptive epidemiology. *Med J Austr* 1988; **148**: 117–23.
20 Bognetti E, Meschi F, Malavasi C, Pastore MR, Sergi A, Illeni MT, Maffeis C, Pinelli L, Chiumello G. HLA antigens in Italian type 1 diabetes patients; role of DR3/DR4 antigens and breast feeding in the onset of the disease. *Acta Diabetol* 1992; **28**: 229–32.
21 Dahlquist G, Savilahti E, Landin-Olson M. An increased level of antibodies to beta lactoglobulin is a risk determinant for early-onset Type 1 (insulin dependent) diabetes mellitus independent of islet cell antibodies and early introduction of cow's milk. *Diabetologia* 1992; **35**: 980–4.
22 Jakobson I, Lindberg T, Benediktson B, Hansson BG. Dietary bovine beta-lactoglobulin is transferred to human milk. *Acta Paediatr Scand* 1985; **74**: 342–5.
23 Tainio V-M, savilahti E, Arjomaa P, Salmenperä L, Perheentupa J, Siimes MA. Plasma antibodies to cow's milk are increased by early weaning and consumption of unmodified milk, but production of IgA and IgM cow's milk antibodies is stimulated even during exclusive breast-feeding. *Acta. Paediatr. Scand.* 1988; **77**: 807–11.
24 Åkerblom HK, Savilahti E, Saukkonen TT, Paganus A, Virtanen SM, Teramo K, Knip M, Ilonen J, Reijonen H, Karjalainen J, Tuomilehto J, and the Childhoold Diabetes in Finland Study Group. The case for elimination of cow's milk in early infancy in the prevention of Type 1 diabetes: the Finnish experience. *Diabetes Metab Rev* 1994; **9**: 456–62.
25 Elliott RB, Martin JM. Dietary protein: a trigger of insulin-dependent diabetes in the BB rat? *Diabetologia* 1984; **26**: 297–9.
26 Daneman D, Fishman, L, Clarson C, Martin JM. Dietary triggers of insulin-dependent diabetes in the BB rat. *Diabetes Res* 1987; **5**: 93–7.
27 Elliott RB, Reddy SN, Bibby NJ, Kida K. Dietary prevention of diabetes in the

non-obese diabetic mouse. *Diabetologia* 1988; **30**: 62–4.

28 Hoorfar J, Buschard K, Dagnaes-Hansen F. Prophylactic nutritional modification of the incidence of diabetes in autoimmune non-obese diabetic (NOD) mice.. *Br J Nutr* 1993; **69**: 597–607.

29 Hoorfar J, Scott F, Cloutier HE. Dietary plant materials and development of diabetes in the BB rat. *J Nutr* 1991; **121**: 908–16.

30 Coleman DL, Kuzava JE, Leiter EH. Effect of diet on incidence of diabetes in nonobese diabetic mice. *Diabetes* 1990; **39**: 432–6.

31 Martin JM, Trink B, Daneman D, Dosch H-M, Robinson BH. Milk proteins in the etiology of insulin-dependent diabetes mellitus (IDDM). *Ann Med* 1991; **23**: 447–52.

32 Beppu H, Winter WE, Atkinson MA, Maclaren NK, Fujita K, Takahashi H. Bovine albumin antibodies in NOD mice. *Diabetes Res* 1987; **6**: 67–9.

33 Dosch H-M, Karjalainen J, Morkowski J, Martin JM, Robinson BH. Nutritional triggers of IDDM. In Laron Z (ed) *Epidemiology and Etiology of Insulin-Dependent Diabetes in the Young*. Basel: Karger, 1992, pp 202–17.

34 Savilahti E, Åkerblom HK, Tainio V-M, Koskimies S. Children with newly diagnosed insulin dependent diabetes mellitus have increased levels of cow's milk antibodies. *Diabetes Res* 1988; **7**: 137–40.

35 Virtanen SM, Saukkonen T, Savilahti E, Ylonen K, Rasanen L, Aro A, Knip M, Tuomilehto J, Akerblom HK, and the Childhood Diabetes in Finland Study Group. Diet, cow's milk protein antibodies and the risk of IDDM in Finnish children. *Diabetologia* 1994; **37**: 381–7.

36 Savilahti E, Saukkonen TT, Virtala ET, Tuomilehto J, Åkerblom HK, and the Childhood Diabetes in Finland Study Group. Increased levels of cow's milk and beta-lactoglobulin antibodies in young children with newly diagnosed IDDM. *Diabetes Care* 1993; **16**: 984–9.

37 Glerum M, Robinson BH, Martin JM. Could bovine serum albumin be the initiating antigen ultimately responsible for the development of insulin dependent diabetes mellitus? *Diabetes Res* 1989; **10**: 103–7.

38 Miyazaki I, Gaedigk R, Hui MF, Cheung RK, Morkowski J, Rajotte RV, Dosch H-M. Cloning of human and rat p69, a candidate autoimmune target in Type I diabetes. *Biochim Biophys Acta* 1994; **1227**: 101–4.

39 Pietropaolo M, Castano L, Babu S, Buelow R, Kuo Yu-Ling S, Martin S, Martin A, Powers AC, Prochazka M, Naggert J, Eisnebarth GE. Islet cell autoantigen 69 Kd (ICA69). Molecular cloning and characterization of a novel diabetes-associated autoantigen. *J Clin Invest* 1993; **92**: 359–71.

40 Karjalainen J, Martin JM, Knip M, Ilonen J, Robinson BH, Savilahti E, Åkerblom HK, Dosch H-M. A bovine albumin peptide as a possible trigger of insulin dependent diabetes mellitus. *N Engl J Med* 1992; **327**: 302–7.

41 Karjalainen J, Saukkonen T, Savilahti E, Dosch H-M. Disease-associated anti-BSA antibodies in Type I (insulin-dependent) diabetes mellitus are detected by particle concentration fluoroimmunoassay but not by enzyme linked immunoassay. *Diabetologia* 1992; **35**: 985–90.

42 Lévy-Marchal C, Karjalainen J, Dubois F, Karges W, Czernichow P, Dosch H-M. Antibodies against bovine albumin and other diabetes markers in French children. *Diabetes Care* 1995; **18**: 67–74.

43 Krokowski M, Caillat-Zucman S, Timsit J, Larger E, Pehuet-Figoni M, Bach JF, Boitard C. Anti-BSA antibodies: genetic heterogeneity and clinical relevance in type I diabetes. *Diabetes Care* 1995; **18**: 170–3.

44 Saukkonen T, Savilahti E, Vaarala O, Virtale ET, Tuomilehto J, Åkerblom HK, and the Childhood Diabetes in Finland Study Group. Children with newly diagnosed

insulin-dependent diabetes mellitus have increased levels of antibodies to bovine serum albumin but not to ovalbumin. *Diabetes Care* 1994; **17**: 970–6.

45 Pigny P, Mortreux G, Racadot A, Stuckens C, Boersma A. Humoral immune response to bovine serum albumin in new onset and established IDDM. *Acta Diabetol* 1995 (in press).

46 Atkinson MA, Bowman MA, Kao K-J, Campbell L, Dush PJ, Shah SC, Simell O, Maclaren NK. Lack of immune responsiveness to bovine serum albumin in insulin-dependent diabetes. *N Engl J Med* 1993; **329**: 1853–8.

47 Karjalainen J, Salmela P, Ilonen J, Surcel H-M, Knip M. A comparison of childhood and adult Type I diabetes mellitus. *N Engl J Med* 1989; **320**: 881–6.

48 Cheung RK, Karjalainen J, VanderMeulen J, Singal D, Dosch H-M. T cells of children with insulin dependent diabetes are sensitized to bovine serum albumin. *Scand. J. Immunol.* 1994; **40**: 623–8.

49 Miyazaki I, Cheung RK, Gaedigk R, Hui MF, Van der Meulen J, Rajotte RV, Dosch H-M. T cell activation and anergy to islet cell antigen in Type 1 diabetes. *J Immunol* 1995; **154**: 1461–9.

50 Blom L, Dahlquist G, Nyström L, Sandström A, Wall S. The Swedish childhood diabetes study—social and perinatal determinents for diabetes in childhood. *Diabetologia* 1989; **32**: 7–13.

51 Dahlquist G, Blom L, Persson LÅ, Sandström A, Wall S. Dietary factors and the risk of developing insulin-dependent diabetes in childhood. *Br Med J* 1990; **300**: 1302–6.

52 Virtanen SM, Räsänen L, Aro L, Ylönen K, Lounamaa R, Tuomilehto J, Åkerblom HK, and the Childhood Diabetes in Finland Study Group. Feeding in infancy and the risk of Type 1 diabetes mellitus in Finland. *Diabetic Med* 1992; **9**: 815–19.

12

Lessons from the Animal Models: the BB Rat

ANNA PETTERSSON,[1] HOWARD JACOB,[2] and
ÅKE LERNMARK[1,3]

[1] Karolinska Institute, Department of Molecular Medicine, Karolinska Hospital, Stockholm, Sweden. [2] Cardiovascular Research Center, Harvard Medical School, Boston, USA. [3] Robert H. Williams Laboratory, University of Washington, Department of Medicine, Seattle, Washington, USA

BRIEF HISTORY OF THE BB RATS

The BB rat was first discovered in a commercial breeding company, BioBreeding Laboratories in Ottawa, Canada. Occasional deaths among weaning rats were observed and the cause was found to be diabetes that closely resembled human insulin-dependent diabetes (IDDM). The initial investigations of the BB rats were published in 1977[1] and since then there are numerous publications and several comprehensive reviews [2-4,5]. The cause of disease was not known. The original diabetes incidence in the BioBreeding colony was approximately 10%, but increased to 25% after selective breeding of diabetic animals[3]. Both males and females were affected although initially the incidence in females was somewhat higher. Microbiological findings were all negative and neighboring rats from other strains were not affected. A simple infectious cause of the disease was unlikely. A genetic component of the diabetic syndrome seemed probable and studies were undertaken to investigate the pattern of inheritance and the degree of heredity of the disease. In parallel with the inbreeding effort, numerous studies were carried out to explore the predictive value of genetic and immune markers (reviewed in references 4, 6–8).[4,6–8]

Early studies on the BB rat focused on the pathology of the islets of

Prediction, Prevention and Genetic Counseling in IDDM. Edited by Jerry P. Palmer.
© 1996 John Wiley & Sons Ltd.

Langerhans and on the symptoms of diabetes. Glucose intolerance was demonstrated at or shortly preceding the clinical diagnosis of hyperglycemia. The classical symptoms of IDDM are summarized in Table 12.1 which compares the BB rat IDDM with that of the human disorder. It is obvious from this table that the similarities are many. There is no effect of gender. The diabetes is truly insulin dependent and associated with a severe ketosis and weight loss. The BB rats will die unless insulin therapy is initiated. The age at onset also conforms with human IDDM. The peak incidence rate occurs during the time of sexual maturation and at maximum weight gain. As in humans[9], genetic factors coded for in the major histocompatibility complex (MHC) seem to be necessary but not sufficient for IDDM[10]. The MHC factors have not yet been identified and the mechanisms are not understood. Recent data suggest that the HLA-DQ homologue, RT1B shows the highest risk for IDDM. Autoantibodies against islet cell antigens have been described (see reference 8 for a review), although the BB rat does not have antibodies which generate the islet cell antibody (ICA) reaction on frozen sections. As in the human IDDM, there is an increased frequency of autoantibodies against antigens in other endocrine organs such as the thyroid and stomach[11]. Lymphocyte antibodies are an unusual feature of the BB rat [12,13]. Dissimilarities to human IDDM include lymphopenia [6,14,15], which represents a complete lack of T lymphocytes at birth affecting both the CD4 and CD8 positive populations. The fact that BB rats have been inbred and that they are reared in specific pathogen free (SPF) conditions represent major but useful differences. Inbreeding was thought by some investigators to result in a loss of diabetes in these rats and our plan to initiate immediate sister–brother breeding in 1980 was questioned. One argument was that the spontaneous diabetes symptoms

Table 12.1. Comparison of BB rat and human IDDM

Similarities
  Weight loss, polyuria, polydipsia
  Rapid onset of hyperglycemia, glycosuria
  Ketoacidosis
  Insulin dependency for life
  Males=females
  Young age at onset
  Islet cells autoantibodies
  Insulitis
  MHC class II association (HLA RT1)
  Association to other autoimmune disorders (thyroid, parietal cell)

Dissimilarities
  Lymphopenia
  Inbred
  Specific pathogen free

---

would be lost and that the so-called inbreeding crisis after 20–24 generations of inbreeding would severely affect these rats. Neither happened since it was possible to demonstrate in crosses between DP and DR rats as well as between DP and other rat strains that IDDM was linked to lymphopenia and dependent on the rat MHC RT1 type inherited according to a Mendelian mode of inheritance[15–17]. Following more than 40 generations of sister–brother breeding, in our colony the rats have been kept SPF since 1989 corresponding to about 10 generations of inbreeding[16,18,19], the age at onset curves seem to have stabilized with the earliest age at onset at 53–55 days of age and 95% of the rats developing IDDM before 100 days of age (Figure 12.1). In SPF conditions there is an almost 100% frequency of diabetes[15,16,19] which makes the BB rat an extremely useful model for IDDM with respect to studies on prediction, the natural history of disease and mechanisms of immune modulation.

During the past several years of inbreeding and also observing animals developing diabetes after different crosses[15], the symptoms of IDDM have not changed. The impression is rather that diabetes-prone BB rats kept in SPF conditions have a shorter time of blood glucose abnormalities before developing hyperglycemia[20]. The disease appears more aggressive and the

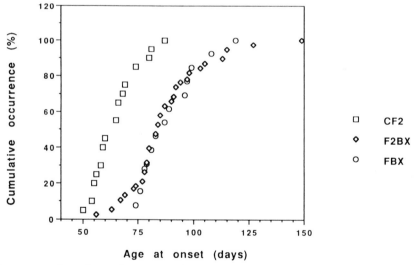

Age at onset (days)

Figure 12.1. Cumulative frequency of insulin-dependent diabetes mellitus in the spontaneously diabetic rat in relation to the age at onset in days. The CF2 animals represent diabetes-prone rats homozygous for the two diabetes genes, *iddm1* (on chromosome 4) and *iddm2* (MHC on chromosome 20) on the BB background. The FBX are *iddm1* and *iddm2* homozygous rats in the (DP × Fischer) × DP backcross and the F2BX rats are homozygous for the same genes in the F2 (DP × Fischer) × DP backcross

necessity of proper insulin management has been accentuated. In studies on diabetes prediction the BB rat is advantageous since the IDDM outcome at around days 60–100 is predictable already at birth. Differences between prone and resistant BB rats are therefore of interest and may reflect the natural history of IDDM which culminates in insulitis and a rapid β-cell destruction.

Diabetes-prone BB rats reared in SPF facilities have a cumulative incidence of IDDM of 60–100%. The variation between colonies is probably explained by differences in degree of inbreeding, type of breeding approach, extent of infections[21] and the subline used for random breeding or sister–brother breeding. The cumulative frequency of IDDM in our colony of genetically characterized diabetes-prone BB rats is shown in Figure 12.1. As is evident from the results, nearly all rats (98%) develop IDDM between 60 and 100 days of age. There is no difference between males and females. The data in Figure 12.1 also illustrate the fact that when two BB genes[15], *iddm1* (lymphopenia on chromosome 4) and *iddm2* (MHC RT1B u/u on chromosome 20) are introgressed on to Fischer in a (DP × Fischer) × DP backcross (FBX in Figure 12.1) or a (DP × Fischer) F2 × DP backcross (F2BX) the cumulative frequency was little affected while there was a delay in the age at onset. These data demonstrate that BB rat IDDM is predictable. All rats among prone animals, i.e. homozygous for *iddm1* and *iddm2* did develop IDDM. The fact that genotyping can now be used to identify diabetes-prone BB rats in the different crosses offers a unique possibility to dissect the sequence of events that results in the spontaneous development of IDDM.

ISLET PATHOLOGY AND IMMUNE ABNORMALITIES

HISTOPATHOLOGY

The histopathology of the BB rat pancreatic islets at the time of clinical diagnosis shows a marked mononuclear cell infiltration in and around the islets of Langerhans[1,22–24]. The loss of beta cells has been estimated at 80–90%[25–27] in keeping with the decrease in the amount of extractable insulin in the pancreas[22,28]. Studies of pancreatic insulitis are mostly descriptive and morphometric evaluations on the progression of infiltration are needed. Insulitis was also quantitated in old non-diabetic BB rats—over 200 days of age—suggesting that other additional insults are necessary for diabetes to be clinically expressed[29]. A major question to be answered is the series of events of cellular infiltrations which take place before insulitis is established. BB rat diabetes may be transferred by spleen cells[30,31] and T cells have subsequently been observed in the islets[6,32]. The ability to predict diabetes by investigating the pancreas and insulitis is, however, poor. Pancreatic biopsies in diabetes-prone BB rats revealed insulitis 10–14 days before clinical diagnosis[23,33,34]. In some rats, IDDM did not develop despite the presence of insulitis. An infiltration of macrophages seems to precede T and B lymphocytes[35-37]. The islet macrophage infiltration seems to involve primarily ED2 positive cells[34] while the focal macrophage infiltration observed in the pancreas of pre-diabetic BB rats includes cells positive for both ED1 and ED2. In addition, in BB DP rats treated with a platelet-activating factor (PAF) inhibitor there was no change in diabetes frequency although the drug was able to protect the β cells in a dose-dependent manner[26]. Severe insulitis was reduced by the PAF inhibitor. Using a more potent PAF inhibitor[38] reduced the frequency of IDDM, increased serum insulin, preserved islet β cells and decreased insulitis compared to the vehicle-treated DP rats. These observations lead to several questions. What is the mechanism that makes bone-marrow-derived macrophages infiltrate islets? Have focal T cell cytotoxic events taken place to initiate beta bell killing and thereby signal macrophages to invade the islets? Are cytokines elaborated from the islets that initiate macrophage infiltration and, finally, how are these functional abnormalities controlled by the IDDM genes, *iddm1* and *iddm2*? What is the positive predictive value of macrophage or cytokine production for IDDM?

MACROPHAGES AND CYTOKINES

MHC class II positive β cells were not observed in insulitis before or at the time of onset of diabetes[36]. Rather, class II positive cells with immunoreactive insulin may be due to the presence of macrophages containing β-cell debris[39]. As summarized in Table 12.2, the presence of class II mRNA did not change in DP BB rats while there was an increase in the class I molecule mRNA levels[40]. Similarly, levels of mRNA detected by RT-PCR or in situ hybridization (Table 12.2) for IL-6, IL-1β and TNF-α were only increased at the time of IDDM onset[41,42]. There was an increased expression of IFN-γ about 10 days before the expected age at onset. This is the same time before onset that diabetes-prone BB rats fail to gain weight[19]. Hence, systemic changes including metabolic alterations perhaps both in feeding behavior and metabolism may be induced by insulitis-associated alterations in cytokine production. This is illustrated by a decreased weight gain following the administration of a large dose of IL-1β which accelerates IDDM onset[43,44]. More importantly, IFN-α expression was up-regulated already at day 37 in BB DP rats[41]. The increased expression of this interferon suggests that an infectious agent may be of importance. Although Kilham virus may be diabetogenic to DR rats[45], this agent is an unlikely explanation for the SPF inbred BB DP rats which are Kilham virus antibody free. The IDDM in the DP BB rat also follows a Mendelian mode of inheritance[16,17] which would be unlikely if the disease was commonly caused by the Kilham virus. The inheritance is also genetically linked to *iddm1* and *iddm2*[15]. It is therefore speculated that the control of the INF-α gene is defective

Table 12.2. MHC and cytokine expression preceding clinical onset of BB rat insulin-dependent diabetes mellitus

MHC				
Class I	Northern blot	40	20	40
Class II	Northern blot	No change		
TCRβ	Northern blot	No change		40
Cytokines				
IFN-α	RT-PCR, ISH	37	35	41
IL-6	RT-PCR, ISH	onset	0	
IL-1β	RT-PCR, ISH	onset	0	
TNF-α	RT-PCR, ISH	onset	0	42
IFN-γ	RT-PCR, ISH	60	10	
Macrophages	Biopsy	40–50	20–30	34
Insulitis	IL-2R gamma camera image	50	10	47

in the BB rat islet β cells. Spontaneous or genetically regulated expression of INF-α may make the islet β cells respond as if they had been infected by a virus. This would lead to severe insulitis involving macrophage infiltration and subsequent lymphocytic infiltration of both CD4 and CD8 T lymphocytes preceding the onset of IDDM. The alternative hypothesis is that macrophage effector cells are brought to the islets of Langerhans by an antibody-dependent cellular cytotoxicity (ADCC) mechanism. The ADCC event would stimulate the β cells to express INF-α due to the cytotoxicity induced by the ADCC reaction. Further studies are necessary to identify the mechanisms and the cells which produce cytokines before macrophages and lymphocytes infiltrate the islets. It would be important to find a marker in the peripheral blood for such alterations. Apart from biopsy studies (Table 12.2), are there predictive markers for islet macrophage infiltration, subsequent insulitis and IDDM?

Cytokine-activated rodent macrophages produce tetrahydrobiopterin (BH4 or biopterin) which may be detectable in serum or urine. Serum biopterin levels were elevated at day 90 in diabetes-prone but not in diabetes-resistant or normal Wistar rats[46]. At earlier ages, serum biopterin did not differ between diabetes-prone and control rats. This biopsy study confirmed an early infiltration of macrophages and the increase in serum biopterin was therefore thought to be due to an acute cell destruction associated with the clinical onset of the disease[46]. The clarification of the natural history of islet pathology is important and is complicated by the fact that all islets may not be affected equally at all time points. Repeated biopsies are difficult to perform and a single biopsy may not be representative. Scanners and imagers may be useful and in a preliminary study of injected ^{123}I-labeled IL-2, an increased uptake in the pancreas was observed[47]. Non-invasive approaches to detect insulitis need further development. In the meantime, a number of markers, cellular and humoral, have therefore been tested in diabetes-prone BB rats in order to evaluate their predictive value for diabetes (Table 12.3).

LYMPHOCYTES

The lymphocytes infiltrating the islets of Langerhans at the time of clinical onset of IDDM have been analyzed by numerous investigators (reviewed in reference 6). The DP BB rats are born with lymphopenia[48,49]. The lymphopenia gene, *lyp*, is located on chromosome 4[15] and in rats homozygous for DP there are markedly reduced numbers of peripheral lymphocytes[18], a deficiency in the expression of the RT6 peripheral T-cell differentiation antigen[50,51], reduced numbers of CD8 positive T cells in the thymus and peripheral blood[52,53] as well as of CD45R positive T lymphocytes[54]. The T-lymphocyte deficiency is associated with reduced T-cell proliferation and cytotoxic responses[52,55–58]. These abnormalities are detected early and are useful in predicting IDDM. However, this relationship is not absolute since some lymphopenic BB rats with these abnormalities do not develop IDDM.

CELLULAR ABNORMALITIES TO PREDICT DIABETES

In BB rats with a cumulative IDDM frequency of 85%, the presence of Ia-positive W3/13 T lymphocytes had a diagnostic sensitivity for IDDM of

Table 12.3. Lymphocyte, autoantibody and other markers in the BB rat

Marker	Sensitivity	Specificity	Days to onset	Reference
Lymphocytes				
1a+ W3/13-cells	85%	83%	20	94
Islet cell autoantibodies				
ICSA	73%	85%	20–30	65, 66
	100%	100%		64, 74
64K antigen	80%	90%		71
Insulin	Not predictive		16	
	89%	0%		95
	38%	95%		72
Cytotoxic antibodies	100%	99%		78
	40%	95%		77
				65
Lymphocyte autoantibodies				
LT	83%	85%	10	13
Other markers				
Serum trypsin	50%	95%		96
Expired pentane	70%	95%		97

85% while the specificity was 83%. In DP by DR rat crosses and an analysis of the 25% F2 rats which develop diabetes as offsprings compared to healthy F1 parents, it was found that coinciding with the time of onset of overt IDDM, there was a large increase in eosinophils, along with smaller increases in neutrophils, monocytes and lymphocytes[18]. Hence, there was a significant leukocytosis at but not before the clinical onset. The eosinophil infiltration of the islets of Langerhans with insulitis is not understood[26] but may be associated with the eosinophilia[18,59]. The acceleration of diabetogenesis in DP rats by IL-1β was associated with increased pre-diabetic levels of monocytes[60].

Utilizing reverse transcription polymerase chain reaction (RT-PCR) to analyze the cytokine mRNA profile of mitogen-activated peripheral T cells derived from BB and BB × Fisher cross rats with and without lymphopenia, it was demonstrated that the cytokine profiles, mostly of recent thymic migrants were linked to *lyp* on chromosome 4[61]. This population of cells may therefore harbor the effector cells required for initiation of IDDM. The identification of the effector cells which govern the infiltration of macrophages followed by CD4 and CD8 positive T-cell subsets[62] and possibly of NK cells[63] is central to the attempts to identify a cellular marker in the peripheral blood which predicts BB rat IDDM. Such a cell is yet to be identified.

HUMORAL AUTOANTIBODIES AND OTHER ABNORMALITIES PREDICT DIABETES

Islet cell antibodies in the BB rat were first detected as islet cell surface antibodies (ICSA) in a radioligand binding assay with insulin-producing cells[12] (Table 12.3). Later this observation was confirmed in studies with indirect immunofluorescence[64,65]. Classical ICA has not been reported in the BB rat (see review in reference 6). In the radioligand binding assays, it was found that diabetes-prone BB rats had both ICSA and lymphocyte antibodies before the onset of diabetes[66] while in the presumably less sensitive immunofluorescence assay, the cell surface antibodies against cell sorter purified β cells as well as lymphocytes were primarily detected at or shortly before the clinical onset of IDDM[65]. The early studies of ICSA in the BB rat have been reviewed previously[8]. Overall, the sensitivity of ICSA for IDDM was 73% and the specificity 85% (Table 12.3). Autoantibodies to the 64K-antigen[67], now identified in humans as glutamic acid decarboxylase[68], the M_r 65 000 isoform[69,70], have been detected in DP BB rats both before and at the clinical onset of diabetes[71]. Further studies are needed using recombinant rat GAD-65 to determine to what extent GAD antibodies predict diabetes in the BB rat.

In tests for insulin autoantibodies as a predictive marker for IDDM the results are highly controversial and variable (Table 12.3). In the first study[72] it was reported that the sensitivity of insulin autoantibodies for IDDM was

100% and the specificity 95%. In subsequent analyses using both ELISA and radioligand binding assays[73,74] these results could not be reproduced (Table 12.3). In humans, insulin autoantibodies are prevalent[75] and the radioligand binding assay has been standardized[76], however, insulin autoreactivity, if any, in the BB rat needs to be fully elicited.

After the observation that ICSA were present in the BB rat before and at the onset of diabetes, it was tested whether ICSA would confer complement-dependent cytotoxicity (Table 12.3). [³H]leucine incorporation into islet proteins and cytotoxicity assays were used[77,78]. In one study[78], the sensitivity for IDDM was as high as 100% and the specificity 99%. In another study[77], the sensitivity was 40%. In some rats the cytotoxic antibodies preceded the onset of overt IDDM by 4–8 weeks while in others the prodrome was only 1–2 weeks[78]. It was speculated that the complement-fixing cytotoxic antibodies may in vivo contribute directly to the destruction of pancreatic islet cells or may attract mononuclear cells to the islets. Lymphocyte antibodies (Table 12.3) were recently analyzed by double immunofluorescence analysis to identify relevant T-cell subsets[13] and it was reported that lymphocytes of the IgM isotope were present before the onset of BB rat IDDM and that their presence predicted IDDM. The presence of such antibodies is unlikely to cause the neonatal lymphopenia and it remains unclear why this type of antibody would serve as a marker for IDDM in the BB rat.

GENETIC PREDICTS DIABETES IN THE INBRED, SPECIFIC PATHOGEN FREE BB RAT

INBREEDING THE BB RAT

Prior to 1980, in several laboratories, diabetic and non-diabetic sibs, as well as parents, were mated and the incidence of diabetes in BB rats was investigated. Based on these results, it was possible to conclude in one colony, that the heredity of the disease was 6.2% and that a single autosomal dominant or recessive model could be excluded[79]. Although inbreeding had not previously been carried out in the BioBreeding laboratories, attempts were then made to breed for increased diabetes frequency. Breeding was designed to obtain lines with a high and predictable incidence of IDDM. Animals belonging to these lines are frequently referred to as "diabetes prone" or DP BB rats, to distinguish them from the control lines with no diabetes or "diabetes resistant" lines. These "control" lines, with no diabetes or very low frequencies were derived at the University of Massachusetts BB rat facility from DP animals in the fifth generation of inbreeding and were continuously selected for diabetes resistance[6]. During the course of breeding, animals were sent out to other laboratories, where strict inbreeding often took place, generating different sub-lines of BB rats[80]. Upon inbreeding, the incidence of IDDM in the BB rat increased dramatically, rendering a penetrance that ranged from approximately 60% to 90% in many colonies throughout the world. Diabetes frequency in DR animals varies between 0.1% and 5%.

Although a genetic factor for the disease was suspected, the nature of this component long remained elusive. Based on findings in human IDDM, the major histocompatibility complex—in the rat called RT1—was a strong candidate for a diabetes susceptibility gene. Indeed, it was shown by Colle and co-workers[28] that IDDM in the BB rat was associated with the RT1 locus and that the allele giving susceptibility with RT1^u, the allele present in the BB rat[28]. Furthermore, diabetes in the BB rat appeared to be associated with lymphopenia, as shown by Guttman and co-workers[81], indicating that the IDDM was somehow connected to the severe immunodeficiency that is present in all DP rats from birth.

SEGREGATION ANALYSES

Segregation analysis implies an attempt to elucidate the mode of inheritance of a disease by studying the pattern of inheritance in a large population. Virtually all segregation analyses attempting to define the mode of inheritance of IDDM in the BB rat have demonstrated an absolute requirement of lymphopenia for overt diabetes. Although it has been suggested that diabetic BB rats need not be lymphopenic[82], breeding experiments between lymphopenic and non-lymphopenic diabetic rats showed that the F1 progeny did not develop IDDM. This indicates that IDDM in non-lymphopenic animals either is of a different genetic origin than that of lymphopenic animals, or it is caused by environmental factors[17]. In fact, it was reported by Markholst and co-workers[16] that diabetes and lymphopenia in crosses between DP and DR animals co-segregate as one single trait. The finding in these inbred SPF rats is that 25% of all F2 rats developed both lymphopenia and IDDM, consistent with the presence of one recessive gene responsible for both phenotypes. The animals had all been housed under SPF conditions with approximately 95% penetrance of diabetes in lymphopenic animals and no occurrences of diabetes in the DR line[16]. These results indicate the presence of one susceptibility gene in addition to the one located in the RT1 complex. Subsequently, it was demonstrated through crosses between DP BB rats and non-diabetic Fischer rats, as well as RT1-congenic ACI rats that there is at least one additional factor influencing diabetes development in the rat[15,83].

CANDIDATE GENES AND SUSCEPTIBILITY LOCI

Genes with unknown functions, which cause genetic disease, can be located and identified through either a candidate gene search or a total genomic search. A candidate gene search has the advantage of allowing one to make assumptions based on known facts about disease pathology and therefore, if successful, greatly reduces the number of loci that need to be analyzed. A likely candidate gene for the disease is selected and subsequently investigated at the DNA level to determine if an association between the genotype and the disease phenotype is present. The disadvantage of this method is that the assumptions made regarding the nature of the disease might not be true, so that the gene may not be one of interest. This is especially true for complex disorders, involving intricate physiological pathways such as glucose regulation and immune response mechanisms. Few candidate gene searches have been successful. The finding of linkage of the glucokinase gene on human chromosome 7 to maturity onset diabetes of the young (MODY) may be an exception[84].

In contrast to a candidate gene search, a total genomic search does not make any assumptions regarding pathology or gene functions. Several polymorphic markers, evenly distributed throughout the genome, are typed and it is determined whether linkage is present between any of the markers and the disease phenotype. This method involves generating a vast amount of genotyping information, but is frequently rewarded with success. Phenotypic traits have been successfully mapped using this method in several different species[15,85–87].

The RT6 cell surface antigen in the rat is present on 60–70% of peripheral T cells, whereas it is absent from bone marrow cells and thymocytes. Both CD4 positive cells and CD8 positive cells possess this antigen, which can be viewed as a maturation antigen, appearing on cells after the expression of CD4 positive and CD8 positive antigens. Greiner and co-workers showed that lymphopenia in the DP BB rat was due in large part to the absence of cells expressing this antigen[50]. It was however not clear whether the association was functional or a secondary phenomenon. Subsequently, it was shown[88] that the RT6 gene, located on rat chromosome 1 close to the albino locus, was not linked to either lymphopenia or diabetes in the BB rat. Using the albino phenotype as a marker, it was determined that the lymphopenic phenotype does not co-segregate with the albino locus and that the absence of RT6 positive cells in lymphopenic rats is most likely a secondary effect of the disease[88].

Bell and co-workers suggested that a polymorphic locus close to the human insulin gene was associated with IDDM[89]. This association has since been found to be present in numerous different study populations, whereas linkage cannot be reproduced[90]. Although four separate alleles of the insulin I gene were identified, it could not be demonstrated that any of these was significantly associated with IDDM in the BB rat[91].

Due to the autoimmune nature of IDDM, genes in the glucose regulatory pathway and genes active for the immune system would be excellent candidates. The severe lymphopenia in the BB rat suggests that genetic factors controlling T-cell development be important. Below, we will discuss the approach to disclose susceptibility loci for IDDM in the BB rat. Although two loci that are linked to the disease have now been identified, the genes underlying these defects are as of this date unknown.

THE MAJOR HISTOCOMPATIBILITY COMPLEX—RT1

After the primary finding that IDDM in the BB rat was associated with the RT1 complex, attempts were made to define the exact region of the complex where the susceptibility gene was located. It has now been shown that the genes responsible for disease map to the class II region of the RT1 complex and that disease can develop irrespective of the genotype in the class I region[4]. In a linkage study, Jacob and co-workers showed that IDDM was not only associated but also linked to the RT1 complex on rat chromosome 20. Results from crosses between DP BB rats and non-diabetic Lewis rats showed that although 25% of F2 progeny still developed lymphopenia, penetrance of IDDM in lymphopenic animals was only approximately 50%. In lymphopenic animals possessing two copies of the RT1u-allele present in the BB rat, the penetrance of IDDM was 80% compared to 15% in animals that were heterozygous in the RT1 locus. This indicates that the RT1 complex holds the only major factor controlling diabetes development in lymphopenic animals and that this factor acts in a semi-dominant fashion. Although at first glance the finding of two susceptibility loci might seem contradictory to Markholst's finding of only one,[16] we shall see that this is in fact not the case. The reason for this is that DP and DR BB rats in this cross[16] have identical MHC[88]. Both diabetes-prone and diabetes-resistant BB rats possess the u-allele in the RT1 locus. Also, importantly, it has shown that MHC class I and class II probes fail to detect any polymorphism between DP and DR that is associated with diabetes[16]. This indicates that DR possesses the RT1 susceptibility gene present in DP and that any gene identified in this cross would be of non-RT1 origin.

Todd and co-workers suggested in 1987 that the region around amino acid 57 in the DQβ locus influences development of IDDM in humans of Caucasian origin[92]. An enrichment of alleles carrying a non-charged amino acid residue, non-aspartate in particular, in position 57 was seen in diabetic subjects compared to controls. Molecular analysis of the BB rat RT1 complex reveals that the region around position 57 in the class II β chains appears to be in common between diabetes-prone BB rats and other non-diabetic rat strains, implying that the position 57 aspartate hypothesis is an oversimplification and does not apply to the BB rat IDDM[93].

THE LYMPHOPENIA GENE

Lymphopenia appears to be required and sufficient for development of IDDM in crosses between DP and DR BB rats[16]. From crosses between DP BB rats and other non-diabetogenic, non-RT1-identical rat strains, it is obvious that although several loci are involved in development of IDDM, lymphopenia segregates as a recessive trait independently of the RT1 complex[16]. Jacob and co-workers mapped this gene to rat chromosome 4, to a region very close to the neuropeptide Y gene. Although strong linkage has been determined, the gene per se has not yet been identified[15].

THE THIRD FACTOR

Whereas two separate factors have been located that control diabetes developed in the BB rat, it has been shown by several different researchers that these may not be sufficient. A third factor was implicated[15]. This third factor has not yet been mapped and its location and function remain unknown.

CONCLUSIONS AND FUTURE DEVELOPMENTS

The etiology and pathogenesis of insulin-dependent diabetes mellitus (IDDM) is not understood—a factor which complicates attempts to predict the disease. Genetic factors are important but not sufficient and the interactions between genetic susceptibility factors and the environment seem crucial. Animals developing diabetes are therefore useful to understand factors, genetic and environmental, which control IDDM development. The BB rat offers a unique possibility to dissect genetic factors which are linked to the development of IDDM. As in other species, humans and the NOD mouse, IDDM is a multifactorial disease. Following more than 30 generations of inbreeding and maintenance in specific pathogen free (SPF) facilities with complete penetrance of the disease, it was possible to develop a line of BB rats with Mendelian mode of IDDM inheritance. In SPF, the diabetes pathogenesis appears programmed to include the spontaneous formation of autoantibodies by days 20–30, infiltration of macrophages in the islets of Langerhans by days 40–50 and a development of insulitis (infiltration of T and B lymphocytes) shortly thereafter. The insulitis is strongly associated with 80–90% loss of beta cells and a subsequent clinical onset of IDDM. In SPF conditions, inbred BB rats homozygous for the diabetes/lymphopenia gene on chromosome 4 (*iddm1*) and for the u/u MHC specificity on chromosome 20 (*iddm2*) there is 100% IDDM at days 60–100. Therefore on the BioBreeding (BB) background only two genes are necessary: *iddm1* is linked to lymphopenia, a recessive phenotype which is necessary but not sufficient for IDDM, and *iddm2* is on chromosome 20 and is tightly linked to the major histocompatibility complex locus coding for the class II molecule genes, RT1.B, a homologue to HLA-DQ in man. The MHC factor for IDDM is semi-dominant. The dissection of these genetic factors in the BB rat allows diabetes to be predicted at birth. In crosses with other inbred strains of rats, it is now possible to dissect the series of events in the pathogenesis which lead to islet autoreactivity and overt diabetes. Such studies may be useful to develop novel means of therapy perhaps applicable to human IDDM.

The BB rat has proven to be an excellent model for human Type 1 diabetes. It develops a spontaneous disease that very closely resembles human IDDM. Among the similarities we find an MHC association with disease, an early age at onset, equal disease frequencies in males compared to females and a propensity for other, organ-specific, autoimmune reactions. High penetrance of IDDM has allowed accurate phenotyping, and linkage studies have therefore been successful. The only marked dissimilarity compared to human IDDM is the occurrence of a severe T lymphopenia, present in all diabetes-prone animals at birth. Lymphopenic animals demonstrate a virtually complete depletion of peripheral T cells containing the RT6 maturation antigen. Although lymphopenia is not apparent in human IDDM, it appears to have a profound effect on IDDM in the BB rat as it gives an otherwise diabetes-resistant animal an almost 100% probability of developing the disease. In addition, the gene responsible for lymphopenia is highly interesting from an immunological point of view as it alone appears to control normal maturation of thymocytes. Two susceptibility loci have so far been identified for BB rat IDDM. One, located on rat chromosome 4, is linked to lymphopenia and alone controls diabetes development in crosses between DP and DR animals. The second susceptibility locus is located on rat chromosome 20, in the RT1 complex, which is the rat MHC. In concordance with human IDDM, this second gene is located within the class II region. Experiments with congenic strains have shown that the genotype in the class I locus is of no or little importance for disease propensity. In addition to the two factors that have previously been identified, at least one other factor that controls diabetes development must be present. This third gene appears to act in a recessive fashion but its exact location has not yet been determined. The location and identification of the three factors that influence diabetes development in the BB rat should shed light on the autoimmune process leading to β-cell destruction and further on IDDM and may be of great importance for the understanding of the pathological mechanisms for insulin-dependent diabetes in man.

ACKNOWLEDGMENTS

The studies in the authors' laboratories were supported by the National Institutes of Health (grant DK 46620), Magn. Bergwall Foundation, the Bald

Trust, the Greenwall Foundation and the Swedish Medical Research Council (19X-10408). Anna Pettersson was supported by a fellowship from the Karolinska Institute. We thank Sue Blaylock for assistance.

REFERENCES

1 Nakhooda AF, Like AA, Chappel CI, Murray FT, Marliss EB. The spontaneously diabetic Wistar rat. Metabolic and morphologic studies. *Diabetes* 1977; 26: 100–12.
2 Marliss EB, Nakhooda AF, Poussier P, Sima AAF. The diabetic syndrome of the "BB" Wistar rat: Possible relevance to type 1 (insulin-dependent) diabetes in man. *Diabetologia* 1982; 22: 225–32.
3 Butler L, Guberski DL, Like AA. The effect of inbreeding on the BB/W diabetic rat. *Metabolism* 1983; 32(7) (Suppl. 1): 51–3.
4 Colle E. Genetic susceptibility to the development of spontaneous insulin-dependent diabetes mellitus in the rat. *Clin Immunol Immunopath* 1990; 59: 1–9.
5 Mordes PP, Desemone J, Rossini AA. The BB rat. *Diabetes Metab Revs* 1987; 3: 725–50.
6 Crisa L, Mordes JP, Rossini AA. Autoimmune diabetes mellitus in the BB rat. *Diabetes/Metab Revs* 1992; 8(1): 9–37.
7 Rossini AA, Greiner DL, Friedman HP, Mordes J. Immunopathogenesis of diabetes mellitus. *Diab Revs* 1993; 1(1): 43–75.
8 Dyrberg T. Humoral autoimmunity in the pathogenesis of insulin-dependent diabetes mellitus. Studies in the spontaneously diabetic BB rat. *Acta Endocrinol.* 1986; 280(Suppl): 1–29.
9 Lernmark Å, Li S, Bækkeskov S, Christie M, Michelsen B, Ursing J, Landin-Olsson M, Sundkvist G. Islet-specific immune mechanisms. *Diabetes/Metab Revs* 1987; 3(4): 959–80.
10 Colle E, Guttman RD, Seemayer TA, Michel F. Spontaneous diabetes mellitus syndrome in the rat. IV. Immunogenetic interactions of MHC and non-MHC components of the syndrome. *Metabolism* 1983; 32(7 Suppl. 1): 54–61.
11 Elder M, Maclaren N, Riley W, McConnell T. Gastric parietal cell and other autoantibodies in the BB rat. *Diabetes* 1982; 31: 313–18.
12 Dyrberg T, Nakhooda AF, Baekkeskov S, Lernmark Å, Poussier P, Marliss EB. Islet cell surface antibodies and lymphocyte antibodies in the spontaneously diabetic BB Wistar rat. *Diabetes* 1982; 31: 278–81.
13 Bertrand S, Vigeant C, Yale J-F. Predictive values of lymphocyte antibodies for the appearance of diabetes in the BB rats. *Diabetes* 1994; 43: 137–42.
14 Jackson RA, Buse JB, Rifai R, Pelletier D, Milford EL, Carpenter CB, Eisenbarth GS, Williams RM. Two genes required for diabetes in BB rats—evidence from cyclical intercrosses and backcrosses. *J Exp Med* 1984; 159: 1629–36.
15 Jacob HJ, Pettersson A, Wilson D, Mao Y-P, Lernmark Å, Lander ES. Genetic dissection of type I diabetes in the BB rat. *Nature Genet* 1992; 2: 56–60.
16 Markholst H, Eastman S, Wilson D, Andreasen BE, Lernmark Å. Diabetes segregates as a single locus in crosses between inbred BB rats prone or resistant to diabetes. *J Exp Med* 1991; 174: 297–300.
17 Guberski DL, Butler L, Kastern W, Like AA. Genetic studies in inbred BB/Wor rats—analysis of progeny produced by crossing lymphopenic diabetes prone rats with non-lymphopenic diabetic rats. *Diabetes* 1989; 38: 887–93.
18 Eastman S, Markholst H, Wilson D, Lernmark Å. Leukocytosis at the onset of diabetes in crosses of inbred BB rats. *Diabetes Res Clin Pract* 1991; 12: 113–23.

19 Markholst H, Eastman S, Wilson D, Fisher L, Lernmark Å. Decreased weight gain in BB rats before the clinical onset of insulin-dependent diabetes. *Diab Res Clin Pract* 1993; **21**: 31–8.

20 Scheurink AJW, Markholst H, Bouritius H, Lernmark Å, Woods SC. Insulin responses to intravenous glucose challenges in pre- and postdiabetic BB rats. (Abstract). *Diabetes* 1991; **40** (Suppl 1): 466A.

21 Like AA, Guberski DL, Butler L. Influence of environmental viral agents on frequency and tempo of diabetes mellitus in BB/Wor rats. *Diabetes* 1991; **40**: 259–62.

22 Seemayer TA, Tannenbaum GS, Goldman H, Colle E. Dynamic time course studies of the spontaneously diabetic BB Wistar rat: III Light microscopic and ultrastructural observations of pancreatic islets of Langerhans. *Am J Pathol* 1982; **106**: 237–49.

23 Logothetopoulos J, Valiquette N, Madura E, Cvet D. The onset of the progression of pancreatic insulitis in the overt, spontaneously diabetic, young adult BB rat studied by pancreatic biopsy. *Diabetes* 1984; **33**: 33–6.

24 Like AA, Rossini AA. Spontaneous autoimmune diabetes mellitus in the BioBreeding/Worcester rat. *Surv Synth Pathol Res* 1984; **3**: 131–8.

25 Löhr M, Markholst H, Dyrberg T, Klöppel G, Oberholzer M, Lernmark Å. Insulitis and diabetes are preceded by a decrease in β-cell volume in diabetes prone BB rats. *Pancreas* 1989; **4**: 95–100.

26 Beck JC, Goodner CJ, Wilson C, Wilson D, Glidden D, Baskin DG, Lernmark Å, Braquet P. Effects of ginkgolide B, a platelet-activating factor inhibitor on insulitis in the spontaneously diabetic BB rat. *Autoimmunity* 1991; **9**: 225–35.

27 Tominaga M, Komiya I, Johnson JH, Inman L, Alam TJM *et al.* Loss of insulin in response to glucose but not arginine during the development of autoimmune diabetes in BB/W rats: relationships to islet volume and glucose transport rates. *Proc. Natl. Acad. Sci. USA* 1990; **83**: 9749–53.

28 Colle ED, Guttman RD, Seemayer T. Spontaneous diabetes mellitus syndrome in the rat. I. Association with the major histocompatibility complex. *J. Exp. Med.* 1983; **154**: 1237.

29 Komyia I, Baetens D, Inman L, Perrelet A, Orci L, Unger RH. Morphometric and functional studies of islets in diabetes-prone BB/W rats that are discordant for overt diabetes. *Diab Nutr Metab* 1989; **2**: 263–7.

30 Bertrand S, de Paepe M, Vigeant C, Yale J-F. Prevention of adoptive transfer in BB rats by prophylactic insulin treatment. *Diabetes* 1992; **41**: 1273–7.

31 McKeever U, Mordes J, Greiner D, Appel MC, Rozing J, Handler ES, Rossini AA. Adoptive transfer of autoimmune diabetes and thyroiditis to athymic rats. *Proc. Natl. Acad. Sci. USA* 1990; **87**: 7618–22.

32 Weringer EJ, Like AA. Diabetes mellitus in the BB/W rat. *Am J Path* 1986; **125**: 107–12.

33 Kolb-Bachofen V, Kolb H. A role for macrophages in the pathogenesis of type 1 diabetes. *Autoimmunity* 1989; **3**: 145–55.

34 Kolb-Bachofen V, Schraermeyer U, Hoppe T, Hanenberg H, Kolb J. Diabetes manifestation in BB rats is preceded by pan-pancreatic presence of activated inflammatory macrophages. *Pancreas* 1992; **7**: 578–84.

35 Lee KU, Kim MK, Amano K, Pak CY, Jaworski MA, Mehta JG, Yoon J-W. Preferential infiltration of macrophages during early stages of insulitis in diabetes-prone BB rats. *Diabetes* 1988; **37**: 1053–8.

36 Dean BM, Walker R, Bone AJ, Baird JD, Cooke A. Pre-diabetes in the spontaneously diabetic BB/E rat: lymphocyte subpopulations in the pancreatic infiltrate and expression of rat MHC class II molecules in endocrine cells. *Diabetologia* 1985; **28**: 464–6.

37 Walker R, Bone A, Cooke A, Baird J. Distinct macrophage subpopulations in

pancreas of prediabetic BB/E rats. Possible role of macrophages in pathogenesis of IDDM. *Diabetes* 1988; **37**: 1301–4.

38 Jobe LW, Ubungen R, Goodner CJ, Baskin DG, Braquet P, Lernmark Å. Protection from BB rat diabetes by the platelet-activating factor inhibitor BN50730. *Autoimmunity* 1993; **16**: 259–66.

39 In't Veld PA, Pipeleers DG. *In situ* analysis of pancreatic islets in rats developing diabetes: Appearance of nonendocrine cells with surface MHC class II antigens and cytoplasmic insulin immunoreactivity. *J Clin Invest* 1988; **82**: 1123–8.

40 Ono SJ, Fuks A, Guttman RD, Colle E. Susceptibility and resistance genes to insulin-dependent diabetes mellitus in the BB rat. *Exp Clin Immunogen* 1989; **6**: 169–78.

41 Huang X, Hultgren B, Dybdal N, Stewart TA. Islet expression of interferon-α precedes diabetes in both the BB rat and streptozotocin treated mice. *Immunity* 1994; **1**: 469–78.

42 Rothe H, Fehsel K, Holb H. Tumour necrosis factor alpha production is upregulated in diabetes prone BB rats. *Diabetologia* 1990; **33**: 573–5.

43 Wilson CA, Jacobs C, Baker P, Baskin DG, Dower S, Lernmark Å, Toivola B, Vertrees S, Wilson D. IL-1β modulation of spontaneous autoimmune diabetes and thyroiditis in the BB rat. *J. Immunol.* 1990; **144**: 3784–8.

44 Vertrees S, Wilson CA, Ubungen R, Wilson D, Baskin DG, Toivola B *et al.* Interleukin-1β regulation of islet and thyroid autoimmunity in the BB rat. *J. Autoimmun* 1991; **4**: 717–32.

45 Guberski DL, Thomas VA, Shek WR, Like AA, Handler ES, Rossini AA, Wallace JE, Welsh RM. Induction of type I diabetes by Kilham's rat virus in diabetes resistant BB/Wor rats. *Science* 1991; **254**: 1010–13.

46 Davies AJ, Bone AJ, Wilkin TJ, Rokos H, Cole DR. Serum biopter in a novel marker for immune activatino during pre-diabetes in the BB rat. *Diabetologia* 1994; **37**: 466–70.

47 Signore A, Parman A, Paolo P, Andreant D, Beverley PCI. Detection of activated lymphocytes in endocrine pancreas of BB/W rats by injection of ^{123}I-interleukin-2: an early sign of type 1 diabetes. *Lancet* 1987; **2**: 537–40.

48 Jackson R, Rassi N, Crump T, Haynes B, Eisenbarth GS. The BB diabetic rat. Profound T-cell lymphocytopenia. *Diabetes* 1981; **30**: 887–9.

49 Poussier P, Nakhooda AF, Falk JA, Lee C, Marliss EB. Lymphopenia and abnormal lymphocyte subsets in the "BB" rat: relationship to the diabetic syndrome. *Endocrinology* 1982; **110**: 1825–7.

50 Greiner DL, Handler ES, Nakano K, Mordes JP, Rossini A. Absence of the RT-6 T-cell subset in diabetes prone BB/W rats. *J. Immunol.* 1986; **136**: 148–51.

51 Haag F, Nolte F, Lernmark Å, Simrell C, Thiele H-G. Analysis of T-cell surface marker profiles during the postnatal ontogeny of normal and diabetes-prone rats. *Transplant Proc* 1993; **25**: 2831–2.

52 Bellgrau D, Lagarde AC. Cytotoxic T-cell precursors with low-level CD8 in the diabetes prone BioBreeding rat: implications for generation of an autoimmune T-cell repertoire. *Proc Natl Acad Sci USA* 1990; **87**: 313–17.

53 Plamondon C, Kottis V, Brideau C, Metroz-Dayer M-D, Poussier P. Abnormal thymocyte maturation in spontaneously diabetic BB rats involves the deletion of CD4–8+ cells. *J Immunol* 1990; **144**: 923–8.

54 Groen H, Van Der Berk JM, Nieuwenhuis P, Kampinga J. Peripheral T-cells in diabetes prone (DP) rats are CD45R-negative. *Thymus* 1989; **14**: 145–50.

55 Woda BA, Like AA, Padden C, McFadden ML. Deficiency of phenotypic cytotoxic-suppressor T lymphocytes in the BB/W rat. *J Immunol* 1986; **136**: 856–9.

56 Georgiou HM, Lagarde A-C, Bellgrau D. T-cell dysfunction in the diabetes-prone BB rat: A role for thymic migrants that are not T-cell precursors. *J Exp Med* 1988;

167: 132–48.
57 Elder M, Maclaren N. Identification of profound peripheral T lymphocyte deficiencies in the spontaneously diabetic BB rat. *J Immunol* 1983; **130**: 1723–31.
58 Bellgrau D, Naji A, Silvers W, Markmann J, Barker C. Spontaneous diabetes in the BB rats: evidence for a T-cell dependent immune response defect. *Diabetologia* 1982; **23**: 359–64.
59 Kürner T, Burkart V, Kolb H. Large increase of cytotoxic/suppressor T lymphoblasts and eosinophils aroend manifestation of diabetes in BB rats. *Diabetes Res* 1986; **3**: 349–53.
60 Jobe LW, Vertrees S, Wilson CA, Jacobs C, Wilson DL, Picha KS, Baker P, Lernmark Å. In vivo effects of interleukin-1β on blood leukocytes in BB rats prone or resistant to diabetes. *Autoimmunity* 1992; **11**: 233–7.
61 Gold D, Shaikewitz ST, Mueller D, Redd JR, Sellins KS, Pettersson A, Lernmark Å, Bellgrau D. T cells from BB-DP rats show a unique cytokine mRNA profile associated with the *Iddm1* susceptibility gene, Lyp. *Autoimmunity* 1995 (in press).
62 Weringer EJ, Like AA. Identification of T cell subsets and class I and class II antigen expression in islet grafts and pancreatic islets of diabetic BioBreeding/Worcester rats. *Am J Path* 1988; **132**: 292–303.
63 Rabinovitch A. Roles of cytokines in IDDM pathogenesis and islet β-cell destruction. *Diab Revs* 1993; **1**: 215–40.
64 Pollard DR, Gupta K, Mancino L, Hynie I. An immunofluorescence study of anti-pancreatic islet cell antibodies in the spontaneously diabetic BB Wistar rat. *Diabetologia* 1983; **25**: 56–9.
65 Pipeleers D, van de Winkel M, Dyrberg T, Lernmark Å. Spontaneously diabetic BB rats have age-dependent islet β-cell-specific surface antibodies at clinical onset. *Diabetes* 1987; **36**: 1111–15.
66 Dyrberg T, Poussier P, Nakhooda F, Marliss EB, Lernmark Å. Islet cell surface and lymphocyte antibodies often precede the spontaneous diabetes in the BB rat. *Diabetologia* 1984; **26**: 159–65.
67 Baekkeskov S, Nielsen JH, Marner B, Bilde T, Ludvigsson J, Lernmark Å. Autoantibodies in newly diagnosed diabetic children immunoprecipitate human pancreatic islet proteins. *Nature* 1982; **298**: 167–9.
68 Baekkeskov S, Aanstoot HJ, Christgau S, Reetz A, Solimena M, Cascalho M, Folli F, Richter-Olesen H, De Camilli P. Identification of the 64K autoantigen in insulin-dependent diabetes as the GABA-synthesizing enzyme glutamic acid decarboxylase. *Nature* 1990; **347**: 151–6.
69 Karlsen AE, Hagopian WA, Grubin CE, Dube S, Disteche CM, Adler DA et al. Cloning and primary structure of a human islet isoform of glutamic acid decarboxylase from chromosome 10. *Proc. Natl. Acad. Sci. USA* 1991; **88**: 8337.
70 Karlsen AE, Hagopian WA, Petersen JS, Boel E, Dyrberg T, Grubin CE, Michelsen BK, Madsen OD, Lernmark Å. Recombinant glutamic acid decarboxylase representing a single isoform expressed in human islets detects IDDM associated 64K autoantibodies. *Diabetes* 1992; **41**: 1355–9.
71 Baekkeskov S, Dyrberg T, Lernmark Å. Autoantibodies to a 64-kilodalton islet cell protein precede the onset of spontaneous diabetes in the BB rat. *Science* 1984; **224**: 1348–50.
72 Wilkin T, Kisel U, Diaz J-L, Burkart V, Kolb H. Autoantibodies to insulin as serum markers for autoimmune insulitis. *Diabetes Res.* 1986; **3**: 173–4.
73 Markholst H, Klaff LJ, Klöppel, Lernmark Å, Mordes JP, Palmer J. Lack of systematically found insulin autoantibodies in spontaneously diabetic BB rats. *Diabetes* 1990; **39**: 720–7.

74 Dean BM, Bone AJ, Varey A-M, Walker R, Baird JD, Cooke A. Insulin autoantibodies, islet cell surface antibodies and the development of spontaneous diabetes in the BB/Edinburgh rat. *Clin. Exp. Immunol.* 1987; **69**: 308–13.

75 Palmer JP. Predicting IDDM—Use of humoral immune markers. *Diab Revs* 1993; **1**: 104–15.

76 Palmer JP, Wilkin TJ, Kurtz AB, Bonifacio E. The Third International Workshop on the Standardization of Insulin Antibody Measurement. *Diabetologia* 1990; **33**: 60–1.

77 Zeigler B, Klöting I, Besch W, Zeigler M, Hahn I-J. Cytotoxic activity of sera from diabetic BB rats against BB rat islet—a functional study. *Diabetes Res.* 1987; **4**: 67–72.

78 Martin DR, Logothetopoulos, J. Complement-fixing islet cell antibodies in the spontaneously diabetic BB rat. *Diabetes* 1984; **33**: 93–6.

79 Chappel CI, Chappel WR. The discovery and development of the BB rat colony: an animal model of spontaneous diabetes mellitus. *Metabolism* 1983; **32**(7 Suppl. 1): 8–10.

80 Prins J-B, Herberg L, Den Bieman M, Van Zutphen L. Genetic characterization and interrelationship of inbred lines of diabetes-prone and not diabetes-prone BB rats. *Frontiers in Diabetes Research. Lessons from Animal Diabets III.* 1990; IA(4): 19–24.

81 Guttman RD, Colle E, Michel F, Seemayer T. Spontaneous diabetes mellitus syndrome in the rat. II. T-lymphopenia and its association with clinical disease and pancreatic lymphocytic infiltration. *J Immunol* 1983; **130**: 1732–5.

82 Like AA, Guberski DL, Butler L. Diabetic BioBreeding/Worcester (BB/Wor) rats need not be lymphopenic. *J Immunol* 186; **136**: 3254–8.

83 Colle E, Fuks A, Poussier P, Eduard P, Guttman RD. Polygenic nature of spontaneous diabetes in the rat—permissive MHC haplotype and presence of the lymphopenic trait of the BB rat are not sufficient to produce susceptibility. *Diabetes* 1992; **41**: 1617–23.

84 Froguel P, Vaxillaire M, Sun F, Velho G, Zouali H, Butel MO *et al.* Close linkage of glucokinase locus on chromosome 7p to early-onset non-insulin-dependent diabetes mellitus. *Nature* 1992; **356**: 162–4.

85 Bell GI, Xiang K-S, Newman MV, Wu S-H, Wright LG, Fajans SS, Spielman RS, Cox NJ. Gene for non-insulin-dependent diabetes mellitus (maturity onset diabetes of the young subtype) is linked to DNA polymorphism on human chromosome 20q. *Proc. Natl. Acad. Sci. USA* 1991; **88**: 1484–8.

86 Todd JA, Aitman TJ, Cornall RJ, Ghosh S, Hall JRS, Hearne CM *et al.* Genetic analysis of autoimmune type 1 diabetes mellitus in mice. *Nature* 1991; **351**: 542–7.

87 Andersson L, Haley CS, Ellegren H, Knott SA, Johansson M, Andersson K *et al.* Genetic mapping of quantitative trait loci for growth and fatness in pigs. *Science* 1994; **263**: 1771–4.

88 Lang F, Kastern W. The gene for the T lymphocyte alloantigen, RT6, is not linked to either diabetes or lymphopenia and is not defective in the BB rat. *Eur J Immunol* 1989; **19**: 1785–9.

89 Bell GI, Horita S, Karam JH. A polymorphic locus near the human insulin gene is associated with insulin-dependent diabetes mellitus. *Diabetes* 1984; **33**: 176–83.

90 Bain SC, Prins JB, Hearne CM, Rodrigues NR, Rowe BR, Pritchard LE *et al.* Insulin gene region-encoded susceptibility to type 1 diabetes is not restricted to HLA-DR4-positive individuals. *Nature Genet* 1992; **2**: 212–15.

91 Winter WE, Beppu H, Maclaren NK, Cooper DL, Bell GI, Wakeland EK. Restriction-fragment-length polymorphisms of 5'-flanking region of insulin I gene in BB and other rat strains—absence of association with IDDM. *Diabetes* 1987; **36**: 193–8.

92 Todd J, Bell JI, McDevitt HO. HLA-DQβ gene contributes to susceptibility and resistance to insulin dependent diabetes mellitus. *Nautre* 1987; **329**: 599–604.

93 Chao NJ, Timmerman L, McDevitt HO, Jacob CO. Molecular characterization of MHC class II antigens (B₁ domain) in the BB diabetes-prone and -resistant rat. *Immunogenetics* 1989; **29**: 231–4.

94 Francfort JW, Naji A, Silvers WK, Barker CF. Elevated levels of a lymphocyte subset accurately predict the diabetic state in the BB rat. *Pancreas* 1986; **2**: 141–5.

95 Diaz J-L, Daneman D, Martin JM, Sochett E, Wilkin TJ. The relationship between insulin autoantibodies and islet cell histology in the diabetes prone BB rat. *Autoimmunity* 1991; **11**: 45–51.

96 Reddy S, Bibby NJ, Smith PA, Elliott RB. Rat trypsin: purification, radioimmunoassay and age-related serum levels in normal and spontaneously diabetic BB Wistar rats. *Aust J Exp Biol Med Sci* 1985; **63**: 667–81.

97 Pitkänen OM, Martin JM, Hallman M, Åkerblom HK, Sariola H, Andersson SM. Free radical activity during development of insulin-dependent diabetes mellitus in the rat. *Life Sci.* 1992; **50**: 335–9.

13

Lessons from the Animal Models: the NOD Mouse

EDWARD H. LEITER

The Jackson Laboratory, Bar Harbor, Maine, USA

INTRODUCTION

The NOD mouse is distinguished from mice of other inbred strains in terms of its unique predisposition to develop autoimmune, insulin-dependent diabetes mellitus (IDDM). Currently the products of over 60 generations of brother × sister matings, NOD mice inherit the same gender-specific set of susceptibility genes through the germ-line. Thus, IDDM development in standard NOD mice is presumably catalyzed by interactions among a fixed set of (homozygous) polygenes. Because of the extensive characterization of the mouse genome, and its extensive homology with the human genome, mammalian geneticists anticipated that the NOD mouse might serve as a potential "Rosetta Stone" for deciphering the complex genetics of IDDM in humans. In Caucasians, the major predisposing role of specific HLA class II *DR* and *DQ* alleles to IDDM susceptibility has been well-established (see Chapter 2). The higher IDDM concordance rate for monozygotic twins versus HLA-identical sibs suggests the requirement for additional non-MHC genes that independently or interactively convert the HLA-encoded predisposition into overt disease. Genetic analysis of IDDM in humans at the population level is confounded by the etiologic heterogeneity of the disease, and by the genetic heterogeneity characteristic of randomly breeding humans. These difficulties can be partially overcome by linkage analysis in affected sib pairs. However, even analysis of sibs in which 50% of the genome is expected to be identical by descent suffers from an inability to control for environmental

Prediction, Prevention and Genetic Counseling in IDDM. Edited by Jerry P. Palmer.

parameters capable of strongly influencing the penetrance of underlying susceptibility genes. NOD mice are inbred and thus are genetically homogeneous. Within the strain, diabetogenesis has a common genetic origin, and the environmental parameters effecting penetrance of the underlying susceptibility genes (provisionally termed *Idd* genes pending precise identification) can be tightly controlled. NOD mice mate at an early age and NOD females produce exceptionally large litters. All 20 NOD chromosomes have been characterized for simple sequence length polymorphisms relative to other standard inbred mouse strains that are IDDM resistant. Hence, the genetic basis for IDDM in NOD mice is particularly amenable to analysis due to the ease of performing segregation experiments entailing large numbers of affected and unaffected progeny whose DNA can be scanned by PCR-based techniques. Further, the contributions of potential *Idd* loci identified by segregation analysis can be confirmed by producing stocks congenic for genetic markers linked to resistance or susceptibility. The congenic approach permits truncation of the congenic segment (by recombination of linked markers) to the minimum length required to maintain the altered phenotype. The *Idd* gene is then amenable to positional cloning, or its product can be identified by differential display analysis, a PCR-based method allowing identification of mRNAs of differentially expressed genes, or of transcripts that vary in size[1]. Optimism that the genes predisposing to IDDM development in NOD mice might facilitate the identification of homologous loci in humans was heightened by the initial demonstration that, as in humans, MHC class II genes within the major histocompatibility complex were major determinants of susceptibility, and that only one or two other loci controlling insulitis development might be required to precipitate diabetogenesis. This chapter will summarize recent findings demonstrating a much more complex genetic control of insulitis and IDDM development in mice, and will discuss the implications of these findings for genetic prediction of IDDM susceptibility in humans.

THE COMPLEX PHENOTYPE OF INSULITIS IN NOD MICE

The NOD mouse has been especially instructive in regard to exploration of the relationship between insulitis development and the ultimate expression of clinical disease. Insulitis in NOD mice entails the selective destruction of beta cells following infiltration of the pancreatic islets by leukocytes (principally macrophages and T and B lymphocytes). In the NOD/Lt colony at The Jackson Laboratory, overt IDDM develops in ~90% of NOD/Lt females between 16 and 24 weeks of age, and in ~50–70% of males between 20 and 30 weeks. A pervasive leukocytic infiltrate emanating from the pancreatic vasculature and secretory ducts is first observed around the time of weaning

(~4 weeks) when the islets are free of lesions. Swelling of the peri-islet vasculature has been observed prior to leukocyte extravasation[2]. Pancreatic islets are concentrated in the perivascular/periductular areas, with the consequence that large numbers of leukocytes aggregate at the periphery of islets (peri-insulitis). The aggregates usually start at one pole, but eventually surround the entire islet perimeter, with increasing numbers of islets affected as the mice age. Widespread insulitis, entailing the erosion of beta cell mass as leukocytes penetrate into the islet core, develops between 5 and 7 weeks in females, and several weeks later in males. However, *this initial increase in insulitis severity is not reflected by a decrease in beta cell mass*. On the contrary, this early insulitis appears to be partially compensated by a period of islet growth, since NOD/Lt islets during the period between 5 and 12 weeks are quite large in comparison to those of the closely related NON/Lt strain despite the heavy leukocytic aggregations surrounding most of the NOD islets. This increase in beta cell mass in the presence of insulitis probably explains why marked decreases in pancreatic insulin content, and impaired responses to glucose tolerance tests, are not demonstrable in most NOD/Lt females prior to 12 weeks of age[3] and several weeks later in males. This would be comparable to an onset in late adolescence in humans, suggesting that many of the leukocytes in the initial infiltrates present in the peripubertal period may not contribute full pathogenic function until after puberty. Most intervention studies must be initiated prior to this abrupt loss of pancreatic insulin content[4]. Introduction of antigens within the thymus that either accelerate or retard the pathogenic activation of leukocytes in the insulitic infiltrate have been correlated with marked changes in the levels of monokine and lymphokine mRNA transcripts[5,6]. Cytotoxic activation of T cells in the insulitic infiltrates has been proposed to reflect a shift in cytokine balance from those associated with CD4+T-helper 2 (Th2) cells secreting IL-4, IL-5, IL-10 that promote humoral responses to those associated with T-helper 1 (Th1) cells secreting and IL-2 and interferon-gamma (IFNγ) that promote cell-mediated immunity[7,8]. A longitudinal analysis of cytokine mRNA profiles of islet-associated leukocytes has indicated a considerably more complex series of changes. Activation of monokine (IL-1 and TNFα) gene transcription in macrophages is an important early step in pathogenic activation[9-11]. With regard to lymphokine gene expression, increased levels of interferon-gamma (IFNγ) mRNA transcripts are consistently seen in islet infiltrating lymphocytes capable of mediating cytopathic damage[12-14]. IL-12 is a cytokine that drives development of IFNγ-producing T-helper 1 cells. Treatment of prediabetic 8-week-old NOD mice with recombinant IL-12 drastically accelerated IDDM onset[15], indicating the pathogenic consequences of IFNγ and monokine production in the vicinity of the islets. Treatment of NOD females with the immunomodulatory reagent, complete Freund's adjuvant (CFA), leads to increased expression in islet associated leukocytes of mRNA for IL-4[13]. Since

CFA protects NOD mice from IDDM development, the hypothesis that cytopathic activation of diabetogenic T cells entails a shift in the balance of Th1 to Th2 cells is logical[16].

Insulitis is also pathognomic of autoimmune IDDM development in humans[17,18]. However, longitudinal assessment of insulitis development in pre-clinical IDDM by surgical pancreatic biopsy normally cannot be done in humans. The design of IDDM prevention trials is based upon the premise that the pre-clinical period is characterized by a progressive spreading of insulitis throughout the islet mass with a constant (linear) loss of beta cell insulin secretory function until a threshold is reached wherein the output of insulin can no longer maintain normoglycemia[19]. As described above, temporal analysis of changes in islet volume and pancreatic insulin content in NOD mice has indicated a more discontinuous relationship between insulitis initiation and beta cell loss. When the NOD/Shi strain was initially described in Japan, males were distinguished from females by a markedly reduced prevalence of IDDM, although insulitis was reported to be equally prevalent in both sexes. Indeed, certain substrains of NOD mice, such as NOD/Wehi, exhibit a high incidence of insulitis in both sexes, but a lower diabetes incidence compared with the NOD/Lt substrain exhibiting a comparable level of insulitis when maintained in the same environment[20]. Interestingly, the NOD/Wehi substrain develops somewhat higher humoral responses to glutamic acid decarboxylase (GAD), a candidate beta cell autoantigen in both humans and NOD mice[21].

As pointed out by J.F. Bach[22], an animal model of IDDM represents the counterpart of a single human individual reproduced in multiple copies. Accordingly, the differential IDDM susceptibility distinguishing NOD/Lt and NOD/Wehi mice illustrates the individual variation in susceptibility that must be extant in humans; both substrains exhibit comparable levels of insulitis, but cytotoxic activation of cells in the infiltrate is more advanced in NOD/Lt. In first degree relatives of IDDM patients, the immunocytochemical demonstration of persistently high autoantibody titers against islet cell cytoplasmic antigens (ICAs), when coupled with autoantibodies against additional beta cell candidate antigens including insulin, GAD, and a 69 kDa protein (ICA69), is highly predictive of incipient IDDM[19]. However, a recent prospective study of IDDM development in high risk siblings in Finland suggests that, as in NOD mice, loss of glucose tolerance is a late (discontinuous) phenomenon in the pre-clinical process that cannot be easily predicted by linear extrapolations based upon humoral measures of islet cell specific autoimmunity[23]. It is noteworthy that the subclinical levels of insulitis present in diabetes-resistant substrains such as NOD/Wehi can be activated by cyclophosphamide[24], a treatment that presumably reduces suppression of autoreactive T-cell effectors. It is unknown whether subclinical insulitis was present in the pancreas of the majority (70%) of high risk siblings of Finnish

IDDM patients reported in the study cited above that had not yet progressed to overt IDDM. It is nonetheless tempting to compare such individuals to NOD/Wehi mice, and to speculate that differential exposure to environmental "triggers" (analogous to cyclophosphamide treatment of NOD/Wehi mice) may have been responsible for cytopathic activation of the islet infiltrates in the 29.8% of the IDDM converters in the study of Knip *et al.*[23] that progressed to clinical disease.

ORIGINS OF INSULITIS IN HEMOPOIETIC STEM CELL DEFECTS

The severe T lymphopenia present in diabetes-prone BB rats is a defect inherent in hemopoietic marrow progenitors, and is central to the etiopathogenesis of IDDM in this model[25]. Although NOD mice are distinguished from T-lymphopenic, diabetes-prone strains of BB rats in terms of increased percentages of peripheral T cells in lymphoid tissues in the former[26], NOD mice are nevertheless immunodeficient in a number of parameters[27-31]. The failure of NOD T cells to acquire and/or maintain tolerance to beta cell autoantigens has been traced to defects in NOD hemopoietic stem cells[32]. These stem cells are the progenitors not only of T cells that mediate autoimmune beta cell destruction, but also of antigen presenting cells, including macrophages, dendritic cells and B lymphocytes. Both MHC and non-MHC genes contribute to a reduced development of functionally mature antigen presenting cells from myeloid precursors in bone marrow. This functional immaturity, in turn, contributes to their failure to activate immunoregulatory functions that maintain T-cell tolerance to beta cells[33]. These immunoregulatory defects controlled by IDDM susceptibility genes probably operate at both intra- and extra-thymic levels. A number of NOD strain-specific characteristics can be proposed that might interact additively or epistatically to initiate the insulitic process. Delayed involution of the thymus and the accumulation of T lymphocytes in peripheral lymphoid organs possibly reflects defects in positive and/or negative selection in the NOD thymus associated with this strain's unique MHC haplotype ($H2^{g7}$)[34], as well as non-MHC controlled genetic defects in apoptotic mechanisms[35]. Release of T cells from peripheral immunoregulatory control is, in part, attributable to defects in the maturation of antigen presenting cells[33]. Extravasation of leukocytes into the peri-insular region, an early stage in the development of destructive insulitis, could reflect NOD strain-specific alterations in vascular permeability[2], increased macrophage arachidonic acid metabolism[36], increased density of intracellular adhesion molecules and integrins on vascular endothelium, or high levels of chemokines in target organs.

GENETICS OF IDDM IN NOD MICE: PREDOMINANT CONTRIBUTIONS OF MHC

Congenic replacement of the diabetogenic $H2^{g7}$ haplotype with a protective MHC haplotype ($H2^b$, $H2^q$, or $H2^{nb1}$) completely eliminates insulitis and spontaneous IDDM development in NOD mice. This fact, coupled with evidence to be described below that no single non-MHC locus has a comparable effect, firmly establishes this complex locus (*Idd1*) as the major component of susceptibility[32]. This MHC-encoded susceptibility entails multiple genes, and includes both the lack of expression of Ea (homologous to DR α in humans) as well as expression of a unique *Ab* locus (histidine at residue 56, serine at 57, homologous to "diabetogenic" HLA-*DQβ* non-aspartic acid 57 containing alleles[37]). The I-A^{g7} peptide binding site is able to selectively bind and present peptides with acidic residues at their C-terminus[38]. NOD T cells exhibit early spontaneous responsiveness to peptides derived from the C-terminus of both isoforms of glutamic acid decarboxylase (GAD-65 and GAD-67), an apparent beta cell autoantigen to which NOD mice fail to develop tolerance[39,40]. The $H2^{g7}$ haplotype (presumably I-A^{g7}) was capable of high affinity binding and presentation of one of these C-terminal peptides (peptide 35, residues 524–543) following priming in vivo whereas the $H2^b$ haplotype was not[41]. Further, antigen presenting cells from NOD mice naturally process both human GAD-65 and coxsackie B5 viral peptide P2-C to produce a common peptide with a seven amino acid sequence homology which is selectively presented by the I-A^{g7} molecule to CD4 positive T cells[42].

In genetic outcross/backcross analyses, heterozygous expression of the diabetogenic $H2^{g7}$ haplotype is permissive for insulitis development, but an insulitic threshold sufficiently severe to produce the clinical phenotype of diabetes is rarely reached in segregants that are not homozygous for this MHC haplotype[43,44]. Thus, if only insulitis induction is considered, the haplotype functions in a co-dominant fashion with other genetic factors in the NOD strain background. However, when development of overt IDDM is considered, recessive components within this haplotype are clearly recognizable. An example of a recessive-like gene effect is the absence of cell surface I-E molecules on antigen presenting cells due to mutation in the Ea locus. NOD mice expressing a Ea^d transgene at high levels are both insulitis- and diabetes-resistant in comparison to standard (I-E null) NOD mice[45,46]. The mechanism of protection primarily entails peripheral suppression rather than intrathymic deletion of autoreactive T cells[47].

Although immunogenetic analysis has concentrated on the diabetogenic contributions of the MHC class II region of the $H2^{g7}$ haplotype, current evidence suggests that the haplotype as a whole should be considered as contributing to susceptibility. The most compelling evidence comes from the congenic transfer of the unique MHC haplotype of the related CTS/Shi strain on to the NOD/Shi genetic background. The MHC ($H2^{ct}$) of CTS mice apparently contains the same class II alleles as NOD, but distinct class I loci, indicating that loci between these markers may differ as well. When this CTS haplotype was transferred on to the NOD inbred background and compared in homozygous state to segregants homozygous for the $H2^{g7}$ haplotype, a lower incidence of diabetes and insulitis was observed in the $H2^{ct}$ homozygous mice than in segregants homozygous for $H2^{g7}$[48]. The reduced diabetogenic potency of the $H2^{ct}$ thus provides strong support for the concept that, while the class II region is clearly important to disease development, other loci within the extended $H2^{g7}$ haplotype also contribute.

Other regions within the MHC both proximal and distal to the H-2^{g7} class II region contain rare or unique alleles that may also contribute to diabetes susceptibility. Among these are a unique heat shock protein 70 (*Hsp70*) allele[49] as well as rare alleles at *Tap1* and *Tap2* (for transporters associated with antigen processing, and until recently designated *Ham1* and *Ham2*)[50]. The *Tap* gene products are members of a superfamily of ATP-dependent transport proteins. They transport antigenic peptide fragments that are generated by intracellular proteolytic mechanisms into the lumen of the endoplasmic reticulum for association with MHC class I molecules[51]. Mouse and human cell lines carrying mutations in *Tap1* or homologous genes lack the ability to form stable MHC class I–peptide complexes[51]. Both this laboratory[50] and another laboratory[52] observed and reported the same unique polymorphism in a non-coding region of the NOD *Tap1* gene. The interpretations placed on the significance of this DNA polymorphism by the other laboratory deserve further comment. Faustman *et al.*[52,53] failed to observe *Tap1* transcripts from NOD spleen by Northern analysis, and further reported that splenocytes from the NOD mice in their colony were expressing diminished constitutive levels of cell surface MHC class I molecules. These diminished class I levels were inferred to be the consequence of a null mutation in the *Tap1* gene. It was further proposed that the low class I expression was the basis for failure of NOD mice to develop immune tolerance to endogenous antigens, and thus represented the molecular basis for the MHC-associated susceptibility. This latter premise was based upon the claim of glucose intolerance in association with low grade islet-associated leukocytic infiltrates in older 129↔C57BL/6 chimeric mice rendered MHC class I deficient by a "knockout" of the β2-microglobulin (*B2m*) gene. These findings could not be replicated by other laboratories. We had no difficulty in showing normal constitutive expression of *Tap1* mRNA or product[50,54]. NOD genomic sequence encoding the *Tap1* ATP binding domain, a critical component for proper loading of peptides on to newly synthesized MHC class I molecules, was found by yet another laboratory to be identical to that of diabetes-resistant BALB/c mice[55]. It was subsequently demonstrated that the affinity for ATP, the kinetics of peptide uptake, and substrate specificity of *Tap* transporters encoded within *H2^{g7}*, do not differ from that of *Tap* transporters encoded within four other MHC haplotypes[56]. That *Tap* gene function is normal in NOD is also supported by the finding that peptides eluted from their H2K^d MHC class I molecules conform to the known motifs of peptides binding to this molecule in non-autoimmune strains[38]. Neither we nor other investigators have been able to replicate the report of low constitutive MHC class I on NOD splenocytes[38,50,57,58] (Pearce, 1995 # 1554). The explanation for the original report of low class I expression on NOD splenocytes was due to the fact that NOD splenocytes are enriched for T lymphocytes which express class I at a lower density than B lymphocytes[54,58]. When splenic leukocytes of NOD and BALB/c were size-matched, no difference in cell surface K^d density was apparent[54]. Although we have observed a defect in IFNγ-stimulated[31,33,49,50] up-regulation of MHC class I in NOD macrophages, this is a *trans*-effect entailing defective signaling via transcriptional activators. This was demonstrated by finding that IFNγ stimulation upregulates MHC class I expression normally in macrophages from NOR/Lt mice, which share the *H2^{g7}* MHC halotype and hence a common *Tap1* sequence with NOD[57]. Although primary associations between human *TAP2* (and not *TAP1*) allelic variants and IDDM have been suggested[59], these appear to result from linkage disequilibrium with diabetogenic class II alleles[60-62].

Although relatively common, the class I genes (e.g. *K^d*, *D^b*) of the *H2^{g7}* haplotype are nevertheless required for diabetogenesis. In contrast to the claim of Faustman *et al.*[52] that the absence of class I expression causes IDDM in *B2m*-"knockout" mice, the inverse holds. We found in two separate vivaria that IDDM failed to develop in stocks of otherwise genetically susceptible NOD mice in which MHC class I expression and CD8 positive T cells were eliminated by congenic transfer of a functionally disrupted *β2m* locus[63,64]. Thus, when expressed in combination with the unusual class II region genes, the common class I gene products of *H2^{g7}* acquire a diabetogenic function, which presumably is to select and target β cell autoreactive CD8 positive T cells. This pathogenic function appears to be dependent upon expression of particular class I alleles, since the incidence of IDDM is reduced in NOD mice congenic for the MHC haplotype of CTS mice, sharing class II and class III, but not the class I alleles with the *H2^{g7}* haplotype[48].

GENETICS OF IDDM IN NOD MICE; NON-MHC GENES

Congenic transfer of *H2^{g7}* onto diabetes-resistant inbred strain backgrounds such as NON/Lt or C57BL/10J (B10) does not elicit IDDM[32,44]. This demonstrates the requirement for additional non-MHC *Idd* genes. Based upon comparative outcrosses of NOD with closely related sister strains (NON, ILI) versus an unrelated strain, C57BL/6J, it was originally inferred that only 1–2 non-MHC genes, in combination with $H2^{g7}$, were responsible for the development of destructive insulitis and IDDM in NOD mice[65–67]. The NOD derived alleles were assumed to be recessive since neither insulitis nor diabetes was observed in F1 hybrids. More recently, NOD outcross to a stock of C57BL/10J (B10) mice congenic for $H2^{g7}$, followed by backcross to NOD, has been analyzed using simple sequence length polymorphisms to mark proximal, medial and distal regions on all segregating chromosomes[68–72]. This detailed genomic scan revealed a considerably more complex genetic control, with the involvement of at least nine non-MHC loci demonstrated. Of these, two susceptibility alleles (*Idd7,Idd8*) were derived from the IDDM-resistant B10 strain.

Collaborative interactions between this laboratory and those of Drs Linda Wicker and Laurence Peterson (Merck, Rahway, NJ), and Dr John Todd (Oxford, UK) have permitted comparative genome scan analysis of the *Idd* genes segregating in an outcross between NOD with the related NON/Lt strain versus those described in outcross to the unrelated B10 strain[73]. The NON/Lt strain was also made congenic for $H2^{g7}$ to increase penetrance of the non-MHC diabetogenic *Idd* alleles (and thus IDDM incidence) in F2 or first backcross (BC1) progeny. The central question was: would a subset of the same genes segregate in the outcross with NON.$H2^{g7}$-congenic mice, or could different polygenic combinations of non-MHC genes interact with the diabetogenic $H2^{g7}$ to elicit IDDM? Both the backcross (BC1) and F1 intercross were performed in the same environment as the comparable B10 crosses were performed, eliminating the possibility of differential environmental contributions[4]. A low frequency of IDDM (1.7%) developed in NON.$H2^{g7}$-congenic females. This established that MHC was the major component of IDDM susceptibility since, on rare occasions, it could override the combined protective action of all the NON-derived resistance loci. IDDM never occurred spontaneously in B10.$H2^{g7}$ congenic mice. Outcrosses of NOD with NON.$H2^{g7}$-congenic mice produced a markedly higher frequency of disease in the F1 (3.7%), F2 (10.9%), and BC1 (38.7%) generations than had been observed in the B10.$H2^{g7}$ outcross (0%, 0.4% and 9.6% in F1, F2 and BC1 respectively). BC1 analysis is well suited to identifying *Idd* loci where the NOD-derived susceptibility allele is dominant with low penetrance, or is recessive. However, fully dominant NOD-derived susceptibility genes cannot be distinguished in backcross analysis since they would contribute equally to diabetogenesis in homozygous and heterozygous segregants. An F2 analysis overcomes this problem by providing a segregation class in which the resistance allele is present in homozygous state. Indeed, the recovery of 40 diabetic mice in the (NOD × NON.$H2^{g7}$) F2 generation permitted us, for the first time, to compare the effects of *Idd* alleles contributed by the outcross partner strain (NON) in both heterozygous and homozygous state. All previous studies were limited to BC1 progeny wherein the contributions of the outcross partner strain could only be assessed in heterozygous state.

Consistent with previous estimates of the numbers of non-MHC genes that might be segregating when NOD was outcrossed with a closely related strain[65–67], the extremely high incidence of IDDM in the (NOD × NON.*H2*^{g7}) BC1 (46% in females, 33% in males) suggested that as few as two NON-derived resistance genes might be segregating. However, a much more complex picture was revealed by analysis of the genotypic frequencies of over 130 polymorphic restriction fragment length variants (RFLV) and microsatellite markers across the genome in NOD × NON.*H2*^{g7} BC1 and F2 progeny. Diabetogenic NOD-derived alleles at *Idd2* (Chr 9), *Idd3* and *Idd10* (both on Chr 3) were detected in BC1, as was an NON-derived susceptibility locus on proximal Chr 7 (*Idd7*). A diabetogenic B10-derived allele at this locus had previously been observed[68]. The NOD mouse is immunodeficient in several respects (e.g. NK cell function deficient, C5 complement deficient), such that certain contributions from more immunocompetent strains may increase the repertoire of immune reactions available to destroy β cells.

In addition to *Idd2* and *Idd3*, other (dominant) NOD susceptibility loci were identified in the F2 cross; these included *Idd9* (Chr 4), and two newly mapped loci, *Idd14* (Chr 13) and *Idd15* (Chr 5). In the F2 cross, the diabetogenic contribution of the NON allele at *Idd7* observed on BC1 could not be discerned, suggesting that expression of its diabetogenic effect required homozygosity for NOD alleles at other loci (epistasis). However, the F2 cross showed that NON was contributing an allele on distal Chr 6, possibly *Idd6*, that was more diabetogenic than the NOD allele in that region. Diabetogenic alleles at *Idd4* (Chr 11) 5, (Chr 1) and 8 (Chr 14), all defined by segregation with IDDM in NOD × B10.*H2*^{g7} outcross/backcross analysis[68], were not significantly associated with IDDM in the NON outcross. Since the NON strain itself was originally selected for high fasting blood glucose levels, it is not surprising that, while resistant to autoimmune IDDM, the strain harbors certain genes predisposing to glucose intolerance not present in the B10 genome. Because of their common origin, it is also likely that NOD and NON share some deleterious *Idd* alleles. Sequence identity between NOD and NON at the natural resistance associated macrophage protein (*Nramp*) gene, a candidate gene for *Idd5* region on Chr 1, supported this possibility. Sequence comparison of NON and NOD alleles of other potential candidate genes (*Il2* for *Idd3*, *Tnfr2* for *Idd9*, *Fcgr1* for *Idd10*), while identifying polymorphisms, did not definitively identify any of these as actual *Idd* genes. Although the high affinity Fc gamma high affinity receptor 1 locus, *Fcgr1*, expressed by macrophages, was suggested as a candidate gene for *Idd10* because of a deletion in the NOD coding sequence[74], the presence of the wild-type allele in the NON genome did not present as a strongly protective factor in the NOD × NON outcross analysis. Indeed, analysis of recombinant mice showing IDDM resistance in Chr 3 congenic stocks[75] may have excluded the mutant NOD *Fcgr1* allele as the *Idd10* candidate (Dr Linda Wicker, personal communication). No single non-MHC *Idd* gene alone was either necessary or sufficient for IDDM development, and the finding that IDDM in outcross progeny could be elicited by different subsets of *Idd* loci then present in the NOD parental strain underscored the etiological heterogeneity of the murine disease. The chromosomal locations and nearest linkage markers for the known murine *Idd* genes are summarized in Table 13.1.

The comparative study described above illustrates that different subsets of non-MHC genes are capable of interacting with a diabetogenic MHC haplotype to achieve a threshold level of genetic susceptibility required for IDDM development. The subsets of non-MHC loci interacting with diabetogenic components of the MHC, and the strengths of these interactions, are a function of the inbred strain used in the outcross analysis. These conclusions are consistent with similar findings for another complex autoimmune disease, systemic lupus erythematosus, where susceptibility was inherited as a threshold genetic liability[76,77]

INSULITIS GENES

Idd loci on three NOD chromosomes have been reported to control the insulitic process directly. Among these, *H2*[87] exerts a co-dominant permissive effect[32,78], while the two NOD-derived loci on Chr 3 (*Idd3*, and to a lesser extent, *Idd10*) affect the frequency and severity of insulitis[69,75]. Separately, B6-derived resistance alleles at *Idd3* and *Idd10* confer only partial resistance to insulitis and IDDM, whereas together both resistance alleles suppress both insulitis and IDDM almost completely[75]. Certain of the defects in functional maturation of marrow-derived NOD macrophages appear to be corrected in NOD mice congenic for B6 resistance alleles at both *Idd3* and *Idd10* as evidenced by normalized growth and functional responses to myeloid growth factors (D.V. Serreze and E.H. Leiter, unpublished observations). Further, marrow from these *Idd3/Idd10* congenic mice does not transfer IDDM into lethally irradiated NOD/Lt mice, unlike standard NOD/Lt marrow. Currently lumped together as "*Idd5*," two loci on Chr 1 (one proximal near the Il-1 receptor (*Il1r*) locus and another more distal, near the *Bcl2* protooncogene also control insulitis and peri-insulitis respectively[35,69]. *Idd* genes on Chr 9 (*Idd2*) and Chr 11 (*Idd4*) appear to act as "timing" genes[69], determining the rate of activation of cytopathic effectors in the insulitic infiltrates rather than the degree of insulitis. Interestingly, the penetrance of *Idd2* is strongly influenced by undefined environmental factors[32]. This locus has been linked to an androgen-responsive gene controlling T-lymphoaccumulation in NOD × NON outcrosses[79]. Similar to the partial resistance to IDDM in the presence of insulitis observed in stocks of NOD mice congenic

Table 13.1. Currently identified *Idd* loci controlling IDDM in NOD mice

Locus (chromosome, linkage marker)	Contribution of NOD allele to IDDM	Comments
Idd1=H2^{g7} (17)	Susceptibility	MHC class I and II loci contribute; unique *Tap* and *Hsp70* alleles
Idd2 (9, *Thy1*)	Susceptibility	Affects timing of IDDM onset; effect more pronounced in outcross with NON than with B10 or B6
Idd3 (3, *Il2*)	Susceptibility	Controls frequency and severity of insulitis; may be the *Il2* gene itself
Idd4 (11, *Acrb*)	Susceptibility	Affects timing of IDDM onset in B10, but not NON outcross analysis
Idd5 (1, *Il1r*) (1, *Bcl2*)	Susceptibility, insulitis Susceptibility, peri-insulitis	*Bcl2* locus may control reduced susceptibility to NOD T cells to apoptotic cell death. Segregates in outcross with C57 strains, but not NON (which also develops peri-insulitis)
Idd6 (6, *D6Mit+14*, 15)	Susceptibility	NON contributes a gene in this region that is more diabetogenic than the NOD allele at *Idd6*. B10 allele is protective
Idd7 (7, *Ckmm*)	Resistance	Both NON and C57BL strains contribute a diabetogenic allele
Idd8 (14, *Plau*)	Resistance	Diabetogenic allele contributed by B10, but not NON
Idd9 (4, *Nppa*)	Susceptibility	Diabetogenic effect clearly demonstrable in F2
Idd10 (3, *Tshb*)	Susceptibility	Protective effect in B10, but negligible in NON outcross
Idd11 (4, *Nhe1*)	Susceptibility	Observed in outcross/backcross with B6 and SJL
Idd12 (14, *Plau*)	Susceptibility	Observed in outcross/backcross with B6 and SJL; possibly the same locus as *Idd8*, but B6 and SJL alleles are not diabetogenic
Idd13 (2, *B2m*, *Il1*)	Susceptibility	Protective allele observed in outcross with related NOR/Lt stock
Idd14 (13, *D13Mit61*)	Susceptibility	Discovered in F2 cross with NON
Idd15 (5, *D5Mit48*)	Susceptibility	Discovered in F2 cross with NON; *Xmv65* a xenotropic proviral locus possibly encoding a defective retrovirus expressed in NOD beta cells

for resistance alleles at either *Idd3* or *Idd10* (but not both), NOD mice congenic for a C57BLKS/J-derived resistance allele at *Idd13* (Chr 2) show a reduced IDDM incidence despite the development of widespread insulitis[80]. Thus, no single non-MHC *Idd* locus associated with control of insulitis is capable of completely suppressing this complex phenotype in the presence of homozygous expression of the diabetogenic *H2^{g7}* haplotype.

It should be noted that, like other autoimmune-prone strains of mice, autoimmunity in NOD mice is not limited to pancreatic beta cells, but instead is characterized by leukocytic infiltration into a wide spectrum of tissues including salivary glands, thyroid, kidney and gut[27]. However, it is the widespread, destructive insulitis that distinguishes autoimmune disease in NOD mice from other inbred mouse strains with autoimmune susceptibilities. Presumably, this reflects, in part, a heightened sensitivity of beta cells to cytokine-mediated damage[81]. It remains an open question as to whether any of the *Idd* genes described above exhibits a beta cell restricted pattern of expression. Humoral responses to endogenous retroviral gene products are typically found in autoimmune-prone strains of mice, including NOD[3,82]. Initiation of insulitis in NOD islets may represent a response to beta cell expression of xenotropic retroviral antigens encoded by two endogenous proviral loci, *Xmv65* and *Xmv66*[3]. The *Xmv65* locus on proximal Chr 5 segregates with IDDM in the (NOD × NON.*H2^{g7}*) F2 cross (*Idd15* marker). *Xmv66* has been mapped just distal to *H2^{g7}* (this laboratory, unpublished), and thus would be present in all F2 segregants. If retroviral gene expression in either NOD β cells or lymphocytes is ultimately associated with IDDM induction, it would lend support to the hypothesis that T cell activation by retroviral-like superantigens may trigger IDDM in humans[83].

Although peri-insulitis is not unique to the NOD strain (it is present in aging NON/Lt mice), the transition of this phenotype to that of a destructive, islet-penetrating insulitic lesion represents a threshold effect entailing both genetic and environmental contributions. The insulitic damage can be restricted to subclinical levels if NOD mice are exposed to environmental pathogens or immunomodulatory substances capable of up-regulating cytokine communication between antigen presenting cells and T cells[4]. This protective up-regulation is relatively non-specific and is not limited to lymphokines associated with Th2 cells, since IL-2 treatment is as effective as IL-4 treatment in preventing progression of insulitis to overt diabetes[84,85]

GENETIC PREDICTION OF IDDM: LESSONS TAUGHT BY THE NOR/Lt MOUSE

NOR/Lt is a recombinant congenic strain (RCS) which has been rendered IDDM resistant by replacement of approximately 12% of the NOD/Lt genome with that from the C57BLKS/J (BKS) strain[80]. Given the currently available genotyping information for NOR, and given the list of known *Idd* susceptibility loci uncovered by NOD outcross to either NON or B10 (Table 13.1), NOR mice would have been predicted to develop insulitis and be IDDM prone (either spontaneously or following cyclophosphamide treatment). Yet they develop only peri-insulitis, and remain resistant to both spontaneous and cyclophosphamide-induced diabetes[86]. The basis for a major component of this IDDM resistance is *Idd13*, a resistance allele at a heretofore unrecognized locus linked closely to the *Il1* structural gene on NOR Chr 2[80]. Since the protection conferred by the BKS allele was recessive, the existence of this locus could only be demonstrated in an F2 cross and confirmed by producing a congenic stock. Several important lessons can be drawn from the difficulty in predicting the susceptibility of the NOR stock on the basis of known *Idd* genes. First, IDDM risk in progeny of NOD mice outcrossed to different inbred strain genomes cannot be accurately predicted by analysis of a limited set of *Idd* susceptibility modifiers based upon outcross with NON or B10. Each outcross would be the equivalent of a different family pedigree in humans. NOD outcross with other strains of mice, such as CBA, SWR, SJL, or with inbred *Mus spretus* can be expected to uncover more *Idd* loci[87,88]. Indeed, in an inter-specific outcross between NOD and *Mus spretus*, undefined genes in the wild-derived *Mus spretus* genome interact with the NOD genome to produce a Type II non-insulin-dependent diabetes mellitus (NIDDM) in backcross males[89]. Since both IDDM and NIDDM appear in human pedigrees, it is not surprising that, in mice, synergism between genes predisposing to Type 1 and to Type II diabetes can occur to elicit syndrome of glucose intolerance distinct from that characterizing the original parental strain. A second important lesson taught by NOR/Lt is that the non-MHC loci are not necessarily "minor" contributors to susceptibility[15] which can only contribute by additive interaction with a host of other "minor" contributory loci. The NOR/Lt genetic background is particularly instructive to the extent that it produces more normal *trans*-regulation of *H2g7*. Peritoneal macrophages from NOD, but not NOR, show an anomalous down-regulation of MHC class I gene expression after exposure to IFNγ in vitro[57]. Since NOD and NOR share *H2g7*, this difference must denote differential *trans*-regulation. Preliminary gel mobility shift assays confirm that IFNγ induces a more normal patter of MHC class I transcriptional activators in nuclear extracts from NOR macrophages compared to NOD[90]. The resistance allele at *Idd13* alone does not confer insulitis resistance, but does retard cytopathic activation of T cells. This may pertain to the fact that T cells from NOR but not from NOD mice can acquire immunoregulatory function in a syngeneic mixed lymphocyte reaction, a measure of potential T-suppressor function deficient in NOD/Lt mice[86].

ENVIRONMENTAL EFFECTS ON PENETRANCE OF *Idd* GENES

No discussion of the genetic control of diabetogenesis in NOD mice would be complete without addressing the issue of environmental effects on gene penetrance. The issue of whether viral or dietary factors (such as cow's milk protein) are diabetogenic triggers in human populations remains controversial. Because the environments in which NOD mice are maintained can be experimentally manipulated, this mouse strain has provided some rather surprising insights into the ability of environmental factors to modulate the expression of the diabetes-prone genotype. Incomplete penetrance of the strongest of the non-MHC *Idd* genes is indicated by the observation that, individually, none is essential for conferring complete IDDM susceptibility or resistance. The NOD mouse has provided researchers with the most compelling evidence to date that environmental factors are important modulators of *Idd* gene functions. Incidence of diabetes in NOD females in most colonies is usually >80% by 30 weeks of age. In contrast, male incidence is highly variable among colonies, commonly varying between <10% and 70%. The environment accounts for a major component of this variation[28,91]. Hence, diabetes incidence in NOD males serves as a useful indicator of the presence of environmental factors affecting the penetrance of this strain's genetic susceptibility to IDDM. Transfer of NOD males from a conventional mouseroom in Japan into germ-free conditions raised the male diabetes incidence from 6% to 70%[92]. Exposure of NOD mice to a variety of murine viruses (encephalomyocarditis virus, lymphocytic choriomeningitis virus, and murine hepatitis virus) prevents diabetes development[93–95]. These infectious agents apparently protect by providing general immunostimulation since treatment of pre-diabetic NOD mice with various types of exogenous immunomodulators, including complete Freund's adjuvant, cytokines (including IL-1, TNFα, IL-2, IL-4), and poly I:C all circumvent diabetes development (reviewed in reference 4). Diabetogenic catalysts are also present in natural ingredient diets which contain lipoidal moieties that are absent or present in low concentration in semi-purified diets[96]. The penetrance of the *Idd2* gene appears to be controlled by undefined environmental factors; a stock of NOD/Lt mice congenic for NON/Lt genome in the *Idd2* region shows a retarded rate of IDDM onset at The Jackson Laboratory, but not in Dr Linda Wicker's vivarium at Merck Research Laboratories[32]. Thus, the diabetic phenotype is not solely determined by the underlying genotype, but also by environmental determinants.

Certain peripheral immunoregulatory functions observed to be defective in NOD mice maintained in specific pathogen-free (SPF) environments can be ameliorated when mice are maintained in pathogen-compromised environments. Defects in the degree of cytokine-elicited differentiation of antigen presenting cells from bone marrow have been associated with inefficient presentation of self-antigens[33,57]. Inefficient presentation of self-antigens by NOD antigen presenting cells may explain not only the defective immunoregulatory functions of these cells as exemplified by defective T-suppressor cell functions measured in vitro, but also the subnormal secretion of monokines by peripheral macrophages in response to lipopolysaccharide stimulation[34]. Presumably, immunomodulatory effects mediated via environmental components serve to up-regulate certain of these defective antigen presenting cell functions, resulting either in more normal thymic elimination of autoreactive T cells, more potent activation of immunoregulatory T cells in the periphery, or both.

FROM NOD MICE TO GENETIC PREDICTION OF IDDM IN HUMANS

In humans, detection of pre-diabetes by testing for autoantibody development to a variety of islet cell autoantigens, coupled with the demonstration of impaired insulin secretory capacity, essentially means that the autoimmune destruction of pancreatic beta cells has already been initiated. The ability to identify a genotype conferring high risk for IDDM in infants at birth would greatly enhance the likelihood that intervention therapy would be successful if initiated prior to the onset of beta cell damage. The established "high risk" HLA class II genes are so prevalent in Caucasian populations that neonatal screening for these genes at a population level would not be especially predictive of future IDDM development. Although detection of "high risk" genotypes such as DQ3.2/DQ2 in individuals with a family history of IDDM can increase the absolute risk of developing IDDM to 1 in 4[97], most new cases of IDDM occur sporadically. In the absence of a history of familial IDDM, the absolute risk conferred by this genotype increases to 1 in 25[97]. Since the studies in NOD mice and BB rats clearly show that diabetogenesis entails an interaction between a diabetes-permissive MHC and other non-MHC genes, the definition of a relatively limited set of high risk non-MHC susceptibility loci in humans might greatly enhance genetic risk assessment of prediabetes in the presence of a "high risk" HLA genotype. The original hope that elucidation of the locations of the major non-MHC *Idd* genes in NOD mice would allow rapid identification of their counterparts in the human genome has not been realized. On the contrary, the disturbing realization has been gained that, following their disruption by outcross, the specific set of diabetogenic susceptibility genes predisposing NOD mice to IDDM need not be completely reconstituted to elicit IDDM in BC1 or F2 segregants. Thus, the NOD genome contains but one subset of a much larger set of potential *Idd* genes predisposing to autoimmune disease. This explains why it has been difficult to establish fixed patterns of inheritance of IDDM genes in humans, since in mice, diabetogenic thresholds can be achieved through the actions of *variable* combinations of MHC-unlinked genes and a diabetogenic MHC haplotype.

Nevertheless, progress has been made in delineating some of the non-MHC loci in humans regulating IDDM susceptibility[98]. Most notably, findings from several laboratories[99-101] indicate that transcription of the insulin gene or a neighboring gene may be influenced by a variable number tandem repeat (VNTR) polymorphism in the 5'-regulatory region of the insulin gene on Chr 11p (*IDDM2*). *IDDM2* may interact epistatically with *IDDM1* (the HLA complex)[98] although additive interaction has been indicated in a different population[102]. *IDDM2* confers susceptibility independently of HLA associated class II risk alleles in French and Norwegian Caucasian populations and in British Caucasian multiplex families[103-105] whereas no significant linkage for this locus with familial clustering of IDDM was observed in either a Tanzanian black or Japanese oriental population study[105]. In Caucasians, diabetogenic alleles at *IDDM1* and *IDDM2* are estimated to account for ~40–50% of the familial clustering of IDDM in multiplex families (Dr John Todd, personal communication). Table 13.2 lists a subset of the non-MHC *IDDM* loci identified by linkage disequilibrium mapping in Caucasian multiplex families[104,106,107] (Todd, 1995 #1609; Copeman, 1995 #1396; Bennett, 1995 #1471). Evidence for putative IDDM linkage at 18 chromosomal regions were initially observed in a genome-wide scan[104]. Eleven of these loci on 9 chromosomes showed linkage of sufficient strength in affected sib pair analysis to be classified as putative *IDDM* loci. In contrast to *HLA* (*IDDM1*), most of these non-MHC loci made relatively weak contributions

Table 13.2. Partial listing of *IDDM* genes in the human genome with reference to known *Idd* genes in the mouse genome

Human locus (Chr)	Marker	Potential NOD *Idd* homolog (Chr)	Marker
IDDM1	*HLA*	*Iddl* (17)	*H2*[87]
IDDM2 (11p15)	VNTR minisatellite in 5' regulatory region of ISN2	None yet identified (distal 7)	
IDDM3 (15q26)	*D15S107*	*?Idd2* (9)	*?Cyp19*
IDDM4 (11q13)	*FGF3*	None yet identified (distal 7)	
IDDM5 (6q25)	*ESR*	None yet identified (proximal 10)	
IDDM6 (18q)	*D18S64*	None yet identified	
IDDM7 (2q31)	*D2S326*	*?Idd5* (1)	*?Il1r/Lsh*
IDDM8 (17p)	*D6S264*		
IDDM9 (3q21-q25)	J. Todd, unpublished		

to IDDM susceptibility, and, as shown in Table 13.2, only a few of those yet described may represent potential human homologs of known NOD *Idd* loci.

The non-MHC genetic markers for IDDM in humans are discussed in detail in Chapter 3 of this volume. There are a number of reasons why the list of human non-MHC *IDDM* loci in Table 13.2 provides so few homologs for the mouse *Idd* loci listed in Table 13.1. Despite striking similarities in organization of the mouse and human genomes, there are nevertheless important genus-specific differences between mice and humans that must be recognized. For example, as discussed previously, the inability to express I-E proteins on NOD antigen presenting cell surfaces represents a component of IDDM susceptibility conferred by the MHC class II region. This inability to produce I-E antigens, however, is not limited to NOD since a number of other inbred mouse strains without autoimmune susceptibility share a common defect in the $E\alpha$ gene that precludes antigen expression. So the lack of I-E expression in NOD mice is diabetogenic only in context of the unique $I-A^{g7}$ in combination with the NOD-specific collection of susceptibility-conferring non-MHC genes[27]. In humans, gene products encoded by *DR* alleles, the homologs of mouse $E\alpha$ and $E\beta$ genes, are always expressed on antigen presenting cells, such that one would not expect to find a DR^{null} homolog in IDDM patients to match the $E\alpha$ gene defect in NOD mice. A further distinction between genetic susceptibility in NOD mice and in humans can be shown when the effect of MHC heterozygosity is considered. Whereas MHC heterozygosity generally prevents spontaneous IDDM development in mice, the greatest susceptibility for IDDM in humans is conferred by *HLA* heterozygosity for specific alleles (e.g. DQ3.2/DQ2).

It is perhaps not surprising that so few of the mouse *Idd* susceptibility loci yet identified have presented as homologs for the human non-MHC *IDDM* loci listed in Table 13.2. Certain of the non-MHC loci implicated in IDDM susceptibility in mice make relatively small and non-mandatory contributions to overall susceptibility. Likewise, when considered individually, none of the human non-MHC *IDDM* loci described in Table 13.2 are either necessary or sufficient for IDDM development. Under such circumstances, human homologs for all of the mouse *Idd* loci listed in Table 13.1, if they do exist, may be exceedingly difficult to detect by linkage disequilibrium analyses. The VNTR polymorphisms defining alleles at the *IDDM2* locus represent the strongest of the non-MHC loci yet detected in human genome wide scans[98]. It might be anticipated that if any non-MHC susceptibility locus were common to NOD mice and Caucasians, it would be this locus. Yet no mouse *Idd* homolog for *IDDM2* in humans has yet been identified in segregation analysis using NOD mice (either on distal Chr 7, the site of the *Ins2* gene which is the homolog of human *INS*, or Chr 19, the site of *Ins1*, the second expressed insulin gene in mice). Interestingly, a locus controlling diet-induced hyperinsulinemia in a

C57BL/6J mouse model of non-insulin dependent diabetes mellitus (NIDDM) has been identified on distal Chr. 7[108].

The search for human non-MHC *IDDM* genes is still at an early stage. As more are identified, and their genetic map positions refined, more loci homologous to known *Idd* regions in the mouse may become apparent. The indication that *IDDM2* may regulate endocrine function of the beta cells rather than immune functions of lymphoid cells illustrates the possibility (probability?) that inheritance of an IDDM-susceptible genotype will entail complex interactions among a broad spectrum of genes, some of which may be equally important in contributing to NIDDM susceptibility. In multi-generational pedigrees showing a history of diabetes (usually cases of both IDDM and NIDDM are present), heterogeneous admixtures of polygenes affecting glucose homeostasis must be reassorting from generation to generation. Although many of these polygenes must be involved in the maintenance of tolerance to self-antigens, certain of them could also regulate endocrine function of a variety of tissues whose products are associated with glucose metabolism. Glucokinase is a key enzyme in the metabolism of glucose in beta cells and liver, and mutations in the glucokinase (*GCK*) gene have been associated with one form of NIDDM. Mutations affecting the normal activity of genes generally associated with susceptibility to development of NIDDM, like the *GCK* gene (or a gene tightly linked to it), may enhance the penetrance of different subsets of polygenes predisposing to development of IDDM as well[109]. This phenomenon is modelled by the remarkably high incidence of IDDM in both F2 and backcross generations following outcross between NOD/Lt and NON/Lt, a strain exhibiting a latent form of NIDDM[28,68]. The penetrance of susceptibility genes within these changing polygenic combinations likely is responsive to different thresholds of intragenic as well as environmental influences. In many instances (perhaps typified by the IDDM-associated variants in the upstream region of the insulin locus), the disease-associated allele may be a common polymorphism that, in the absence of other genetic/environmental risk factors, is not particularly deleterious. In the NOD mouse, the contribution of a putative *Idd* susceptibility locus to development of insulitis and IDDM, and elucidation of its function, can be achieved by construction of congenic stocks into which the resistance allele from a diabetes-resistant donor strain has been introgressed. Further, the studies in mice can be done under strictly controlled environmental conditions so that the influence of environment of gene penetrances can be assessed. Human geneticists have no such advantages. Under these circumstances, it remains to be seen whether the small additional risk associated with diabetogenic alleles at individual non-MHC *IDDM* loci will provide sufficient additional predictive power to permit intervention studies at the earliest preclinical phase.

In conclusion, it appears that the MHC-non-MHC gene interactions underlying diabetogenesis in a randomly breeding human population will certainly be as complex as was demonstrated in the breeding studies with NOD mice. This complexity does not bode well for the notion that genetic prediction of non-MHC IDDM susceptibility in humans will simply be a matter of identifying human homologs for the NOD's non-MHC *Idd* loci. Nevertheless, early identification of important IDDM- predisposing genes in children by genome-wide scan procedures, coupled with a better understanding of what environmental factors modulate their penetrance, may stimulate the development of new therapies that will retard or prevent the eventual development of this disease.

ACKNOWLEDGMENTS

This chapter has been supported by NIH grants DK 36175 and DK27722, and a grant from The Juvenile Diabetes Foundation, International. The author thanks Drs David Serreze, Len Shultz, Linda Wicker, and John Todd for helpful discussions.

REFERENCES

1 Liang P, Averbouck L, Pardee AB. Distribution and cloning of eukaryotic mRNAs by means of differential display: refinements and optimization. *Nuc. Acids. Res.* 1993; 21: 3269–75.
2 Jansen A, Homo-Delarche F, Hooijkaas H, Leenen PJ, Dardenne M, Drexhage HA. Immunohistochemical characterization of monocytes-macrophages and dendritic cells involved in the initition of the insulitis and β-cell destruction in NOD mice. *Diabetes* 1994; 43: 667–75.
3 Gaskins H, Prochazka M, Hamaguchi K, Serreze D, Leiter E. Beta cell expression of endogenous xenotropic retrovirus distinguishes diabetes susceptible NOD/Lt from resistant NON/Lt mice. *J. Clin. Invest.* 1992; 90: 2220–7.
4 Bowman M, Leiter E, Atkinson M. Autoimmune diabetes in NOD mice: a genetic programme interruptible by environmental manipulation. *Immunol. Today* 1994; 15: 115–20.
5 Gerling IC, Atkinson, MA, Leiter EH. The thymus as a site for evaluating the potency of candidate β cell autoantigens in NOD mice. *J. Autoimmun* 1994; 7: 851–8.
6 Gerling I, Peck A, Cornelius J, Leiter E. Acceleration of IDDM by intrathymic (IT) injection of a glutamic acid decarboxylase (GAD) derived peptide. *Diabetes* 1994: 43 (suppl 1): 93A.
7 Shehadeh NN, LaRosa F, Lafferty KJ. Altered cytokine activity in adjuvant inhibition of autoimmune diabetes. *J. Autoimmun.* 1993; 6: 291–300.
8 Rabinovitch A. Immunoregulatory and cytokine imbalances in the pathogenesis of IDDM: therapeutic intervention by immunostimulation? *Diabetes* 1994; 43: 613–21.
9 Anderson J, Cornelius J, Jarpe A, Winter W, Peck A. Insulin-dependent diabetes in the NOD mouse model. II. β cell destruction in autoimmune diabetes is a Th2 and not a Th1 mediated event. *Autoimmunity* 1993; 15: 113–22.

10 Mueller C, Held W, Imboden MA, Carnaud C. Accelerated beta-cell destruction in adoptively transferred autoimmune diabetes correlates with an increased expression of the genes coding for TNF-alpha and granzyme a in the intra-islet infiltrates. *Diabetes* 1995; **44**: 112–17.

11 Welsh M, Welsh N, Bendtzen K, Mares J, Strandell E, Öberg C, Sandler S. Comparison of mRNA contents of interleukin-1β and nitric oxide synthase in pancreatic islets isolated from female and male nonobese diabetic mice. *Diabetologia* 1995; **38**: 153–60.

12 Toyoda H, Formby B, Magalong D, Redford A, Chan E, Takei S, Charles MA. In situ cytokine gene expression during development of type I diabetes in the non-obese diabetic mouse. *Immunol Lett* 1994; **39**: 283–8.

13 Rabinovitch A, Suarezpinzon WL, Sorensen O, Bleackley RC, Power RF. IFN-gamma gene expression in pancreatic islet-infiltrating mononuclear cells correlates with autoimmune diabetes in nonobese diabetic mice. *J Immunol* 1995; **154**: 4874–82.

14 Muir A, Peck A, Claire-Salzier M, Song Y, Cornelius J, Luchetta R, Krischer J, Maclaren N. Insulin immunization of nonobese diabetic mice induces a protective insulitis characterized by diminished intraislet interferon- transcription. *J Clin Invest* 1995; **95**: 628–34.

15 Trembleau S, Penna G, Bosi E, Mortara A, Gately MK, Adorini L. Interleukin 12 administration induces T helper type 1 cells and accelerates autoimmune diabetes in NOD mice. *J Exp Med* 1995; **181**: 817–21.

16 Liblau RS, Singer SM, McDevitt HO. Th1 and Th2 CD4(+) T cells in the pathogenesis of organ-specific autoimmune diseases. *Immunol Today* 1995; **16**: 34–8.

17 Gepts W. Pathologic anatomy of the pancreas in juvenile diabetes mellitus. *Diabetes* 1965; **14**: 619–33.

18 Santamaria P, Nakhleh RE, Sutherland DE, Barbosa JJ. Characterization of T lymphocytes infiltrating human pancreas allograft affected by isletitis and recurrent diabetes. *Diabetes* 1992; **41**: 53–61.

19 Eisenbarth GS, Verge CF, Allen H, Rewers MJ. The design of trials for prevention of IDDM. *Diabetes* 1993; **42**: 941–7.

20 Baxter A, Koulamanda M, Mandel T. High and low diabetes incidence nonobese diabetic (NOD) mice. Origins and characterization. *Autoimmunity* 1991; **9**: 61–7.

21 De Aizpurua HJ, French MB, Chosich N, Harrison LC. Natural history of humoral immunity to glutamic acid decarboxylase in non-obese diabetic (NOD) mice. *J. Autoimm* 1994; **7**: 643–53.

22 Bach J-F. Insulin-dependent diabetes mellitus ans an autoimmune disease. *Endocr Revs* 1994; **15**: 516–42.

23 Knip M, Vahasalo P, Karjalainen J, Lounamaa R, Akerblom HK, Childhood Diabetes in Finland Study Group 1994. Natural history of preclinical IDDM in high risk siblings. *Diabetologia* 1994; **37**: 388–93.

24 Baxter A, Mandel T. Accelerated diabetes in non-obese diabetic (NOD) mice differing in incidence of spontaneous disease. *Clin. Exp. Immunol* 1991; **85**: 464–8.

25 Crisa L, Mordes J, Rossini A. Autoimmune diabetes in the BB rat. *Diabetes/Metab. Rev.* 1992; **8**: 9–38.

26 Serreze D, Leiter E. Insulin dependent diabetes mellitus (IDDM) in NOD mice and BB rats: origins in hematopoietic stem cell defects and implications for therapy. In Shafrir E (ed), *Lessons from Animal Diabetes*, Vol V. London: Smith-Gordon, 1995; pp 59–73.

27 Leiter EH. The NOD mouse meets the "Nerup Hypothesis". Is diabetogenesis the result of a collection of common alleles present in unfavorable combinations? In Vardi P, Shafrir E. (eds), *Frontiers in Diabetes Research: Lessons from Animal Diabetes*,

Vol III. London: Smith-Gordon, 1990; pp 54–8.

28 Leiter E. The nonobese diabetic mouse: a model for analyzing the interplay between heredity and environment in development of autoimmune disease. *ILAR News* 1993; **35**: 4–14.

29 Baxter A, Cooke A. Complement lytic activity has no role in the pathogenesis of autoimmune diabetes in NOD mice. *Diabetes* 1993; **42**: 1574–8.

30 Serreze DV, Leiter EH. Genetic and pathogenic basis for autoimmune diabetes in NOD mice. *Current Opin Immunol* 1994; **6**: 900–6.

31 Shultz LD, Schweitzer PA, Christianson SW, Gott B, Birdsall-Maller I, Tennent B, McKenna S, Mobrauten L, Rajan TV, Greiner DL, Leiter EH. Multiple defects in innate and adaptive immunological function in NOD/LtSz-*scid* mice. *J Immunol* 1995; **154**: 180–91.

32 Leiter EH, Serreze DV. Antigen presenting cells and the immunogenetics of autoimmune diabetes in NOD mice. *Regional Immunol.* 1992; **4**: 263–73.

33 Serreze DV, Gaedeke JW, Leiter EH. Hematopoietic stem cell defects underlying abnormal macrophage development and maturation in NOD/Lt mice: defective regulation of cytokine receptors and protein kinase C. *Proc Natl Acad Sci USA* 1993; **90**: 9625–9.

34 Serreze D. Autoimmune diabetes results from genetic defects manifest by antigen presenting cells. *FASEB J* 1993; **7**: 1092–6.

35 Garchon H-J, Luan J-J, Eloy L, Bédossa P, Bach J-F. Genetic analysis of immune dysfunction in non-obese diabetic (NOD) mice: mapping of a susceptibility locus close to the *Bcl-2* gene correlates with increased resistance of NOD T cells to apoptosis induction. *Eur J Immunol* 1994; **24**: 380–4.

36 Lety MA, Coulaud J, Bens M, Dardenne M, Homo-Delarche F. Enhanced metabolism of arachidonic acid by macrophages from nonobese diabetic (NOD) mice. *Clin Immunol Immunopath* 1992; **64**: 188–96.

37 Todd JA, Acha-Orbea H, Bell JI, Chao N, Fronek Z, Jacob CO, McDermott M, Sinha AA, Timmerman L, Steinman L, McDevitt HO. A molecular basis for MHC class II-associated autoimmunity. *Science* 1988; **240**: 1003–9.

38 Reich E-P, von Grafenstein H, Barlow A, Swenson KE, Williams K, Janeway CA. Self peptides isolated from MHC glycoproteins of non-obese diabetic mice. *J Immunol* 1994; **152**: 2279–88.

39 Kaufman DL, Clare-Salzler M, Tian J, Forsthuber T, Ting GSP, Robinson P, Atkinson MA, Sercarz EE, Tobin AJ, Lehmann PV. Spontaneous loss of T-cell tolerance to glutamic acid decarboxylase in murine insulin-dependent diabetes. *Nature* 1993; **366**: 69–72.

40 Tisch R, Yang X-D, Singer S, Liblau R, Fugger L, McDevitt H. Immune response to glutamic acid decarboxylase correlates with insulitis in non-obese diabetic mice. *Nature* 1993; **366**: 72–5.

41 Chen S-L, Whiteley PJ, Freed DC, Rothbard JB, Peterson LS, Wicker LS. Responses of NOD congenic mice to a glutamic acid decarboxylase-derived peptide. *J. Autoimmune* 1994; **7**: 635–41.

42 Tian J, Lehmann PV, Kaufman DL. T cell cross-reactivity between Coxsackie and glutamate decarboxylase is associated with a murine diabetes susceptibility allele. *J. Exp. Med.* 1994; **180**: 1979–84.

43 Prochazka M, Serreze DV, Worthen SM, Leiter EH. Genetic control of diabetogenesis in NOD/Lt mice: development and analysis of congenic stocks. *Diabetes* 1989; **38**: 1446–55.

44 Wicker LS, DeLarto NH, Pressey A, Peterson LB. Genetic control of diabetes and insulitis in the nonobese diabetic mouse: analysis of the NOD.H-2^b and B10.H-2^{nod}

strains. In: Alt F, Vogel H (eds), *Molecular Mechanisms of Immunological Self-recognition.* New York: Academic Press, 1993; 173–81.

45 Uehira M, Uno M, Kurner T, Kikutani H, Mori K, Inomoto K, Uede T, Miyazaki J, Nishimoto H, Kishimoto T, and Yamamura K. Development of autoimmune insulitis is prevented in Ea^d but not in Aβ^k NOD transgenic mice. *Int Immunol* 1989; 1: 209–13.

46 Lund T, O'Reilly L, Hutchings P, Kanagawa O, Simpson E, Gravely R, Chandler P, Dyson J, Picard JK, Edwards A, Kioussis D, Cooke A. Prevention of insulin-dependent diabetes mellitus in non-obese diabetic mice by transgenes encoding modified I-A β-chain or normal I-E a-chain. *Nature* 1990; 345: 727–9.

47 Parish NM, Chandler P, Quartey-Papafio R, Simpson E, Cooke A. The effect of bone marrow and thymus chimerism between non-obese diabetic (NOD) and NOD-E transgenic mice, on the expression and prevention of diabetes. *Eur J Immunol* 1993; 23: 2667–75.

48 Ikegami H, Makino S, Yamato Y, Ueda H, Sakamoto T, Takekawa K, Ogihara, T. Identification of a new susceptibility locus for insulin dependent diabetes mellitus by ancestral haplotype congenic mapping. *J Clin Invest* 1995; 96: 1936–42.

49 Gaskins HR, Prochazka MP, Nadeau JH, Henson VW, Leiter, EH. Localization of a mouse heat shock protein Hsp70 gene within the H-2 complex. *Immunogenetics* 1990; 32: 286–9.

50 Gaskins HR, Monaco JJ, Leiter EH. Intra-MHC transporter (*Ham*) genes in diabetes susceptible NOD/Lt mice. *Science* 1992; 256: 1826–8.

51 Monaco JJ. A molecular model of MHC class I-restricted antigen processing. *Immunol Today* 1992; 13: 173–9.

52 Faustman D, Li X, Lin HY, Fu Y, Eisenbarth G, Avruch J, Guo J. Linkage of faulty major histocompatibility complex class I to autoimmune diabetes. *Science* 1991; 254: 1756–61.

53 Faustman D. Mechanisms of autoimmunity in Type 1 diabetes. *J Clin Immunol* 1993; 13: 1–7.

54 Pearce RB, Trigler L, Svaasand EK, Chen HM, Peterson CM. Levels of Tap-1 and Tap-2 mRNA and expression of K^d and D^b on splenic lymphocytes are normal in NOD mice. *Diabetes* 1995; 44: 572–9.

55 Pearce RB, Trigler L, Svaasand EK, Peterson CM. Polymorphism in the mouse *Tap-1* gene. *J. Immunol* 1993; 151: 5338–47.

56 Schumacher TNM, Kantesaria DV, Serreze DVV, Roopenian DC, Ploegh HL. Transporters from *H-2^b*, *H-2^d*, *H-2^s*, *H-2^k*, and *H-2^{2g7}* (NOD/Lt) haplotype translocate similar sets of peptides. *Proc Natl Acad Sci USA* 1994; 91: 13004–8.

57 Serreze DV, Gaskins HR, Leiter EH. Defects in the differentiation and function of antigen presenting cells in NOD/Lt mice. *J Immunol* 1993; 150: 2534–43.

58 Wicker L, Podolin P, Fischer P, Sirotina A, Boltz R, Peterson L. Expression of intra-MHC transporter (Ham) genes and class I antigens in diabetes-susceptible NOD mice. *Science* 1992; 256: 1828–30.

59 Caillat-Zucman S, Bertin E, Timsit J, Boitard C, Assan R, Bach J-F. TAP1 and TAP2 transporter genes and predisposition to insulin dependent diabetes mellitus. *CR and Acad Sci Paris* 1992; 315: 535–9.

60 Ronningen KS, Undlien DE, Ploski R, Maouni N, Konrad RJ, Jensen E, Hornes E, Reijonen H, Colonna M, Monos, DS, Strominger JL, Thorsby E. Linkage disequilibrium between TAP2 variants and HLA class II alleles; no primary association between TAP2 variants and insulin dependent diabetes mellitus. *Eur J Immunol* 1993; 23: 1050–6.

61 Kawaguchi Y, Ikegami H, Fukuda M, Takekawa K, Fujioka Y, Fujisawa T, Ueda H,

Ogihara T. Absence of association of TAP and LMP genes with type 1 (insulin dependent) diabetes mellitus. *Life Sci* 1994; **54**: 2049–53.

62 Esposito L, Lampasona V, Bosi E, Poli F, Ferrari M, Bonifacio E. HLA DQA1-DQB1-TAP2 haplotypes in IDDM families: no evidence for an additional contribution to disease risk by the TAP2 locus. *Diabetologia* 1995; **38**: 968–74.

63 Serreze DV, Leiter EH, Christianson GJ, Greiner D, Roopenian DC. MHC class I deficient NOD-$B2m^{null}$ mice are diabetes and insulitis resistant. *Diabetes* 1994; **43**: 505–9.

64 Wicker LS, Leiter EH, Todd JA, Renjilian RJ, Peterson E, Fischer PA, Podolin PL, Zijlstra M, Jaenisch R, Peterson LB. $\beta2$ microglobulin-deficient NOD mice do not develop insulitis or diabetes. *Diabetes* 1994; **43**: 500–4.

65 Makino S, Muraoka Y, Kishimoto Y, Hayashi Y. Genetic analysis for insulitis in NOD mice. *Exp Anim* 1985; **34**: 425–32.

66 Prochazka M, Leiter EH, Serreze DV, Coleman DL. Three recessive loci required for insulin-dependent diabetes in NOD mice. *Science* 1987; **237**: 286–9.

67 Hattori M, Fukuda M, Ichikawa T, Baumgartl H-J, Katoh H, Makino, S. A single recessive non-MHC diabetogenic gene determines the development of insulitis in the presence of an MHC-linked diabetogenic gene in NOD mice. *J. Autoimmunity* 1990; **3**: 1–10.

68 Todd JA, Aitman TJ, Cornall RJ, Ghosh S, Hall JRS, Hearne CM, Knight AM, Love JM, McAleer MA, Prins J-B, Rodrigues N, Lathrop M, Pressey A, DeLarato NH, Peterson LB, Wicker LS. Genetic analysis of autoimmune type 1 diabetes mellitus in mice. *Nature* 1991; **351**: 542–7.

69 Ghosh S, Palmer S, Rodrigues N, Cordell H, Hearne C, Cornall R, Prins J-B, McShane P, Lathrop G, Peterson L, Wicker L, Todd J. Polygenic control of autoimmune diabetes in nonobese diabetic mice. *Nature Genet* 1993; **4**: 404–9.

70 Risch N, Ghosh S, Todd JA. Statistical evaluation of multiple-locus linkage data in experimental species and its relevance to human studies: application to nonobese diabetic (NOD) mouse and human insulin-dependent diabetes mellitus (IDDM). *Am J Human Genet* 1993; **53**: 702–14.

71 Chestnut K, Shie J-X, Cheng I, Muralidharan K, Wakeland E. Characterization of candidate genes for IDD susceptibility from the diabetes-prone NOD mouse strain. *Mammal Genome* 1993; **4**: 549–54.

72 Rodrigues N, Cornall R, Chandler P, Simpson E, Wicker L, Peterson L, Todd J. Mapping of an insulin dependent diabetes locus, *Idd-9* in NOD mice to Chromosome 4. *Mammal Genome* 1994; **5**: 167–70.

73 McAleer MA, Reifsnyder P, Palmer SM, Prochazka M, Love JM, Copeman JB, Powell EE, Rodrigues NR, Prins J-B, Serreze D V, DeLarto NH, Wicker LS, Peterson LB, Todd JA, Leiter EH. Crosses of NOD mice with the related NON strain: a polygenic model for type I diabetes. *Diabetes* 1995; **44**: 1186–95.

74 Prins J-B, Todd J, Rodriques N, Ghosh S, Hogarth P, Wicker L, Gaffney E, Podolin P, Fischer P, Sirotina A, Peterson L. Linkage on chromosome 3 of autoimmune diabetes and defective Fc receptor for IgG in NOD mice. *Science* 1993; **260**: 695–8.

75 Wicker LS, Todd JA, Prins J-B, Podolin PL, Renjilian RJ, Peterson LB. Resistance alleles in two non-MHC-linked insulin dependent diabetes loci on chromosome 3, *Idd3* and *Idd10*, protect NOD mice from diabetes. *J Exp Med* 1994; **180**: 1705–13.

76 Morel PA, Dorman JS, Todd JA, McDevitt HO, Trucco M. Aspartic acid at position 57 of the HLA-DQβ chain protects against type 1 diabetes: a family study. *Proc. Natl. Acad. Sci., USA* 1988; **85**: 8111–15.

77 Kono DH, Burlingame RW, Owens, DG, Kuramochi A, Balderas RS, Balomenos D, Theofilopoulos AN. Lupus susceptibility loci in New Zealand mice. *Proc. Natl.*

Acad. Sci., U.S.A. 1994; **91**: 10168–72.

78 Wicker LS, Miller BJ, Fischer PA, Pressey A, Peterson LB. Genetic control of diabetes and insulitis in the nonobese diabetic mouse. Pedigree analysis of a diabetic H-$2^{nod/b}$ heterozygote. *J Immunol* 1989; **142**: 781–4.

79 Pearce RB, Formby B, Healy K, Peterson CM. Association of an androgen-responsive T cell phenotype with murine diabetes and *Idd2*. *Autoimmunity* 1995; **20**: 247–58.

80 Serreze DV, Prochazka M, Reifsnyder PC, Bridgett M, Leiter E. Use of recombinant congenic and congenic strains of NOD mice to identify a new insulin dependent diabetes resistance gene. *J Exp Med* 1994; **180**: 1553–8.

81 Mandrup-Poulsen T, Zumsteg U, Reimers J, Pociot F, Mørch L, Helqvist S, Dinarello CA, Nerup J. Involvement of interleukin 1 and interleukin 1 antagonist in pancreatic β-cell destruction in insulin-dependent mellitus. *Cytokine* 1993; **5**: 185–91.

82 Serreze DV, Leiter EH, Kuff EL, Jardieu P, Ishizaka K. Molecular mimicry between insulin and retroviral antigen p73. Development of cross-reactive autoantibodies in sera of NOD and C57BL/KsJ-*db/db* mice. *Diabetes* 1988; **37**: 351–8.

83 Conrad B, Weidmann E, Trucco G, Rudert WA, Behboo R, Ricordi C, Rodriquezrilo H, Finegold D, Trucco M. Evidence for superantigen involvement in insulin-dependent diabetes mellitus aetiology. *Nature* 1994; **371**: 351–5.

84 Serreze DV, Hamaguchi K, Leiter EH. Immunostimulation circumvents diabetes in NOD/Lt mice. *J Autoimmunity* 1990; **2**: 759–76.

85 Rapoport M, Zipris D, Lazarus A, Jaramillo A, Serreze D, Leiter E, Cyopick P, Delovitch T. IL-4 reverses thymic T cell anergy and prevents the onset of diabetes in NOD mice. *J Exp Med* 1993; **178**: 87–99.

86 Prochazka M, Serreze DV, Frankel WN, Leiter EH. NOR/Lt; MHC-matched diabetes-resistant control strain for NOD mice. *Diabetes* 1992; **41**: 98–106.

87 Morahan G, McClive P, Huang D, Little P, Baxter A. Genetic and physiological association of diabetes susceptibility with raised Na+/H+ exchange activity. *Proc Natl Acad Sci USA* 1994; **91**: 5898–902.

88 De Gouyon B, Melanitou E, Richard M, Requarth M, Hahn I, Guenet J, Demenais F, Julier C, Lathrop G, Boitard C, Avner P. Genetic analysis of diabetes and insulitis in an interspecific cross of the nonobese diabetic mouse with *Mus spretus*. *Proc Natl Acad Sci USA* 1993; **90**: 1877–81.

89 Hattori M, Yamato E, Hirokawa KJ, Petruzzelli M, Makino S, Chapman VM. Male backcross mice of NOD with *Mus spretus* Strain predominantly develop diabetes regardless of MHC homozygosity and heterozygosity. *Diabetes* 1992; **41**: 93A.

90 Serreze D, Chapman H, Leiter E. MHC class I trans-regulatory defects in autoimmune diabetes prone NOD mice. *J Cell Biochem* 1995; Suppl 21A: 154.

91 Leiter EH. The role of environmental factors in modulating insulin dependent diabetes. In de Vries R, Cohen I, van Rood JJ (eds), *Current Topics in Immunology and Microbiology. The Role of Microorganisms in Non-infectious Disease.* Berlin: Springer-Verlag, 1990, pp 39–55.

92 Suzuki T, Yamada T, Takao T, Fujimura T, Kawamura E, Shimizu ZM, Yamashita R, Nomoto K. Diabetogenic effects of lymphocyte transfusion on the NOD or NOD nude mouse. In Rygaard J, Graem N, Sprang-Thomsen M (eds) *Immune-Deficient Animals in Biomedical Research.* Basel: Karger, 1987, pp 112–16.

93 Oldstone MBA. Prevention of type 1 diabetes in nonobese diabetic mice by virus infection. *Science* 1988; **23**: 500–2.

94 Wilberz S, Partke HJ, Dagnaes-Hansen F, Herberg, L. Persistent MHV (mouse hepatitis virus) infection reduces the incidence of diabetes mellitus in non-obese diabetic mice. *Diabetologia* 1991; **34**: 2–5.

95 Hermite L, Vialettes B, Naquet P, Atlan C, Payan M-J, Vague P. Paradoxical

lessening of autoimmune processes in non-obese diabetic mice after infection with the diabetogenic variant of encephalomyocarditis virus. *Eur J Immunol* 1990; 20: 1297–303.

96 Coleman DL, Kuzava JE, Leiter EH. Effect of diet on the incidence of diabetes in non-obese diabetic (NOD) mice. *Diabetes* 1990; 39: 432–6.

97 Nepom GT. Class II antigens and disease susceptibility. *Annu Rev Med* 1995; 46: 17–25.

98 Todd J. Genetic analysis of type 1 diabetes using whole genome approaches. *Proc. Natl. Acad. Sci., USA* 1995; 92: 8560–5.

99 Bennett ST, Lucassen AM, Gough SCL, Powell EE, Undlien DE, Pritchard LE, Merriman ME, Kawaguchi Y, Dronsfield MJ, Pociot F, Nerup J, Bouzekri N, Cambonthomsen A, Ronningen KS, Barnett AH, Bain SC, Todd JA. Susceptibility to human type 1 diabetes at IDDM2 is determined by tandem repeat variation at the insulin gene minisatellite locus. *Nat Genet* 1995; 9: 284–92.

100 Kennedy GC, German MS, Rutter WJ. The minisatellite in the diabetes susceptibility locus IDDM2 regulates insulin transcription. *Nat Genet* 1995; 9: 293–8.

101 Undlien DE, Bennett ST, Todd JA, Akselsen HE, Ikaheimo I, Reijonen, H, Knip M, Thorsby E, Ronningen KS. Insulin gene region-encoded susceptibility to IDDM maps upstream of the insulin gene. *Diabetes* 1995; 44: 620–5.

102 She JX, Bui MM, Tian XH, Muir A, Wakeland EK, Zorovich B, Zhang LP, Liu MC, Thomson G, Maclaren NK. Additive susceptibility to insulin-dependent diabetes conferred by HLA-DQB1 and insulin genes. *Autoimmunity* 1994; 18: 195–203.

103 Lucassen A, Julier C, Beressi J-P, Boitard C, Froguel P, Lathrop M, Bell J. Susceptibility to insulin dependent diabetes mellitus maps to a 4.1kb segment of DNA spanning the insulin gene and associated VNTR. *Nature Genet* 1993; 4: 305–9.

104 Davies JL, Kawaguchi Y, Bennett ST, Copeman JB, Cordell HJ, Pritchard LE, Reed PW, Gough SCL, Jenkins SC, Palmer SM, Balfour KM, Rowe BR, Farrall M, Barnett AH, Bain SC, Todd JA. A genome-wide search for human type 1 diabetes susceptibility genes. *Nature* 1994; 371: 130–6.

105 Undlien DE, Hamaguchi K, Kimura A, Tuomilehto-Wolf E, Swai ABM, McLarty DG, Tuomilehto J, Thorsby E, Ronningen KS. IDDM susceptibility associated with polymorphism in the insulin gene region. A study of blacks, Caucasians, and orientals. *Diabetologia* 1994; 37: 745–9.

106 Field LL, Tobias R, Magnus T. A locus on chromosome 15q26 (IDDM3) produces susceptibility to insulin dependent diabetes mellitus. *Nature Genet* 1994; 8: 189–94.

107 Hashimoto L, Habita C, Beressl JP, Delepine M, Besse C, Cambon-Thomsen A, Deschamps I, Rotter JI, Djoulah S, James MR, Froguel P, Welssenbach J, Lathrop GM, Juller C. Genetic mapping of a susceptibility locus for insulin-dependent diabetes mellitus on chromosome 11q. *Nature* 1994; 371: 161–4.

108 Seldin MF, Mott D, Bhat D, Petro A, Kuhn CM, Kingsmore SF, Bogardus C, Opara E, Feinglos MN. Glycogen synthase: a putative locus for diet-induced hyperglycemia. *J Clin Invest* 1994; 94: 269–76.

109 Rowe RE, Wapelhorst B, Bell GI, Risch N, Spielman RS, Concannon P. Linkage and association between insulin-dependent diabetes mellitus (IDDM) susceptibility and markers near the glucokinase gene on chromosome 7. *Nat Genet* 1995; 10: 240–2.

14

Current Status and Future Prospects for Prediction of IDDM

POLLY J. BINGLEY and EDWIN A. M. GALE
Department of Diabetes and Metabolism, St Bartholomew's Hospital, London, UK

INTRODUCTION

Prediction in science usually starts with pattern recognition and ends with understanding. The movements of the planets across the night sky could be predicted long before they were known to move around the sun. Our attempts at prediction of Type 1 diabetes bear some resemblance to the efforts of the old astronomers (or astrologers?), i.e. we can make increasingly accurate use of our observations to guess at what *will* happen, but not *why*.

Future editions of this book will, we predict, be able to concentrate more on the science of prediction, based on understanding of the underlying disease mechanisms. This chapter, however, will concentrate on the phenomenology of diabetes prediction—how it can be achieved, how success can be measured, the limits of current approaches, and possible ways in which these might be overcome.

OVERVIEW OF CURRENT STATUS

Prediction may be relatively novel in the context of pre-Type 1 diabetes, but it increasingly forms part of the basis of modern medicine. Assessing the risk associated with blood pressure, cholesterol and other potential markers of

Prediction, Prevention and Genetic Counseling in IDDM. Edited by Jerry P. Palmer.
© 1996 John Wiley & Sons Ltd.

vascular disease is now routine and many more otherwise healthy middle-aged individuals are offered treatment for cholesterol or hypertension than would ever (untreated) have suffered myocardial infarction or stroke. If a young person is overweight, smokes heavily, has a high cholesterol and a family history of early onset ischemic heart disease, we would be justified in assigning a high risk of a coronary heart attack, but would scarcely claim to be able to *predict* that one will occur. The term prediction is however now entrenched in the diabetes literature, implying rather more precision and prescience than we actually possess, but we should not fall victim to our own rhetoric. Essentially we are using the same processes to assign risk as those used in other areas of medicine, and our estimates are stochastic, relating to populations and probabilities rather than to individuals and certainties.

Having pointed out the similarities in the methods of risk assessment, it is only fair to add that few areas of medicine can offer as much prognostic certainty as Type 1 diabetes. For example, a child of 10 with an affected sibling and an ICA titer of ≥ 20 JDF units has a 60% risk of insulin treatment within 5 years, rising to 80% or more by 10 years, even before other markers of risk are applied[1]. But, since most IDDM occurs in individuals without a family history of IDDM, only a minority of future cases of diabetes can be predicted with this degree of certainty. Risk could be visualized as a pyramid. At the tip, individual risk is very high, but a high proportion of future cases will come from those at the base of the pyramid who, individually, are at much lower degrees of risk. The ultimate goal of risk assessment is to identify all future cases from the general population (with the ideal of achieving 100% sensitivity and 100% specificity), but at present the task is simply to maximize both.

Diabetes prediction still rests largely upon detection of antibodies directed against beta cell antigens, and an enormous number of candidates have been identified in recent years (Table 14.1). In the 1980s controversy proliferated concerning the value of markers such as ICA and IAA, often based around lack of standardization. The Immunology of Diabetes Workshops (IDW) did a great deal to move science forward in this area, supplemented by clinical initiatives such as ICARUS. As a result novel markers such as antibodies to

Table 14.1. Islet autoantigens 1995

*GAD-65	*Glucose transporter
*GAD-67	*Ca^{2+} channel protein
*Insulin	*GM2-1
*Proinsulin	*Sulfatides
*Carboxypeptidase H	*Hsp 65
*ICA 69	*ICA 512
*38 000 M_r	*52 000 M_r
*37 000/40 000 M_r tryptic fragments	*Bovine serum albumin
	*PTP-IA2

GAD-65 (GADA) have moved rapidly towards standardization. Problems of analysis and interpretation remain with us, however, and papers are still published which reveal lack of understanding of the limitations and appropriate use of the statistical methods available for assessing risk.

In this chapter we will concentrate on the way in which markers are interpreted and applied, and will outline current methods of analysis and their limitations. One major theme will be that *the significance of a marker depends heavily upon the context in which it is employed.* The differences that emerge will often resolve into applications of Bayes's theorem, which at its most simple affirms that the level of risk conferred by a given marker reflects pre-existing risk. It is self-evident that a high cholesterol will be more predictive of myocardial infarction in a 40-year-old with angina and a positive family history than in an asymptomatic individual of the same age. Although the same principles apply it is however less intuitive that, for example, GADAs are less predictive in the general population than in the unaffected monozygotic co-twin of a child with Type 1 diabetes. Finally, the future directions for diabetes prediction will be determined by the natural history of the disease process. The great majority of cases will come from those with no family history of the disease. Some 25% of childhood cases present under the age of 5 years[2], while children diagnosed under 10 bear the brunt of the excess morbidity and mortality associated with Type 1 diabetes[3]. It follows that predictive measures need to be developed and refined within the general population, and applied at the earliest possible age, if they are to lead to effective strategies of intervention.

MARKERS OF RISK

ANTIBODY MARKERS

In this chapter we will briefly discuss the potential importance of some of these markers, which are described at more length elsewhere, before going on to consider how they may contribute to our overall ability to predict IDDM.

ICA

Cytoplasmic islet cell antibodies were first described in patients with IDDM and other organ-specific autoimmune disease[4]. These antibodies to islet antigens that are still incompletely characterized are present in the serum of about 80% of newly diagnosed patients, falling to about 30% 5 years after diagnosis[5]. The observation that ICA can be found in individuals who, many months or years later, develop the typical clinical features of insulin-dependent diabetes forms the basis of the concept of the long prodrome of Type 1 diabetes[6]. Prospective studies in family members, in patients with polyendocrine autoimmunity and in the general population have shown that risk of IDDM is directly proportion to the level of ICA detected[7-10]. Measurement of these antibodies is not easy; in spite of a 10 year programme of IDW workshops and proficiency programmes, assay performance still varies considerably between laboratories. Problems persist both in terms of assay sensitivity and quantification of antibody levels in standardized international (JDF) units[11]. They have however repeatedly proved themselves to be robust markers of risk with amazingly similar survival curves being produced in many family studies[7,8,12]. ICAs are the initial entry criterion in both current major intervention studies, ENDIT and DPT-1. Even with all their technical limitations, their performance as predictive markers will be difficult to surpass.

Heterogeneity within ICA

It is apparent that ICAs are heterogeneous and there are subgroups which carry different prognostic significance according to the staining pattern of the antibodies. Some ICAs stain predominantly beta cells within islets (*beta cell selective* or *restricted* pattern) and are associated with a markedly lower risk of progression to diabetes than ICAs that stain all type of islet cells (*whole islet* or *nonrestricted* pattern)[13-15]. ICAs of the beta cell selective pattern are completely blocked by pre-incubation with rat brain homogenate and this inhibition is prevented by pre-clearing the rat brain with sheep anti-GAD antibodies or a serum with selective ICAs, but not if a serum with whole islet ICAs is used[13]. These findings suggest that the antibodies which give this pattern of staining are directed against GAD.

Other Antigens Involved in the ICA Response

The islet antigens against which ICAs are directed remain uncertain. There are probably several components to the response, each with a different prognostic significance. In early 1995, the major candidates are GADA, antibodies to 37/40K-antigen, ICA 512, and IAA, but the list of possibilities may well have changed by the time of publication.

GADA

Identification of the 64K-antigen as glutamate decarboxylase, the subsequent cloning of the antigen and development of relatively simple immunoprecipitation assays have set the scene for this to become the first anti-islet antigen to be widely investigated. GADAs are associated with increased risk of IDDM in family members[16,17] and in pregnant women[18]. The ease and precision of the test is such that it is tempting to suggest that this should now be used as the primary screening measure, but GADAs alone currently appear insufficiently sensitive for this purpose, particularly in young children. Thus, Bonifacio and colleagues found that the overall sensitivity of GADAs in newly diagnosed patients was 70% compared with 88% for ICAs ≥ 2 JDF units, but GADAs were only found in 65% of children aged under 15 years at diagnosis while ICAs were found in 95%[19]. In certain contexts high titers of GADAs and/or GAD-specific ICAs appear protective. This has been observed in polyendocrine patients[20], while Yu *et al.* report more rapid progression to IDDM in relatives with lower levels of GADAs than in those with high titers and GAD-absorbable ICAs[21].

Harrison and colleagues measured GAD autoimmunity in 31 ICA positive relatives, and observed an inverse relationship between concentrations of circulating antibodies and a proliferative response of peripheral T cells following exposure to the central region of recombinant GAD-67[22]. This observation suggested that the in vivo immune response to GAD is bipolar, favoring either humoral or cellular immune responses. Those with a predominantly humoral response would, on this analysis, have high circulating levels of antibodies to GAD but a weak cellular response, and would therefore be unlikely to develop IDDM.

IAA

Insulin was the first islet antigen to be characterized[23]. IAAs are age-specific markers, almost invariably present in children diagnosed under the age of 5, but relatively uncommon in adults[24]. They appear to identify a high risk subgroup within family members with high levels of ICA, but are of limited predictive value used in isolation[25]. Multiple regression analysis suggests that the effect of IAA is independent, and not simply a consequence of its association with young age[12]. Its future role will most probably be as a useful component of a panel of autoantibodies used in screening for risk of diabetes, but at present its value is limited by the lack of a satisfactory miniaturized assay that can be applied on a large scale.

Antibodies to 37/40K-antigen

Antibodies to the 37 000/40 000 M_r fragments of 64K islet antigens[26] have been found in around 50–70% of future cases is prospective studies[1,17,20]. They are highly predictive in ICA positive family members, discordant monozygotic twins, polyendocrine patients and school children[1,17,20,27], although the complex nature of the assay has limited full evaluation of their specificity.

In the study referred to above, Bonifacio and colleagues used sensitive assays for ICA, GADA and antibodies to 37/40K to examine the combinations of antibodies detected at diagnosis in 100 patients. ICAs ≥ 2 JDF units were found in 88%, GADAs in 70% and antibodies to 37/40K in 54%. All patients with ICAs had either GADAs or antibodies to 37/40K, suggesting that it may eventually be possible to replace ICA measurement by a combination of antibodies to known antigens that could more easily be standardized and applied on a large scale[19]. In this study antibodies to 37/40K segregated strongly with high titer ICA, and their prevalence was increased in children under the age of 10, many of whom were negative for GADA. A similar age-specificity has also been reported from a study of French children with newly diagnosed IDDM[28].

ICA512

This is a recombinant human antigen that was isolated from an islet cDNA expression library by screening with sera from a patient with IDDM. Immunoprecipitation and ELISA assays for antibodies to ICA512 have been developed with reported sensitivity of around 50% at diagnosis[29]. Preliminary reports (E. Bonifacio, G. Eisenbarth, personal communications) suggest that these are valuable new markers with a performance comparable to that of antibodies to 37/40K. Their current advantage over these is that, since ICA512 has already been cloned and DNA is available, it can be incorporated into assays based on immunoprecipitation of in vitro translated antigen similar to those in widespread use for the measurement of GADA[30].

The Cellular Immune Response

Antibodies do not appear to be directly involved in the destruction of beta cells, which is a T-cell mediated phenomenon. It is therefore surprising that they give us such accurate information about the destructive process. This may be due to the fact that antibodies pass freely throughout the circulation, while the T cells that are of greatest interest are confined to the pancreas. Could T-cell characteristics therefore provide better predictive markers? As yet no T-cell marker has an established role in the repertoire of predictive tests. Changes in peripheral blood lymphocytes have been described prior to diagnosis but have been difficult to reproduce in other studies. Most tests are difficult to perform, depend on nonspecific markers of activation and are not standardized. Perhaps the most promising are studies into the dominant T-cell subtype activated in response to a specific antigen. As already noted[22], a proliferative T-cell response to epitopes of GAD may give a better indication of future diabetes than autoantibody titers, but this has yet to be confirmed.

Metabolic Testing

Testing pancreatic function, mainly in terms of the first phase insulin response to an intravenous glucose bolus, is used as a marker of the degree of beta cell destruction. While there is no question that complete loss of the first phase insulin response (FPIR) to below 50 mU l⁻¹ is strongly predictive of early progression to IDDM[31], in the ICARUS dataset differences between lesser degrees of loss of FPIR were of lower significance[12]. Loss of FPIR is useful in staging the disease process and for recruitment for intervention trials, but it is difficult to standardize in multicenter trials. In addition, abnormalities do not become apparent until the late stages in the destructive process (end-stage pre-diabetes) while the logical aim is to intervene before this.

Multiple Antibody Markers

While several antibody markers used in isolation can achieve good prediction in relatives, we would clearly not be making optimal use of the data available if we failed to consider all risk markers in conjunction. Further, it seems likely that combined analysis will allow us to improve on the specificity of markers such as ICA without undue loss of sensitivity, and thus form the basis for more flexible predictive strategies. Antibodies to insulin, GAD and 37/40K were measured in the initial samples taken from 101 family members with ICA ≥ 10 JDF units followed for up to 14 years, 18 of whom subsequently developed IDDM. The overall risk of diabetes within 10 years was 43%. As expected, the addition of IAA, GADA or antibodies to 37/40K each resulted in some increase in cumulative risk at the expense of loss of sensitivity. When, however, all these markers were combined, we found that risk was largely concentrated in the subgroup with multiple antibodies. One-third of the cohort had ICA only, and had a risk of diabetes of only 8% within 10 years. Another 38 individuals had ICA and one other antibody; their 10 year cumulative risk was 27%. Twenty-seven family members had ICA with at least two other antibodies. In this group, from which 14 of the 18 cases came, the cumulative risk of diabetes within 10 years was 88%[1]. The type of antibodies appeared to be associated to the likely time to diabetes. Eight of the nine family members with antibodies to 37/40K developed diabetes within 5 years, whilst those with ICA/GADA/IAA in the absence of antibodies to 37/40K generally developed diabetes after longer follow-up. Another group have since adopted a similar approach initially using antibodies to insulin, GAD and ICA69 and found that 55 of 65 family members who developed IDDM had at least two antibodies, compared with 3 of 52 family members who remained non-diabetic[32]. More recently they have achieved similar results using IAA, GADA and antibodies to ICA512 (G. Eisenbarth, personal communication).

This strategy also looks promising in the general population. We tested IAA, GADA and antibodies to 37/40K in 81 school children with ICA ≥ 4 JDF units and found that 68 had ICA alone and only 7 had either of the other antibodies in addition. Both ICA positive children who subsequently developed diabetes had antibodies to 37/40K and one of them also had IAA and GADA[27]. The presence of multiple autoantibody markers appears both specific and sensitive. Most large-scale testing has been carried out using ICA and GADA and it appears that only a small minority of individuals with either ICA or GADA will have both. In our own study in school children, using comparable thresholds for ICA and GADA (just below the third percentile), we found that only 1 in 30 antibody positive children (0.18% of the whole population) had both ICA and GADA (unpublished data). On the other hand, around 70% of patients with newly diagnosed diabetes have both antibodies[19,33]. The positive predictive value of the combination would therefore be expected to be high. The mechanisms underlying this observation can only be guessed at. Presumably sustained immune attack on beta cells of the type likely to result in IDDM exposes other antigens and leads to a secondary autoantibody response. Whatever the underlying reason, this approach does seem to offer considerable promise of *early* accurate identification of high risk individuals for inclusion in trials of intervention before the major part of the beta cell mass has been destroyed.

Non-progressors

Another possible means of improving prediction of diabetes is to identify combinations of genetic or immune markers conferring protection rather than susceptibility. One promising avenue is identification of individuals positive for DBQ*0602, which appears to confer considerable protection against early progression to IDDM. It is possible that the VPH haplotype on the insulin gene may also have a protective role, at least within the UK population[34] (see below). Detailed investigation of non-progressors in terms of gene markers, humoral and cellular immunity may yield useful information concerning the nature of the immune responses in those who possess markers such as ICA yet do not progress, and consequently may point us towards a better understanding of the disease process in those who do.

MEASURES OF RISK

The two principal questions involved in estimating risk of IDDM are "What is the chance that a given individual will develop IDDM?" and "What proportion of future cases will we be able to identify within a given population?". The methods used are essentially simple, the principles are widely used, but the situation is slightly unusual. In other fields the main consideration is that of *risk*—for example the risk that a smoker will develop cancer—but most of the tests we use identify pathological processes that are already under way. Thus we are really setting out to describe *prognosis*, disease progression rather than disease initiation. For this reason many of the methods we use are derived from the field of oncology.

Certain limitations should always be borne in mind when considering our current ability to derive accurate risk assessments. Relatively few people have been studied—even the pooled data from the ICARUS register are based on fewer than 500 subjects. Analysis has therefore been predominantly univariate although it is becoming increasingly obvious that we are dealing with a complex interaction of risk markers. The length of follow-up in most studies is limited, and many have been carried out in highly selected populations, unrepresentative of the population from which most future cases will arise. Our ability to stage the disease process leading to IDDM remains very limited. For example, autoantibody levels that are raised on initial testing do not usually change during follow-up[35]; we do not therefore know at what stage in the process the individual stands. Metabolic testing may allow us to detect "end-stage pre-diabetes", but from the point of view of prevention this may already be too late.

SENSITIVITY AND SPECIFICITY

The performance of a diagnostic test can be broken down into the proportion of cases of disease it will identify (sensitivity), and the proportion of non-diseased people who will be correctly identified (specificity) (Table 14.2). Even these simple measures are used in a slightly idiosyncratic way in pre-diabetes. As generally applied, they are used to evaluate tests made at a single time-point to identify *existing* disease, as compared with a gold standard—for example a circulating tumor marker as against a biopsy. They therefore require some qualification if applied to tests used to assess risk of *future* disease. They should only be applied to a defined time interval; for example to determine the sensitivity and specificity for disease within 5 years, the whole cohort must have been followed for that time. Instead many studies quote sensitivity and specificity within prospective studies in which there is a

Table 14.2. Sensitivity, specificity and predictive values

	Disease	No disease
Test positive	A	B
Test negative	C	D

Sensitivity=/A+C
Specificity=/B+D
Positive predictive value=A/A+B
Negative predictive value=D/C+D

wide range of length of follow-up. Problems also commonly arise from failure to acknowledge the effects of using small samples. The estimates produced by a study can only be as precise as the number of observations allows. The precision of the estimate is easily shown by providing confidence intervals but these are often omitted, particularly if embarrassingly wide!

Sample size is of prime importance in determining the specificity of predictive markers. To be really useful, a disease marker must have a low prevalence in the normal population. It follows that very large sample sizes are essential if precise estimates are to be obtained. For example, a recent paper found GADA in none of 100 controls. The authors concluded that this was a highly specific marker and that the results were "sufficiently good for the assay to be used prospectively as a screening test to detect individuals at risk of developing IDDM"[18]. The confidence intervals around this estimate of specificity were however so wide (0–3.6%), that their conclusion could reasonably be considered invalid[36].

PREDICTIVE VALUES

These describe the *proportion of people with a positive test who will have disease and of those with a negative test who will not have disease* (the positive and negative predictive values). As with sensitivity and specificity, predictive values must be quoted for a defined time and must include only individuals followed for the whole of that time. These methods do not therefore make full use of the data available: some individuals will have dropped out from the study and others will have been followed in the study for a shorter time. These incomplete data are termed *censored*.

RATES

Rates of development of disease, e.g. cases per person-year of follow-up, can also be used to summarize risk. They are simple but convey no idea of differences over time. For example, a 5 year rate of 50% might mean that all the cases occurred within year one, and that the risk thereafter was zero.

SURVIVAL ANALYSIS

Survival (life table) analysis is a method that makes efficient use of all the available data, allowing for variation in the length of follow-up. In spite of its name its use is not restricted to life and death but can be applied to any dichotomous outcome that occurs only once, for example diagnosis of IDDM. In the analysis "the chance of surviving to any point in time is estimated from the cumulative probability of surviving each of the time intervals that preceded it"[37]. This can be illustrated with a simple example: if half the cohort develop disease in the first year of follow-up, and half of the remainder develop disease in the second year of follow-up, the cumulative risk of disease within two years is 75% (50% in the first year + (50% × 50%) in the second). The points on the curve provide the best estimate of the probability of survival, but here again the precision of each estimate depends on the number of observations on which it is based. This precision, or lack of it, can be illustrated by confidence intervals but these often tend to be omitted. Even in large studies the number of unaffected individuals falls rapidly during follow-up. The Gainesville Family Study screened 4015 relatives and identified 125 with ICA ≥ 10 JDF units, only 24 of whom had completed 5 years' follow-up without diabetes[8]. By definition this problem of falling numbers is worst for the most highly predictive markers, since these identify those individuals most likely to develop diabetes.

MISUSE OF LIFE TABLES

Estimates of risk derived from life table analysis have been used to design both the major intervention trials in pre-diabetes, ENDIT and DPT-1. Considerable caution is needed when applying these estimates prospectively, and we should acknowledge how precarious they are. The ability to detect a treatment effect depends on the rate of progression to disease in the control group, and relatively small errors in calculation can have major implications for the success or failure of the study.

Here we consider some only of the potential pitfalls:

1. *The point of entry may not be comparable*   Life tables are usually constructed from the point of first screening. Some groups, however, have shifted individuals between groups according to the results of repeated testing. Individuals analyzed in this way effectively disappear from one risk category and reappear in another. This can potentially increase or decrease the cumulative risk. Repeated ICA estimation in the same population will tend to recruit borderline positives (those who just fell below the screening threshold at first testing, but exceeded this threshold subsequently); the effect will be to dilute the level of risk within the ICA positive category as a whole. Alternatively, repeated testing for loss of FPIR may exaggerate the significance of the test by transferring the individuals most likely to develop diabetes out of "low risk" categories.

2. *There is distortion involved in applying retrospective data prospectively*   Historical studies estimate risk from time of first screening, but an intervention trial must estimate risk from the time of intervention. The entry points are therefore not comparable, and since the intervention trial will need to confirm eligibility by repeat testing, there will typically be a delay of several months from the first time of testing. This will inevitably mean that

the study group will be depleted of those individuals at highest risk (e.g. those with loss of FPIR) by the time of study entry. The historical study will therefore show a higher yield of progressors (and possibly also of individuals with low FPIR) than the prospective study. Minor alterations in the early part of follow-up may have a profound effect on later risk, and when intervention is contemplated the delay in each group *must* be similar.

3. *Other selection criteria may not be identical*   To give a hypothetical example, the historical analysis may attribute risk to ICA or loss of FPIR in individuals who did not have an OGTT at the same time. Some may therefore have had impaired glucose tolerance (IGT) when entered in the predictive model. If the prospective study were to involve an OGTT and exclusion of IGT, this might be expected to introduce significant variation from the historical model.

METHODS OF COMBINED ANALYSIS AND THE DECISION TREE MODEL

COMBINED ANALYSIS

Markers of high risk tend to cluster together. Insulin antibodies and risk of diabetes are both inversely related to age in first degree relatives[24]. In the Bart's–Oxford study, ICA positive children under 13 years of age were more likely to have high levels of ICA, IAA, antibodies to 37/40K and multiple antibodies—each individually associated with high risk of IDDM[1]. Analysis of the pattern of association (covariation) of many predictive variables has the obvious potential to improve risk assessment. Small sample size has limited this type of analysis and this aspect of risk estimation is in its infancy. The simplest method is to stratify the subjects according to more than one variable at a time (e.g. age and ICA level). As the number of strata is increased, however, the group sizes decrease very rapidly and there is a high probability of type II error. Multiple logistic regression makes it possible to adjust to several prognostic factors at the same time. However, it can only be applied to uncensored data[38]. The dual parameter model used linear regression to estimate time to diabetes but, since the original model was based on data only from those progressing to diabetes, it cannot be used to assess risk, merely the time to insulin requirement if the individual is destined to develop diabetes[39]. The Cox regression model can be used for multivariate survival analysis including censored data, providing the assumptions of the model are fulfilled[40]. This can allow the most predictive combination of markers to be identified. The power of the analysis depends on the number of end-points that occur, and spurious results may be produced if too many predictor variables are analyzed.

DECISION TREE ANALYSIS

This came into medicine as a way of formalizing and improving the process of thought of a clinician confronted with a complex clinical problem. The likelihood of a given outcome can be set out in the form of a stepwise selection procedure, with progressively increasing probability that a given outcome will (or will not) occur. The likely yield from additional diagnostic steps can be evaluated in the light of information already available, and the approach therefore represents a comprehensive application of Bayes's rule. If the pre-existing level of risk is already high, the new test will have a high yield of true positives, few false positives, and a high positive predictive power. Conversely, if risk is low true positives fall and the false positive rate will rise, with a corresponding reduction in predictive power.

The decision tree provides a simple and easily visualized framework within which it is possible to summarize and link a vast and evolving mass of data. The approach forces the user to be explicit, and steps based on scanty data readily become apparent. Potential disadvantages are that it imposes dichotomy in situations where this may not be appropriate. For example, age should be considered as a continuous variable rather than in relation to a given threshold. Further, the decision tree does not allow for interaction between markers of risk except within the context of an imposed hierarchy. Techniques such as multiple regression analysis would be needed to explore this type of interaction.

Applied to Type 1 diabetes, the decision points of paramount importance are family history (a 15-fold increase in risk), age under 40, and ICA. Age justifies an early appearance on the pathway for two reasons. First, it is simple, accurate and cheap to measure. Second, predictive measures seem to lose discriminant value rapidly over the age of 40 and both ENDIT (40 years) and DPT-1 (45 years) exclude older individuals from therapy on the basis of overall decrease in risk. ICAs remain the only marker sufficiently well validated and tested to act as the next step, although we may see alternative tests taking over within the next year or so. In our previous description of the decision tree model[41] we selected a titer of ≥ 20 JDF units, which would confer a 40–45% risk of progression in 5 years in non-diabetic relatives of IDDM patients under 40 years of age. This threshold, however, entails considerable loss of sensitivity, and we would now lower it to ≥ 10 JDF units. The step beyond this will be testing for other autoantibody specificities, particularly GADA and antibodies to 37/40K and/or ICA512. Following this would come identification of potential protective factors, including possession of DBQ*0602, and possibly also now of the VPH haplotype in the insulin gene, which (at least in a UK population) confers a relative risk of 0.28 for IDDM[34]. Long-term risk of insulin treatment may well be established by this stage of the sequence, but metabolic testing will have the added benefit of staging the disorder, with an indication of probability that the disease will or will not develop within the next 5 years (Figure 14.1).

The main limitation of this formulation, already mentioned, is that age behaves more as a continuous variable even within the age-range up to 40 years. A child under 10 years with a first degree family history and ICA is already at such high risk that the additive effect of other markers, although statistically impressive, is actually of limited practical value. As data accumulate, it should be possible to adapt the model to each decade of life to allow for the powerful effect of age. A further comment is that this scheme should not be interpreted as implying that prediction is either impossible or unhelpful in those over 40. High levels of prediction should be possible within this age category, but the yield of such high risk individuals will be much lower than in younger age groups. The cost–benefit ratio of screening within this age category is therefore unlikely to be favorable.

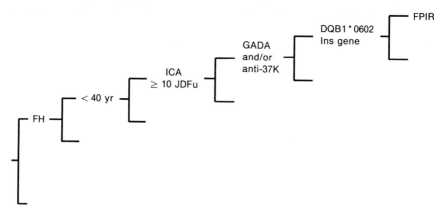

Figure 14.1. The decision tree 1995

Sequential analysis of probability means that it is highly unlikely that any "magic marker" with 100% specificity and 100% sensitivity will be identified. Further it emphasizes that the prognostic significance of any marker varies in populations at differing levels of risk. It demonstrates that adding in further tests has a limited yield once high specificity has been achieved by the preceding steps in the analysis, so that, for example, genetic testing has limited utility in relatives with high titers of ICA. The main test for this type of analysis is in the application of predictive models in populations at very different levels of risk.

RISK ESTIMATION IN THE GENERAL POPULATION

Effective risk estimation is already possible in families, but in order to have a real impact on the frequency of disease we need to be able to predict and prevent within the general population. There are major practical difficulties about this, not least the relatively low level of awareness of IDDM and motivation to do something about it, in the general population as compared with families. A further problem is that much larger numbers of people have to be studied in order to obtain useful results.

The overall risk of developing diabetes before age 20 is 10–15 times lower in the general population than in siblings of children with IDDM and, as already emphasized, the predictive value of a test is greatly influenced by the population in which it applied. We would therefore expect that, even if a marker is highly predictive in family members, it would yield a large proportion of false positives in the general population where the disease is rare. This principle is illustrated by the examples in Table 14.3 in which a hypothetical test with sensitivity 80%, specificity 99% is applied to 1000 individuals from two populations with different disease prevalence. Table 14.3(a) shows a population with a 20% prevalence of disease. The sensitivity of 80% means that the test is positive in 160 out of 200 individuals with disease, and the 99% specificity that the test is negative in 792 out of 800 individuals without disease. The remaining 8 have a positive test in the absence of disease. The positive predictive value of the test in that population (the proportion of those with a positive test who have disease) is 95% (160/168). Table 14.3(b) shows a population with a 1% disease prevalence. In this situation, the total number of true positives is lower while the number of individuals with a false positive test is slightly higher. The predictive value of a positive test is then only 44% (8/18). Similar constraints would be expected

Table 14.3. The effect of disease prevalence on positive predictive value
(a) Population 1 (disease prevalence 20%)

	Individuals with disease	Individuals without disease	Total
Test positive	160	8	168
Test negative	40	792	832
Total	200	800	1000

Positive predictive value=160/168=95% (test positive with disease/total test positive)

(b) Population 2 (disease prevalence 1%)

	Individuals with disease	Individuals without disease	Total
Test positive	8	10	18
Test negative	2	980	982
Total	10	990	1000

Positive predictive value=8/18=44%

to apply whatever test is used, and could only be overcome if the specificity of the test were considerably higher in the low risk population. In this example the specificity in the low risk population would have to be greater than 99.5% to achieve the same positive predictive value as that observed in the high risk group.

In IDDM, with risk around 5% in family members and 0.5% in the general population, we could potentially achieve equivalent levels of positive predictive value if we found a marker that was present in 5% of family members but only 0.5% of the general population. Unfortunately, none of the markers examined to date, including GAD and ICA, has been found to have a 10-fold lower prevalence in the general population than in families.

The specificity of a marker is the major determinant of its positive predictive value, but it is difficult to determine this accurately if the prevalence of the marker is low. An apparently small difference in the background prevalence of a marker can dramatically effect its positive predictive value (Table 14.4). It is therefore essential to reach precise estimates, and this in turn requires large samples. For example, to be 95% certain that the prevalence of a marker is less than 0.5%, we need to test more than 3000 subjects if it is detected in 0.2%, and around 40 000 if it is found in 0.4%! If markers are to be applied in the general population, it is therefore essential to ensure that proper control populations have been studied and to appreciate the implications of failing to do so.

The primary purpose of risk assessment in family studies is the identification of family members at increased risk in order to *test* potential interventions. In this situation sensitivity is less important than specificity. In contrast, the ultimate reason for risk assessment in the general population will be to identify subjects to *treat* in order to reduce the frequency of disease in the community. Any screening strategy is going to be expensive and difficult. Even if the treatment is extremely safe and cheap, the cost–benefit ratio will only be favorable if the sensitivity of the screening programme is high—probably at least 90%. The initial test in any program of serial testing must therefore aim to pick up almost all future cases. The risk pathway is delineated in Figure 14.2.

Table 14.4. The effect of changes in marker prevalence on positive predictive value

Marker	Sensitivity	Prevalence	PPV
1	80%	1.2%	20%
2	80%	0.8%	30%
3	80%	0.4%	60%

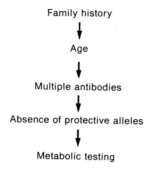

Family history

↓

Age

↓

Multiple antibodies

↓

Absence of protective alleles

↓

Metabolic testing

Figure 14.2. The risk pathway

POSSIBLE STRATEGIES

For the reasons outlined above, the evaluation of predictive markers in the general population is considerably less advanced than in family members, and is subject to many of the problems encountered in family studies in the 1970s and 1980s. Most studies have only recently started and, worldwide, the number of individuals identified in general population studies and followed up to the development of diabetes is probably less than 100. Many of the early studies were undertaken before measurement of ICA and other autoantibodies were standardized, and inclusion criteria vary considerably. Potential strategies are, therefore, for the most part, theoretical rather than prospectively tested.

SCREENING FOR GENETIC SUSCEPTIBILITY

Screening for markers of genetic susceptibility offers a potentially sensitive means of identifying individuals at increased risk but studies large enough to quantify and stratify risk have previously been difficult to perform because typing techniques could not easily be applied on a large scale. Interpretation of studies is therefore limited by the size of samples that have been tested, and also by failure to ensure that controls are rigorously selected from the same population as the cases. Many potential markers have been identified, but few studies allow accurate assignment of risk. Some general conclusions are however possible. Susceptibility alleles are quite common in the general population and only a small minority of genetically susceptible children will develop disease. Thus, the most specific combination of HLA and non-HLA genetic markers is only associated with a 6% lifetime risk of disease[42]. Further, this combination is present in only 30% of cases, so that even this degree of specificity results in considerable loss of sensitivity. A gradient of risk can be defined and, as with autoantibodies, a "threshold" of genetic susceptibility will have to be set to achieve the balance of sensitivity and specificity that is most appropriate for a particular purpose. In a recent population-based Swedish study the highest risk DQ genotype (four susceptibility alleles) was found in 48% of patients and 6% of controls, conferring an absolute risk of IDDM of approximately 3%. Another 38% of patients had three susceptibility alleles. The absolute risk associated with this was 10 times less than that of the most potent combination of DQ alleles, but was still significantly higher than in the background population[43]. Different allele combinations may also be associated with varying age of diagnosis. In a Belgian population-based study the highest risk combination was found in 54% of patients under 10 years of age at diagnosis, but only 30% of those aged 10–19[44]. A Finnish study reported that a panel of DQB markers could be used that identified 82% of cases and was only found in 3% of the background population[45]. These findings have not been confirmed in other populations and illustrate that risk estimates can only be applied in the population in which they were derived. Accurate quantification of genetic risk should soon be possible but will have to await the results of much larger population-based studies than have hitherto been performed.

IMMUNE MARKERS ALONE

The prevalence of ICA in school children has been reported to be greater than the expected cumulative incidence of IDDM in several studies[46–50] although two prospective studies have reported positive predictive values that are not significantly different from those in family members of children with diabetes[10,51]. In our own studies, ICAs ≥ 4 JDF units were detected in 2.8% of 2925 school children aged 9–13 years in the Oxford region. Our incidence data showed that 0.2% of the school children would be expected to develop diabetes within 10 years[46]. ICAs ≥ 4 JDF units were also found in 88% of children with newly diagnosed IDDM in the same region (unpublished observation). We would therefore estimate that less than 6% of the children with ICAs ≥ 4 JDF units would develop diabetes in the next 10 years. We compared this group with 272 age-matched siblings of children with IDDM from the same region. Of these 6.6% had ICAs ≥ 4 JDF units and 2.8% would be expected to develop IDDM within 10 years, so that we estimate that more than 40% of those with ICAs ≥ 4 JDF units would go on to diabetes within this time. This indirect estimate of the difference in predictive value of ICA ≥ 4 JDF units in the general population versus relatives of IDDM patients is similar to prospective data from siblings and school children in Finland[52], and indeed accords well with the theoretical estimate derived from Bayes's rule. The Gainesville group has undertaken a prospective study comparing the prognostic significance of ICA in school children and relatives[10]—a study that illustrates some of the difficulties of undertaking prospective studies in the general population. Life table analysis revealed no difference in risk by 7 years but, as can be seen by the 95% confidence intervals around the cumulative risk at that time (15–74% in school children versus 22–63% in relatives), the power of the study to detect a significant difference was low, in spite of starting out with screening populations of 9696 school children and 2959 relatives. Differences may also have been minimized by the fact that the life table was drawn from the time that ICA $\geq$ 10 JDF units were first detected rather than from initial testing since all ICA negative siblings but only a minority of ICA negative school children underwent repeated testing. Siblings at the lower levels of risk therefore had a greater chance of being included than school children in the same category. It seems reasonable to conclude that, in theory, single markers will not be sufficient to identify individuals at high risk in the general population. Prospective studies have so far failed to address this issue satisfactorily and have produced conflicting results so that very large, carefully designed prospective studies are essential.

COMBINED TESTING: GENETIC AND IMMUNE MARKERS

We have proposed a theoretical model for prediction of IDDM using combined analysis of genetic and immune markers that could potentially overcome the inevitable effect of low overall disease prevalence on the predictive value of individual tests and offer levels of prediction equivalent to those achieved in family members. In this strategy, markers of genetic susceptibility are used to identify a subgroup of the general population whose risk of IDDM is higher than baseline and other markers are applied within that group. Markers of genetic susceptibility are, in effect, substituting for the assumed genetic susceptibility reflected in a positive family history, and a decision tree approach can be adopted. Our estimates were based on the Finnish study which used a panel of four sequence-specific oligonucleotide probes to identify susceptible and protective DQ alleles, thus achieving the best segregation of patients and controls subjects yet described in IDDM. DQ8, in the absence of a protective DQ allele, was found in 82% of patients with IDDM compared with 3% of control subjects, giving a lifetime absolute risk in that population of 13.7%[45]. As explained above, in the general childhood population in Oxford, the expected positive predictive value of ICAs $\geq$ 4 JDF units for developing IDDM within 10 years is about 6%. If, however, ICA testing were confined to those already identified as genetically susceptible by DQ typing (applying the Finnish oligonucleotide screen), in whom the absolute risk of IDDM within 10 years would be 5.5%, the calculated positive predictive value for IDDM within 10 years would rise to more than 50%. This approach obviously needs testing, bearing in mind that the panel of genetic markers can only be applied to the population within which it was developed[41].

COMBINED TESTING: MULTIPLE ANTIBODIES

As in families, the detection of multiple antibodies in children in the general population seems to provide a specific marker of high risk of IDDM. The combination of antibodies to GAD-65 with ICA in the prospective study of Dutch school children gave a positive predictive value of 67% (95% CI 22–96%) compared with 50% (CI 16–84%) with ICA alone[53]. We measured ICA and GADA in newly diagnosed patients and school children from the same region. The combination of ICA (≥ 5 JDF) and GADA was present in 68% of patients and only 0.18% of school children, giving an estimated risk of progression to IDDM before age 20 greater than 80%. One limitation of this strategy is its relatively low sensitivity—less than 70%—probably insufficient for a large-scale screening programme. This approach looks promising but needs to be tested prospectively and the stability of ICA and GADA levels over time needs to be confirmed.

FUTURE PROSPECTS

Our ability to predict diabetes is currently improving in a relentless manner with each passing year. At present we continue to favor the decision tree approach to prediction, and there is still no other easily visualized way of outlining the whole pathway to prediction in different populations. According to the 1995 version of this model, family history and age form the basis of risk stratification, and low titer ICAs remain the most useful initial screening step in the process of prediction. Use of antibody markers in combination has greatly enhanced our ability to predict the disease. For example, in our original formulation of the decision tree the predictive power of ICA *alone* appeared so limited in the general population (a view we still consider correct) that genetic markers were introduced into the model as a surrogate for a positive family history. Although this remains a valid route to prediction, we have since come to appreciate that combinations of antibody markers are sufficiently potent to render genetic testing unnecessary even in this situation—except perhaps for exclusion of those with protective haplotypes. This view has been outlined earlier in the chapter. Therefore a single diabetes pathway can be outlined for all population groups and ages, although the levels of predictive power reached at the end of the pathway will still inevitably represent an amplification of the level of risk at entry.

SECONDARY PREVENTION

What will the future hold for diabetes prediction as an adjunct to intervention trials? In the first place, the obsolescence of ICA appears imminent. This difficult and imprecise test will almost certainly be replaced by automated measurement of several autoantibodies, performed on a few microliters of serum. The autoantibodies most likely to be of use in this situation are GADA and antibodies to 37/40K and/or ICA512. The ability to screen large numbers of individuals simply and cheaply for risk of IDDM may however prove a mixed blessing, and the social and ethical consequences of this could easily prove unpalatable. These issues will be discussed later. Genetic screening may have a limited role in identifying the minority who will be likely non-progressors, but its possible role in this respect still requires clarification. Metabolic testing remains the only way of introducing staging into the process of beta cell damage, but it is important not to overemphasize its discriminant power. In the ICARUS database, for example, an FPIR under 50 Mu l^{-1} was highly predictive of rapid progression—or as we would say, "end-stage pre-diabetes"—but there was overlap of the 95% confidence intervals of higher levels of FPIR, even in this extensive database. Our view is that interventions should be introduced before loss of first phase insulin secretion, and we believe that multiple antibody testing will be able to identify sufficiently high levels of risk to justify intervention. In other words, the ultimate role of metabolic testing may be in interpretation of outcome, not in terms of selection for entry.

Further considerations apply particularly to evaluation of intervention trials. At present the necessary end-point for all trials in pre-diabetes is insulin treatment. The search for possible surrogate end-points which could give early indications of efficacy is likely to continue. As yet no really strong candidates for this role have emerged. Another point of considerable interest is non-progression in marker-positive individuals. Not only will it be helpful to exclude these people from intervention trials, but they are most assuredly telling us something important about the disease process, and possible ways of aborting it.

SECONDARY PREVENTION IN THE GENERAL POPULATION

We have seen that risk assessment is in theory quite possible in the general population, but that this should be based on evaluation of multiple markers of risk. The predictive power of multiple antibody markers is such that genetic testing—at least at our current level of understanding—does not appear to be essential. Screening children in adequate numbers using automated measurement of combinations of antibody markers will soon be a practical proposition, and indeed a nicotinamide trial in school children is under way using a combination of ICA and metabolic testing. There are however major difficulties involved. The numbers needed for screening will be large, and awareness of diabetes and motivation to participate will be less than in family members. Acceptance of lifestyle changes and unwanted effects of treatment will be correspondingly lower. The ethical issues involved in the screening and labeling process will be considerable. Finally, risk estimation in the general population is still based on theory, rather than observation. It is therefore our view that secondary prevention should be tested in first degree relatives before being extended to the general population.

PRIMARY PREVENTION

In the longer term view, secondary prevention will probably be seen as nothing more than a stop-gap. By the time antibody combinations are present in the circulation, we may be reasonably certain that the disease process has been active for several years, and that the full resources of the immune system are being mobilized—however slowly—to destroy beta cells and their antigens. The logical way forward would be to aim to intervene at an earlier stage, either before the immune response was initiated or, failing that, before it was fully established. This in turn implies intervention in the first few years of life. Antibody markers will have little role in recruitment to such primary prevention studies, since the aim will be to intervene before they have even appeared. Antibody markers may well find a role as end-points rather than as entry criteria.

The future of diabetes prevention therefore seems to lie in neonatal screening and intervention, or, if the intervention were to prove safe and simple, in blanket treatment of the whole neonatal population without preliminary screening. Safety would then assume prime importance. Vaccination or induction of oral tolerance would be potential options, although questions concerning nature, dose and presentation of the antigenic stimulus would need to be resolved first. Avoidance of cow's milk antigens would be another acceptable strategy, provided the rationale for this approach could be more securely established, but would probably prove difficult to implement in practice. Strategies such as this would need to be tested in higher risk groups before extension to the population as a whole, and genetic screening at birth and treatment of the subgroup at greatest risk would be one potential strategy. Evaluation could, as already indicated, be initially in terms of induction of an antibody response, although no public health measure is likely to be adopted without evidence of effect upon actual disease incidence.

Therefore we anticipate that future developments will include better definition of genetic risk within a given population, further analysis of the initiation and sequence in which islet autoantibodies appear in the circulation, and perhaps better understanding of gene–antibody interactions. A potential spin-off of this approach is that it may prove simpler to identify adverse neonatal environmental influences in those children who develop antibody responses in early life than in the minority of these who progress to childhood onset diabetes some years later. Definition of gene mutations, and of the products of such mutated genes, may also help to pinpoint the search for environmental influences.

OTHER LIKELY DEVELOPMENTS

The pragmatic ability to predict is not enough. In the longer term, we must strive for a more knowledge-based approach. It is for example something of a paradox that antibody combinations should promise such accurate disease prediction in a disease that is commonly agreed to be T-cell mediated. We need therefore to examine the T-cell correlates of antigen spreading in order to achieve a better understanding of the disease process. We can assume that means of studying T cells and their function will improve rapidly over the coming years. Diabetes prediction based on antibody combinations is already so good that T-cell markers may have only a limited contribution to make, but there remains the hope that they will provide information of value in staging the disease process, and possibly even in evaluating the effects of forms of therapy.

One basic gap in our understanding of IDDM is the inaccessibility of the pancreas. We are forced to infer the course of events within the human pancreas based either on analogy with the NOD mouse—which might be misleading—or on the limited data from post-mortem pancreatic material. The latter give clear indications that human IDDM can develop in the absence of histological features of insulitis[54], particularly over the age of 15–20 years. Further, Bottazzo and colleagues have reported absence of insulitis in the pancreata of two individuals known to have been ICA positive over many years[55]. These observations challenge our understanding of the disease process itself. There is, however, some hope that it may prove possible to image lymphocytic infiltration of the pancreas externally, for example by injecting a radiolabelled IL-2, which binds in situ to activated lymphocytes[56]. Insulitis appears to be a constant finding under the age of 15[54], so that this approach, if successful, could provide useful information concerning the diabetes prodrome, and the effects of therapy, in children at least.

ORGANIZATIONAL AND ETHICAL ISSUES

It is not the purpose of this chapter to explore the ethical and social implications of recent work in diabetes prediction, but these have to be mentioned. Automated, relatively cheap large-scale screening for genetic and immune markers of IDDM is almost upon us. Given the availability of the technology, some unwanted consequences of our research activities will become virtual certainties. The first is that some individuals or organizations will offer IDDM screening outside the context of research studies, without proper counseling, and without adequate understanding of the limitations of the methods being used. The second is that ad hoc treatment will be offered to marker-positive individuals, whether on an individual basis, or else under the banner of research even when considerations such as sample size may render scientific evaluation impossible. The third inevitability is that health or insurance organizations will in time make use of the new technology to identify high risk individuals—to the individuals' considerable disadvantage. It is true that none of these issues is restricted to IDDM, but on the other hand the rate of progress in our area is such that we may unintentionally provide the test-bed for some of these wider issues. It is our view that researchers in this area, as in other areas of science, cannot disclaim social responsibility for the consequences of their actions. Researchers and diabetes organizations should issue very clear guidelines concerning use of these technologies. Equally, it is vital that the scientific community does not offer a platform for those who carry out studies that are poorly designed, of inadequate statistical power, or use unsafe forms of intervention. Finally, it is essential that we monitor the social consequences of our actions, while ensuring that data from research studies are never used to the personal disadvantage of those who volunteer to take part.

REFERENCES

1 Bingley PJ, Christie MR, Bonifacio E, Bonfanti R, Shattock M, Fonte MT, Bottazzo GF, Gale EAM. Combined analysis of autoantibodies improves prediction of IDDM in islet cell antibody-positive relatives. *Diabetes* 1994; **43**: 1304–10.
2 Metcalfe MA, Baum JD. Incidence of insulin dependent diabetes in children under 15 years in the British Isles during 1988. *Br Med J* 1991; **302**: 443–7.
3 Borch-Johnsen K Kreiner, S, Deckert T. Mortality of Type 1 (insulin-dependent) diabetes mellitus in Denmark: a study of relative mortality in 2930 Danish diabetic patients diagnosed from 1933–1972. *Diabetologia* 1986: **29**; 767–72.
4 Bottazzo GF, Florin-Christensen A, Doniach D. Islet-cell antibodies in diabetes mellitus with polyendocrine disease. *Lancet* 1974; **ii**: 1279–83.
5 Lendrum R, Walker G, Gamble DR. Islet-cell antibodies in juvenile diabetes mellitus of recent onset. *Lancet* 1975; **i**: 880–3.
6 Gorsuch AN, Spencer KM, Lister J, McNally JM, Dean BM, Bottazzo GF, Cudworth AG. Evidence for a long prediabetic period in Type 1 (insulin-dependent) diabetes mellitus. *Lancet* 1981; **ii**: 145–7.
7 Bonifacio E, Bingley PJ, Dean BM, Shattock M, Dunger D, Gale EAM, Bottazzo GF. Quantification of islet-cell antibodies and prediction of insulin-dependent diabetes. *Lancet* 1990; **335**: 147–9.
8 Riley WJ, Maclaren NK, Krischer J, Spillar RP, Silverstein J, Schatz DA, Schwartz S, Malone J, Shah S, Vadheim C, Rotter JI. A prospective study of the development of diabetes in relatives of patients with insulin-dependent diabetes. *New Engl J Med* 1990; **323**: 1167–72.
9 Bosi E, Becker F, Bonifacio E, Wagner R, Collins P, Gale EAM, Bottazzo GF. Progression to Type 1 (insulin-dependent) diabetes in autoimmune endocrine patients with islet cell antibodies. *Diabetes* 1991; **40**: 977–84.

10 Schatz D, Krischer J, Horne G, Riley W, Spillar R, Silverstein J, Winter W, Muir A, Derovanesian D, Shah S, Malone J, Maclaren N. Islet cell antibodies predict insulin dependent diabetes in United States school age children as powerfully as in unaffected relatives. *J Clin Invest* 1994; **93**: 2403–7.

11 Lernmark A, Molenaar J, van Beers WAM, Yamaguschi Y, Nagataki S, Ludvigsson J, Maclaren NK. The Fourth International Serum Exchange Workshop to standardize cytoplasmic islet cell antibodies. *Diabetologia* 1991; **34**: 534–5.

12 Bingley PJ. Prediction of diabetes: interaction of risk markers in islet cell antibody positive family members: The first analysis of the ICARUS dataset. *Diabetologia* 1994; **37**: A55. (Abstract)

13 Genovese S, Bonifacio E, Dean BM, McNally JM, Wagner R, Bosi E, Gale EAM, Bottazzo GF. Distinct cytoplasmic islet cell antibodies with different risks for Type 1 (insulin-dependent) diabetes mellitus. *Diabetologia* 1992; **35**: 385–8.

14 Gianani R, Pugliese A, Bonner-Weir S, Schiffrin A, Soeldner JS, Erlich HA, Awdeh Z, Alper CA, Jackson RA, Eisenbarth GS. Prognostically significant heterogeneity of cytoplasmic islet cell antibodies in relatives of patients with Type 1 diabetes. *Diabetes* 1992; **41**: 347–53.

15 Timsit J, Caillat-Zucman S, Blondel H, Chedin P, Bach JF, Boitard C. Islet cell antibody heterogeneity among Type 1 (insulin-dependent) diabetic patients. *Diabetologia* 1992; **35**: 792–5.

16 Thivolet CH, Tappaz M, Durand A, Petersen J, Stefanutti A, Chatelain P, Viallettes B, Scherbaum W, Orgiazzi J. Glutamic acid decarboxylase (GAD) autoantibodies are additional predictive markers of Type 1 (insulin-dependent) diabetes in high risk individuals. *Diabetologia* 1992; **35**: 570–6.

17 Christie MR, Tun RYM, Lo SSS, Cassidy D, Brown TJ, Hollands J, Shattock M, Bottazzo GF, Leslie RDG. Antibodies to GAD and tryptic fragments of the islet 64K antigen as distinct markers for development of IDDM: studies with identical twins. *Diabetes* 1991; **41**: 782–7.

18 Tuomilehto J, Zimmet P, Mackay IR, Koskela P, Vidgren G, Toivanen L, Tuomilehto-Wolf E, Kohtamaki K, Stengard J, Rowley MJ. Antibodies to glutamic acid decarboxylase as predictors of insulin-dependent diabetes melitus before clinical onset of disease. *Lancet* 1994; **343**: 1383–5.

19 Bonifacio E, Genovese S, Braghi S, Bazzigaluppi E, Lampasona V, Bingley PJ, Rogge L, Pastore MR, Bognetti E, Bottazzo GF, Gale EAM, Bosi E. Islet autoantibody markers in IDDM: strategies risk assessment yielding high sensitivity. *Diabetologia* 1995; **38**: 816–22.

20 Christie MR, Genovese S, Cassidy D, Bosi E, Brown TJ, Lai M, Bonifacio E, Bottazzo GF. Antibodies to islet 37k antigen but not to glutamate decarboxylase discriminate rapid progression to insulin-dependent diabetes mellitus in endocrine autoimmunity. *Diabetologia* 1994; **43**: 1254–9.

21 Yu L, Gianini R, Eisenbarth GS. Quantitation of glutamic acid decarboxylase autoantibody levels in prospectively evaluated relatives of patients with type 1 diabetes. *Diabetes* 1994; **43** 1229–33.

22 Harrison LC, Honeyman MC, DeAizpurua HJ, Schmidli RS, Colman PG, Tait BD, Cram DS. Inverse relation between humoral and cellular immunity to glutamic acid decarboxylase in subjects at risk of insulin-dependent diabetes. *Lancet* 1993; **341**: 1365–9.

23 Palmer JP, Asplin CM, Clemons P, Lyen K, Tatpati O, Raghu PK, Paquette TL. Insulin antibodies in insulin-dependent diabetes before insulin treatment. *Science* 1983; **222**: 1337–9.

24 Vardi P, Ziegler AG, Mathews JH, Dib S, Keller RJ, Ricker AT, Wolfsdorf JI,

Herskowitz RD, Rabizadeh A, Eisenbarth GS, Soeldner JS. Concentration of insulin autoantibodies at onset of Type 1 diabetes. Inverse log-linear correlation with age. *Diabetes Care* 1988; **11**: 736–9.

25 Ziegler AG, Ziegler R, Vardi P, Jackson RA, Soeldner JS, Eisenbarth GS. Life-table analysis of progression to diabetes of anti-insulin autoantibody-positive relatives of individuals with Type 1 diabetes. *Diabetes* 1989; **38**: 132–5.

26 Christie MR, Hollands JA, Brown TJ, Michelsen BK, Delovitch TL. Detection of pancreatic islet 64,000 Mr autoantigens in insulin-dependent diabetes distinct from glutamate decarboxylase. *J Clin Invest* 1993; **92**: 240–8.

27 Genovese S, Bingley PJ, Bonifacio E, Christie MR, Shattock M, Bonfanti R, Foxon R, Gale EAM, Bottazzo GF. Combined analysis of IDDM-related autoantibodies in healthy schoolchildren. *Lancet* 1994; **344**: 756.

28 Ongagna JC, Levy-Marchal C. Anti-37kDa antibodies are associated with the development of IDDM in individuals with islet cell antibodies. *Diabetologia* 1995; **38**: 370–5.

29 Rabin DU, Pleasic SM, Shapiro JA, Yoo-Warren H, Oles J, Hicks JM, Goldstein DE, Rae PM. Islet cell antigen 512 is a diabetes-specific islet autoantigen related to protein tyrosine phosphatases. *J Immunol* 1944; **152**: 3183–8.

30 Peterson JS, Hejnaes KR, Moody A, Karlsen AE, Marshall MO, Hoier-Madsen M, Boel E, Michelsen BK, Dyrberg T. Detection of GAD65 antibodies in diabetes and other autoimmune diseases using a simple radioligand assay. *Diabetes* 1994; **43**: 459–67.

31 Vardi P, Crisa L, Jackson RA. Predictive value of intravenous glucose tolerance test insulin secretion less than or greater than the first percentile in islet cell antibody positive relatives of Type 1 (insulin-dependent) diabetic patients. *Diabetologia* 1991; **34**: 93–102.

32 Pietropaolo M, Yu L, Eisenbarth GS. Combined anti-islet autoantibody determination. *Diabetologia* 1994; **37**: A56.

33 Verge CF, Howard NJ, Rowley MJ, Mackay IR, Zimmet PZ, Egan M, Hulinska H, Hulinsky I, Silvestrini RA, Kamathm S, Sharp A, Arundel T, Silink M. Anti-glutamate decarboxylase and other antibodies at the onset of childhood IDDM: a population-based study. *Diabetologia* 1994; **37**: 1113–20.

34 Bennett ST, Lucassen AM, Gough SCL, Powell EE, Undlien DE, Pritchard LE, Merriman ME, Kawaguchi Y, Dronsfield MJ, Pociot F, Nerup J, Bouzekri N, Cambon-Thomsen A, Ronningen KS, Barnett AH, Bain SC, Todd JA. Susceptibility to human type 1 diabetes at IDDM2 is determined by tandem repeat variation at the insulin gene minisatellite locus. *Genetics* 1995; **9**: 284–92.

35 Leslie RDG, Elliott RB. Early environmental events as a cause of IDDM (evidence and implications). *Diabetes* 1994; **43**: 843–50.

36 Bingley PJ, Bonifacio E, Gale EAM. Antibodies to glutamic acid decarboxylase as predictors of insulin-dependent diabetes. *Lancet* 1994; **344**: 266.

37 Fletcher RH, Fletcher SW, Wagner EH. *Clinical Epidemiology*. Baltimore: Williams and Wilkins, 1988.

38 Armitage P, Berry G. *Statistical Methods in Medical Research*. Oxford: Blackwell Scientific Publications, 1987, pp. 117–20.

39 Colman PG, Eisenbarth GS. Immunology of Type 1 diabetes—1987. In Alberti KGGM, Krall LP (eds), *Diabetes Annual*, Vol 4. Amsterdam: Elsevier, 1988, pp. 17–45.

40 Christensen E. Multivariate survival analysis usings Coxs regression model. *Hepatology* 1987; **7**: 1346–58.

41 Bingley PJ, Bonifacio E, Gale EAM. Can we really predict IDDM? *Diabetes* 1993; **42**: 213–20.

42 Todd JA, Bain SC. A practical approach to identification of susceptibility genes for IDDM. *Diabetes* 1992; **41**: 1029–34.

43 Sanjeevi CB, Lybrand TP, DeWeese C, Landin-Olsson M, Kockum I, Dahlquist G, Sundqvst G, Stenger D, Lernmark A. Polymorphic amino acid variations in HLFA-DQ are associated with systematic physical property changes and occurrence of insulin-dependent diabetes. *Diabetes* 1995; **44**: 125–31.

44 Vandewalle CL, Decraene T, Schuit FC, De Leeuw IH, Pipeleers DG, Gorus FK, The Belgian Diabetes Registry. Insulin antibodies and high titre islet cell antibodies are preferentially associated with the HLA DQA*0301-LDQB1*0302 haplotype at clinical onset of Type 1 (insulin-dependent) diabetes mellitus before age 10 years, but not at onset between age 10 and 40 years. *Diabetologia* 1933; **36**: 1155–62.

45 Reijonen H, Ilonen J, Knip M, Akerblom HK. HLA-DQB1 alleles and absence of Asp 57 as susceptibility factors of IDDM in Finland. *Diabetes* 1991; **40**: 1640–4.

46 Bingley PJ, Bonifacio E, Shattock M, Gillmor HA, Sawtell PA, Dunger DB, Scott RDM, Bottazzo GF, Gale EAM. Can islet cell antibodies predict IDDM in the general population? *Diabetes Care* 1993; **16**: 45–50.

47 Levy-Marchal C, Tichet J, Fajardy I, Gu XF, Dubois F, Czernichow P. Islet cell antibodies in normal French schoolchildren. *Diabetologia* 1992; **35**: 577–82.

48 Karjalainen J. Islet cell antibodies as predictive markers for IDDM in children with high background incidence of disease. *Diabetes* 1990; **39**: 1144–50.

49 Boehm BO, Manfras B, Seissler J, Schoffling K, Gluck M, Holzberger G, Seidl S, Kuhnl P, Trucco M, Scherbaum WA. Epidemiology and immunogenetic background of islet cell antibody-positive nondiabetic schoolchildren. Ulm-Frankfurt Population Study. *Diabetes* 1991; **40**: 1435–9.

50 Muntoni S, Loviselli A, Martino E, Velluzzi M, Shattock M, Balestrieri A, Songini M, Muntoni S, Bottazzo GF. High prevalence of islet cell antibodies (ICA) in healthy schoolchildren in Sardinia. *Diabetologia* 1992; **35**: A32. (Abstract)

51 Bruining GJ, Molenaar JL, Grobbee DE, Hofman A, Scheffer GJ, Bruining HA, de Bruyn AM, Valkenburg HA. Ten-year follow-up study of islet cell antibodies and childhood diabetes mellitus. *Lancet* 1989; **i**: 1100–3.

52 Knip M, Vahasalo P, Karjalainen J, Lounamaa R, Akerblom HK, The Study Group on Childhood Diabetes in Finland. Natural course of pre-type 1 diabetes in high risk individuals. *Diabetologia* 1992; **35**: A32.

53 Aanstoot HJ, Sigurdsson E, Jaffe M, Shi Y, Christgau S, Grobbee D, Bruining GJ, Molenaar JL, Hofman A, Baekkeskov S. Value of antibodies to GAD65 combined with islet cell cytoplasmic antibodies for predicting IDDM in a childhood population. *Diabetologia* 1994; **37**: 917–24.

54 Pipeleers DG, Ling Z. Pancreatic beta cells in insulin-dependent diabetes. *Diabetes/Metab Revs* 1992; **8**: 209–27.

55 Wagner R, McNally JM, Bonifacio E, Genovese S, Foulis AK, McGill M, Christie MR, Betterle C, Bosi E, Bottazzo GF. Lack of immunohistological changes in the islets of nondiabetic, autoimmune, polyendocrine patients with B-selective GAD-specific islet cell antibodies. *Diabetes* 1994; **43**: 851.

56 Signore A, Chianelli M, Ferretti E, Toscano A, Britton K, Andreani D, Gale EAM, Pozzilli P. New approach for in vivo detection of insulitis in type 1 diabetes: activated lymphocyte targeting with 123I-labelled interleukin 2. *Eur J Endocrinol* 1994; **131**: 431–7.

Part 3

PREVENTION

15

Cyclosporine and Azathioprine for IDDM

JEFFREY L. MAHON and JOHN DUPRE
University of Western Ontario, Ontario, Canada

INTRODUCTION

Reports of immunotherapy for human insulin-dependent diabetes mellitus (IDDM) first appeared in the early 1980s[1,2]. These initiatives were justified on two grounds. First, it was strongly suspected that the main pathophysiological problem in IDDM was immune-mediated loss of pancreatic beta cells[3]. Second, conventional management of IDDM did not forestall an immense personal and societal burden of suffering[4]. At the time of writing, over a dozen different immunotherapies have been given to persons with presumed immune-mediated beta-cell loss either shortly after onset of overt IDDM or in the disease's subclinical phase[5]. In most cases clear conclusions regarding biological and clinical effects have not been possible because the studies used small numbers of subjects and observational methodology. Immunosuppression with cyclosporine and azathioprine for patients with newly diagnosed IDDM remain the most rigorously tested approaches thus far. Nicotinamide has also been carefully studied[6] and is discussed elsewhere in this volume.

Despite unequivocal evidence that cyclosporine and azathioprine favorably affect the natural course of beta-cell destruction in IDDM, the adverse effects of both drugs have made it impossible to justify their long-term use for the disease. Nevertheless, the experience with these drugs, and especially observations from randomized control trials, have been pivotal to further efforts to prevent IDDM through immunotherapy. In this chapter, we will summarize the randomized trials with cyclosporine and azathioprine for

Prediction, Prevention and Genetic Counseling in IDDM. Edited by Jerry P. Palmer.
© 1996 John Wiley & Sons Ltd.

newly diagnosed IDDM. We will then review the importance of this experience to the understanding of the pathogenesis of human beta-cell loss and to future trials of immunotherapy to prevent IDDM and its sequelae.

THE RANDOMIZED TRIALS OF CYCLOSPORINE AND AZATHIOPRINE FOR ESTABLISHED IDDM

Assessment of cyclosporine and azathioprine for newly diagnosed IDDM followed the paradigm of exploratory non-randomized trials[7-14] to more definitive randomized control trials[15-20]. In both types of studies, determination of efficacy used insulin dosage, markers of glycemic control including blood glucose and glycosylated hemoglobin (GHb) levels, and insulin secretion by connecting-peptide (C-peptide) blood levels. These variables are subject to many influences, including factors under the control of patients and physicians. Thus, the non-randomized trials carried a strong risk for bias through confounding and cointervention, making random allocation, and, where possible, placebo controls and double-blinding essential for definitive conclusions. An early example of such a trial which, while negative, deserves recognition because it set the methodological standard, was a Finnish study of alpha-interferon for IDDM of recent onset[21]. For the randomized trials, a priori estimates of sample sizes sufficiently large to reliably detect minimal differences of clinical importance were also highly desirable[15,16].

Six randomized trials[15-20] of cyclosporine and azathioprine have been reported in the English literature and are listed in Table 15.1.

THE CYCLOSPORINE TRIALS

The French Randomized Trial

The first randomized, placebo-controlled, double-blind trial of cyclosporine for IDDM came from a multicenter French group[15]. One hundred and twenty-two patients (age range 15 to 40 years old) with a mean duration of symptomatic hyperglycemia of 10 weeks were randomized to cyclosporine or placebo. Insulin dosage was minimized provided blood glucose levels did not exceed 7.8 mM before meals and 11.1 mM after meals. A "complete remission" occurred if glucose levels were maintained in these ranges with a GHb level ≤7.5% (upper limit of normal = 5.8%) in the absence of insulin therapy. "Partial remission" required the same glycemic parameters and an insulin dosage of <0.25 U kg^{-1} day^{-1}.

All patients were followed to 6 months and 106 patients were followed to 9 months. Glycosylated hemoglobin levels at 6 months were not significantly different between the two groups. Cyclosporine therapy resulted in higher

Table 15.1. Randomized control trials of cyclosporine and azathioprine for recent-onset IDDM

Trial (Ref) Design	Subject N	Follow-up	Main results	
French Cyclosporine[15]	Double-blind, placebo-controlled	122	9 months	Cyclosporine increased the rate of clinical remissions
Canadian–European Cyclosporine[16]	Double-blind, placebo-control	188	1 year	Cyclosporine increased the rate of clinical remissions and preserved insulin secretion
Miami Cyclosporine[17]	Double-blind, placebo-controlled	23	1 year	Cyclosporine preserved insulin secretion but had no effect on clinical remissions
Denver Cyclosporine[18]	Open	43	3 years	Cyclosporine therapy for 4 months had no effect on clinical remissions or insulin secretion
Australian Azathioprine[19]	Double-blind, placebo-controlled	49	1 year	Azathioprine enhanced insulin secretion over the first 3 months but had no effect on clinical remissions
American Azathioprine– Corticosteroid[20]	Open	46	1 year	Azathioprine and corticosteroid improved metabolic status and insulin secretion

rates of complete remission at 9 months (cyclosporine 24% versus placebo 6%, $p < 0.01$) and higher combined rates of complete and partial remissions at 6 months (cyclosporine 46% versus placebo 29%, $p = 0.05$) and 9 months (cyclosporine 37% versus placebo 14%, $p < 0.01$). Although insulin secretion was not evaluated and compared between the treatment arms within the framework of the clinical trial, a subsequent report showed that cyclosporine-treated patients had a higher mean C-peptide level versus historical controls[13].

Several post hoc subgroup analyses were done. Within the cyclosporine group, complete remissions at 9 months were associated with whole-blood cyclosporine trough levels $\geqslant 300$ ng ml^{-1} over the first 3 months of treatment. Also, complete remissions in both groups were associated with shorter duration of symptoms and greater body weight at entry. Formal statistical assessment for an interaction between these variables, treatment group and remissions was not done.

The Canadian–European Randomized Trial

A second randomized, double-blind, placebo-controlled trial of cyclosporine for IDDM was performed in Canada and Europe[16]. One hundred and eighty-eight patients (age range 10 to 35 years old) were randomized within 14 weeks of symptom onset and 6 weeks of starting insulin therapy. Blinding was maintained to 1 year, during which patients were assessed every 3 months for clinical response and insulin secretion by glucagon-stimulated C-peptide levels. Insulin therapy was systematically minimized provided capillary blood glucose levels did not exceed 7.8 mM before meals. Two end-points were defined in advance. A "non-insulin receiving remission" (NIR) required these glycemic targets without insulin therapy for at least 2 weeks. A second, compound end-point required either a NIR or a glucagon-stimulated C-peptide level of at least 0.6 nM (a value attained in 90% of normal subjects).

Glycemic control by GHb level was not significantly different between the groups through 1 year. At the same time, NIR remissions were more frequent in the cyclosporine group at 6 months (cyclosporine 39% versus placebo 19%, $p = 0.03$) and 12 months (cyclosporine 24% versus placebo 10%, $p = 0.009$). Furthermore, the cyclosporine group had a higher mean glucagon-stimulated C-peptide level at 90 days, which was maintained to 1 year, whereas the mean value in the placebo group fell progressively after 3 months. At 1 year, the mean stimulated C-peptide level was higher in the cyclosporine group (0.46 Nm versus placebo 0.35 Nm, $p < 0.002$).

In this trial, a strong interaction between treatment group, duration of disease, and NIR remissions was demonstrated by a post hoc subgroup analysis. The NIR remission rate at 12 months among patients with short duration disease, where the definition of short duration was not data-driven and was ≤6 weeks of symptoms before entry with ≤2 weeks of insulin therapy, was significantly different (cyclosporine 32% versus placebo 3%, $p = 0.001$). On the other hand, a difference in NIR remissions at 12 months among patients with long-duration disease was not seen (cyclosporine 19% versus placebo 15%, $p = 0.55$). An interaction between earlier intervention and treatment group was also suggested in respect to insulin secretion: the rates of remission at 12 months by the compound end-point among short duration patients were 40% for the cyclosporine group and 16% for the placebo group ($p = 0.02$), whereas the respective rates among patients with long-duration disease were 28% and 24% ($p = 0.58$). When the baseline variables of sex, age, body mass index, and C-peptide level were controlled for through multiple logistic regression, only duration of disease continued to show an interaction between treatment and response. Specifically, the adjusted difference in efficacy of cyclosporine between short- and long-duration patients for both end-points was statistically significant at 6 months (NIR, $p = 0.003$; compound end-point, $p = 0.02$) and showed clear trends at 12 months (NIR, $p = 0.06$; compound end-point, $p = 0.15$).

The American Randomized Trials

Two smaller randomized control trials of cyclosporine in recent-onset IDDM were completed in Miami and Denver[17,18].

In a trial from Miami, 23 patients (age range 9 to 38 years old) with IDDM of 6 weeks or less were randomized to cyclosporine or placebo for 1 year under double-blind conditions[17]. Insulin was minimized provided weekly capillary glucose levels did not exceed 6.7 mM before meals, 10 mM 1 hour after meals and at 3 AM, and 7.8 mM 2 hours after meals. Insulin secretion in response to three secretogogues (glucagon, intravenous glucose and a standardized mixed meal) was serially assessed at 3–6 month intervals for 1 year. Cyclosporine treatment was associated with significantly higher meal-stimulated C-peptide levels through this time. Similar responses to the other stimuli were not seen, nor was a difference found between groups in clinical remission rates. As acknowledged by the investigators, however, the probability of a type II statistical error was high because of the small sample size.

In an open trial from Denver, 43 patients (age range, 8 to 36 years old) with IDDM of up to 2 weeks' duration were randomized to receive cyclosporine for 4 months or no immunosuppression[18]. Glucagon-stimulated C-peptide levels were done at approximately 4, 12 and 36 months after entry. A remission was defined as a period of no insulin treatment for at least 7 days with concurrent fasting and 2 hour post-prandial blood glucose levels <7.25 mM and no ketonuria. No differences were seen between the two groups over 3 years in GHb levels, remissions or C-peptide secretion. Again, however, the small sample size meant the study had a low probability to detect realistic effects in respect to clinical remission. The lack of an apparent effect of cyclosporine on insulin secretion may have been a result of the short duration of therapy. Also, the investigators chose to analyze C-peptide level as a categorical rather than continuous variable (high production $\geqslant 0.3$ pM, some production > 0.1 pM, or no production $\leqslant 0.1$ pM) which further limited the study's power.

THE AZATHIOPRINE TRIALS

The Australian Randomized Trial

A randomized, double-blind, placebo-controlled trial of azathioprine for newly diagnosed IDDM was reported from Australia in 1989[19]. This trial followed a promising but smaller open trial from the same group in which adult IDDM patients were sequentially allocated to azathioprine or no treatment[14]. In the subsequent trial, 49 patients (age range 2–20 years) with a median duration of symptomatic IDDM of 20 days were randomized and followed for 1 year. C-peptide levels before and 1 hour after a standard meal breakfast were measured every 3 months for 1 year. Insulin was given to maintain home capillary blood glucose levels in near-normal range ($\leqslant 8$ mM). A "complete remission" was defined as the restoration of normal carbohydrate tolerance without dietary or other treatments. A "partial remission" occurred if the GHb level was below the upper limit of normal ($\leqslant 7.9\%$) and pre-meal home capillary glucose levels were $\leqslant 8$ mM while taking insulin at a dose of $\leqslant 0.5$ U kg^{-1} day^{-1}.

Complete remissions were not seen in either group, nor were significant differences found between groups in mean GHb level, insulin dosage and rates of partial remissions at 6 and 12 months. A statistically significant ($p < 0.04$) increase in fasting C-peptide over the first 3 months occurred in azathioprine-treated but not placebo-treated patients and was maintained to 6 months. However, no apparent differences were seen between groups in fasting C-peptide levels at 9 and 12 months or in stimulated C-peptide levels at any point.

The American Randomized Trial of Azathioprine and Corticosteroids

In a study from Gainesville, 46 patients (age range 4 to 33 years) with symptomatic IDDM of up to 150 days were randomized to open therapy with azathioprine for 1 year plus corticosteroids (intravenous methylprednisolone for four doses followed by a 10 week tapering course of prednisone) or no immunosuppression[20]. Fasting and meal-stimulated C-peptide levels were determined every 3 months and insulin dosage was minimized in both groups provided pre-prandial capillary blood glucose levels did not exceed 6.7 mM.

Through 1 year, mean GHb levels did not differ between the two groups. At the same time, the mean insulin dosage was higher among immunosuppressed patients ($p < 0.001$) and this was associated with a higher stimulated C-peptide level (mean C-peptide level at 1 year: azathioprine group = 0.52 Nm versus control group = 0.26 Nm; $p < 0.03$). Although more patients receiving immunosuppression ($N = 10$) than controls ($N = 2$) discontinued insulin for at least 1 week over 12 months, this difference was not significant. At 1 year, three patients receiving immunosuppression had normal blood glucose and GHb levels without insulin therapy whereas all control patients were receiving insulin.

Post hoc analyses showed that better metabolic status (defined by a composite index using GHb level, insulin dosage and ratio of stimulated C-peptide to glucose levels) and older age at entry was associated with improved metabolic status at 1 year among patients receiving immunosuppression. A lower lymphocyte count during azathioprine therapy was also associated with enhanced metabolic status at 1 year.

The side-effects of steroids precluded double blinding in this trial and raised the possibility that the apparent improvement in metabolic response among the immunosuppressed patients was not a result of the treatment but some other factor. However, the comparable approach to decisions concerning insulin in both groups and the lack of an apparent difference in GHb levels over the year made this unlikely.

THE IMPORTANCE OF THE CYCLOSPORINE AND AZATHIOPRINE TRIALS TO CONTINUING EFFORTS TO PREVENT IDDM

Improved treatment for IDDM did not emerge from the trials of cyclosporine and azathioprine for overt IDDM. This is because the perceived risk–benefit ratio of both drugs for patients with newly diagnosed IDDM was unacceptably high. Concerning risk, it was apparent from the non-randomized trials, and confirmed in the subsequent randomized trials, that efficacy in terms of insulin secretion and clinical remissions would probably require long-term drug administration[8,12–14,18–20]. The major risks included drug-specific effects (irreversible nephrotoxicity for cyclosporine[22] and bone marrow suppression and hepatotoxicity for azathioprine[23]) and general effects from chronic immunosuppression (severe infection and neoplasia[24]). While these complications either did not occur (neoplasia and severe infection[7–20]) or appeared to be avoidable through close monitoring of laboratory markers (nephrotoxicity[23], bone marrow suppression and hepatotoxicity[14,19,20]), the marginal clinical benefit seen in the randomized trials could not justify these potential risks. Enhancing efficacy through long-term use of either agent in persons with greater beta-cell reserve, that is, in the subclinical prodrome of IDDM, has also not emerged as a testable option, in part because of the additional difficulty of needlessly treating a proportion of persons not destined to become overtly diabetic. For both strategies, the recognition that children would comprise at least half of the target population further accentuated concerns about toxicity.

Despite this roadblock, the clinical trials of these agents have been vital to continuing efforts to identify safe and effective immunotherapy for IDDM. The trials' importance arises from the broad implications they bring to biological inferences on the pathogenesis of human beta-cell destruction and to the design and conduct of future clinical trials to prevent IDDM and its sequelae. A summary of some of the more important of these implications now follows.

Beta-cell Loss in Human IDDM is Immune-mediated

The main contribution from the randomized trials of cyclosporine and azathioprine for IDDM was provision of definitive proof that an immune-mediated process causes beta-cell loss in human IDDM. All other laboratory and clinical observations before these trials could only yield circumstantial evidence for this conclusion. For this reason, these trials remain the strongest existing argument for further efforts to identify effective, safe immunotherapy for IDDM.

The strength of the randomized trials in proving causation arises from the capacity of randomization to protect against known and, especially, unknown confounding. The use of double blinding in the cyclosporine trials and the Australian azathioprine trial afforded further protection to the validity of this conclusion by limiting the potential for cointervention bias. Although for both agents the randomized trials generally confirmed the non-randomized trials' finding that immunosuppression defers or prevents beta-cell loss, the latter trials[8,9,11,14] tended to overestimate treatment effects relative to the former[15,16,19,20]. This observation, which is not new[25], reinforces the methodological demands that must be met before novel immunotherapeutic strategies for IDDM at any stage, including primary and secondary prevention, can be accepted as standard clinical practice.

It should be acknowledged that the demonstration of this cause and effect relationship is limited to pathogenetic events around the time of onset of overt IDDM. There is a strong temptation to generalize the finding to earlier stages of beta-cell loss. However, this remains speculative pending results of current randomized control trials of immunotherapy for non-diabetic subjects with subclinical beta-cell destruction[6,26,27].

T-lymphocytes Play a Central Role in Human Beta-cell Loss

A second observation from the randomized trials concerned the mechanism of beta-cell loss in human IDDM. In view of the major actions of cyclosporine and azathioprine[28,29], it was reasonable to conclude that a T-lymphocyte directed process mediates beta-cell destruction. As above, these inferences are greatly strengthened by the randomized control methodology but may not bear upon earlier events in beta-cell destruction. Nevertheless, the efficacy of at least one mechanism of action has been established which bears consideration in designing future studies.

Two subsequent reports involving subsets of patients from the Canadian–European cyclosporine randomized trial explored the relationships between humoral immunity, clinical and biological responses, and immunosuppression[30,31]. In one report, expression of islet cell antibodies and insulin antibodies was inhibited by cyclosporine, yet presence of these antibodies at baseline was not associated with clinical remissions or insulin secretion at 1 year in either cyclosporine- or placebo-treated patients[30]. In a second study[31], expression of glutamic acid decarboxylase antibodies (GADA) was not inhibited by cyclosporine, yet GADA positivity at baseline was associated with a significantly greater decline in insulin secretion among placebo-treated, but not cyclosporine-treated, patients at 9 and 12 months. These observations are also consistent with the conclusion that humoral mechanisms are not of primary significance in the pathogenesis of human beta-cell loss.

Insulin Sensitivity is Important

A third observation from the experience with cyclosporine and azathioprine for IDDM drew attention to the importance of accounting for insulin action when assessing clinical efficacy in future preventive trials. In randomized trials of both agents[16,20], and in the non-randomized trials of cyclosporine[8,11], glycemic control was lost despite preservation of endogenous insulin secretion by immunosuppression. Moreover, the levels of insulin secretion that were maintained during immunosuppression in several of the randomized and non-randomized trials were not trivial[8,12,16,20]. They approached values seen in non-diabetics[16] and exceeded the threshold (a stimulated C-peptide level of at least 0.2 nM) that was associated with lower GHb levels and lower daily doses of insulin in a large representative cohort of long-standing insulin-dependent diabetics[32]. Neither cyclosporine not azathioprine has been convincingly shown to affect insulin action, making independent changes in insulin resistance the probable explanation for this discrepancy. Direct measurement of insulin sensitivity in cyclosporine-treated insulin-dependent diabetics enrolled in non-randomized trials subsequently supported this hypothesis[13,33].

This observation has at least two implications. First, further clinical trials of immunotherapy for IDDM, including trials testing primary and secondary prevention strategies, should evaluate insulin action in addition to the usual markers of clinical (glycemic control) and biological (endogenous insulin secretion) response. Second, it sharpens the emerging interest in assessment of insulin sensitivity in the subclinical prodrome of IDDM, and adds impetus to the question of whether changes in insulin action improve existing predictive models for subsequent IDDM[34].

There is a Cause and Effect Relationship Between Insulin Secretion and Glycemic Control

A fourth important finding from the randomized trials of cyclosporine and azathioprine was to demonstrate conclusively a cause and effect relationship between improved endogenous insulin secretion and improved glycemic control. Prior to the randomized trials, studies in patients with well-established IDDM had shown an association between higher C-peptide levels and more-normal glycemic control[32,35-37]. However, these data were observational and could therefore not prove cause and effect. In the Canadian–European cyclosporine trial, maintenance of endogenous insulin secretion with cyclosporine led to significantly fewer insulin-dependent diabetics receiving insulin through one year without an increase in glycated hemoglobin level[16]. This difference could not be accounted for by cointervention bias given the double-blind methodology[16]. A similar relationship between enhancement of insulin secretion and improved glycemic control was also shown in the American azathioprine–corticosteroid randomized trial[20].

At face value, this conclusion is self-evident. Indeed, the cardinal features of IDDM—loss of insulin secretion followed by elevated blood glucose levels—come close to prima facie evidence for cause and effect in the first place. Furthermore, in isolation this conclusion has little apparent clinical or biological significance to further efforts to prevent IDDM and its sequelae. The observation's importance becomes clear when the causal chain is extended from enhanced insulin secretion causing improved glycemic control leading, in turn, to a major aim of all preventive initiatives in IDDM—specifically, prevention of chronic end-organ complications. The Diabetes Control and Complications Trial (DCCT) definitively established the second half of this causal sequence. In that trial, insulin-dependent diabetics randomized to an experimental program designed to attain a GHb as close to normal as safely possible showed relative risk reductions for each of retinopathy, nephropathy and peripheral neuropathy of about 50% when compared to patients having higher GHb levels during conventional management[38].

An inverse association between endogenous insulin secretion and chronic complications (mainly microvascular complications and neuropathy) has not been a consistent finding in other studies[39-47]. However, this does not weaken the inference that more-normal endogenous insulin secretion causes fewer structural complications. Explanations for the contradictory results include different methods of assessing endogenous insulin secretion and complications, and use of small sample sizes with resultant type II statistical errors. Perhaps of more importance are the facts that these studies used observational methodology and evaluated patients with long-standing IDDM having levels of insulin secretion that are extremely low relative to those that could be attained through immunotherapy when more substantial beta-cell function is present. The main limitation of the observational studies is that they cannot definitely address confounding variables. The most obvious confounder is disease duration. Multivariate analysis that assesses the association between C-peptide levels and complications while controlling for disease duration may be unable to disentangle the independent relationship of either variable with complications because disease duration and C-peptide levels are highly correlated[42].

In principle, the problems of confounding and relative insulinopenia can only be fully addressed by a randomized trial that: (a) enters subjects having relatively high levels of endogenous insulin secretion to begin with, for example, subjects at a stage prior to onset of overt IDDM; (b) isolates and maintains insulin secretion as the experimental variable; and (c) follows both groups to an end-point of structural complications. In fact, such a trial will likely never be done for two reasons. First, the sample size required for a primary or secondary prevention trial using structural complications as the primary outcome measure will be impracticably large. Second, if the test therapy is effective in maintaining insulin secretion, it will also likely defer exogenous insulin treatment. The unacceptable situation would then arise of ignoring a reduction in the rate of the surrogate end-point of exogenous insulin dependence in order to follow subjects to the "harder" end-point of structural complications.

Thus, the recognition that structural diabetic complications are reduced by improved glycemic control (as shown in the DCCT) and that improved glycemic control results from enhanced endogenous insulin secretion (as shown in the cyclosporine and azathioprine trials for IDDM) serves to strengthen an otherwise untestable but key rationale behind continuing primary and secondary preventive trials for IDDM. These considerations also renew interest in the question of whether preserving insulin secretion by immunotherapy at the relatively late stage of onset of overt IDDM can still result in clinically important benefit. The DCCT has made normalization of blood glucose levels a major aim for many patients with IDDM. However, current strategies to normalize GHb levels in insulinopenic IDDM patients are labor-intensive, associated with significant hypoglycemia, and require highly compliant patients for success[38]. A treatment that preserves the low levels of endogeneous insulin secretion that are present within the first year of diagnosis could greatly facilitate glycemic control in the longer term. This approach, however, demands that the treatment have a proven record of minimal toxicity (potential examples are nicotinamide and bacille Calmette–Guérin) and requires unequivocal demonstration that the treatment is effective through placebo-controlled randomized trials of at least medium- to long-term duration (5 to 10 years).

The Intensity of Beta-cell Destruction May Fluctuate

A fifth observation from the Canadian–European cyclosporine randomized trial has a bearing upon the chronology of beta-cell loss. It had previously been thought that this process was one of unremitting decline[48]. The Canadian–European trial demonstrated a large difference in remission rates according to length of symptomatic disease of less than or more than six weeks[16]. This was an extremely short time relative to the potential duration of beta-cell autoimmunity[49] and suggested that, in at least a subset of IDDM patients, beta-cell loss was greatly accelerated near the time of onset of overt disease. Glucose toxicity did not explain the differential response because glycemic control was not different between the treatment groups in that trial[16]. Concern that the validity of this interaction was jeopardized by use of a post-hoc subgroup analysis can be counterbalanced by the consistency of similar associations seen in the non-randomized trials of cyclosporine[7,11], by avoidance of a data-driven approach when choosing the subgroups, and by the high level of statistical significance seen in the difference in remission rates between short- and long-duration subjects[16].

This observation accords with findings in identical twins discordant for disease in which the non-diabetic twin showed evidence of beta-cell autoimmunity not progressing to IDDM[50]. Further, the possibility is raised that a less toxic approach of intermittent immunotherapy, even with broadly direct immunosuppressives such as azathioprine or cyclosporine, during active periods of autoimmunity in the subclinical phase of IDDM phase may be sufficient to prevent further beta-cell loss. Critical to such a strategy, however, and as yet not clearly at hand, is the need for completely reliable markers of active beta-cell destruction in the prodromal period.

CONCLUSION

Although for many it has been a disappointment that the trials of cyclosporine and azathioprine for IDDM have not resulted in safe, effective means of preventing the disease, the experience with these agents has been extremely important. The trials have confirmed the immune basis for beta-cell loss in human IDDM and have reaffirmed the value of randomized control trials in assessing novel therapies. We are optimistic that current and future efforts will build upon this experience and make prevention of IDDM and its sequelae a reality.

REFERENCES

1 Elliot RB, Berryman CC, Crossley JR, James AG. Partial preservation of pancreatic beta-cell function in children with diabetes. *Lancet* 1981; 2: 1–4.
2 Mistura L, Beccaria L, Meschi F, D'Arcais A, Pellini C, Puzzovio M, Chiumello G. Prednisone treatment in newly diagnosed type 1 diabetic children: 1 year followup. *Diabetes Care* 1981; 10: 39–43.
3 Nerup J, Lernmark A. Autoimmunity in insulin-dependent diabetes mellitus. *Am J Med* 1981; 70: 135–41.
4 Cahill GF, McDevitt HO. Insulin-dependent diabetes mellitus: the initial lesion. *N Engl J Med* 1981; 304: 1454–65.
5 Atkinson MA, Maclaren NK. The pathogenesis of insulin-dependent diabetes mellitus. *N Engl J Med* 1994; 331: 1428–36.
6 Mandrup-Poulsen T, Reimers JI, Andersen HU, Pociot F, Karlsen AE, Bjerre U, Nerup J. Nicotinamide treatment in the prevention of insulin-dependent diabetes mellitus. *Diabetes Metab Revs* 1993; 9: 295–309.
7 Stiller CR, Dupre J, Gent M, Jenner MR, Keown P, Laupacis A, Martell R, Rodger NW, von Graffenried B, Wolfe BMJ. Effects of Cyclosporine immunosuppression in insulin-dependent diabetes mellitus of recent onset. *Science* 1984; 223: 1362–7.
8 Dupre J, Stiller CR, Gent M, Donner A, von Graffenried B, Murphy G, Heinrichs D et al. Effects of immunosuppression with Cyclosporine in insulin-dependent diabetes mellitus of recent onset: the Canadian open study at 44 months. *Transplant Proc* 1988; 20: 184–92.
9 Assan R, Feutren G, Debray-Sachs M, Quiniou-Debrie MC, Laborie C, Thomas G, Chatenoud, Bach JF. Metabolic and immunological effects of cyclosporin in recently diagnosed type 1 diabetes mellitus. *Lancet* 1985; i: 67–71.
10 Levy-Marchal C, Czernichow P. Effect of different doses of cyclosporine A (CsA) on the early phase of overt insulin-dependent diabetes mellitus (IDDM) in children. *Transplant Proc* 1985; 18: 1543–4.
11 Bougneres PF, Carel JC, Castano L, Boitard C, Gardin JP, Landais P, Hors J et al. Factors associated with early remission of type 1 diabetes in children treated with Cyclosporine. *N Engl J Med* 1988; 318: 663–70.
12 Bougneres PF, Landais P, Boisson C, Carel JC, Frament N, Boitard C, Chassain JL, Bach JF. Limited duration of remission of insulin dependency in children with recent overt type 1 diabetes treated with low-dose cyclosporin. *Diabetes* 1990; 39: 1264–72.
13 Assan R, Feutren G, Sirmai J, Laborie C, Boitard C, Vexiau P, Du Rostu H et al. Plasma C-peptide levels and clinical remissions in recent-onset type 1 diabetic patients treated with cyclosporine A and insulin. *Diabetes* 1990; 39: 768–74.
14 Harrison LC, Colman PG, Dean B, Baxter R, Martin FIR. Increase in remission rate in newly diagnosed type 1 diabetic subjects treated with azathioprine. *Diabetes* 1985; 34: 1306–8.

15 Feutren G, Papoz L, Assan R, Vialettes B, Karsenty G, Vexiau P, Du Rostu H *et al.* Cyclosporin increases the rate and length of remissions in insulin-dependent diabetes of recent onset. *Lancet* 1986; 2: 119–23.

16 The Canadian–European Randomized Control Trial Group. Cyclosporin-induced remission of IDDM after early intervention. *Diabetes* 1988; 37: 1574–82.

17 Skyler J, Rabinovitch A. Cyclosporine in recent onset type 1 diabetes mellitus. Effects on islet beta-cell function. *J Diab Comp* 1992; 6: 77–88.

18 Chase HP, Butler-Simon N, Garg SK, Hayward A, Klingensmith GJ, Hamman RF, O'Brien D. Cyclosporine A for treatment of new-onset insulin-dependent diabetes mellitus. *Paediatrics* 1990; 85: 241–5.

19 Cook JJ, Hudson I, Harrison LC, Dean B, Colman PG, Werther GA, Warne GL, Court JM. A double-blind controlled trial of azathioprine in children with newly diagnosed type 1 diabetes. *Diabetes* 1989; 38: 779–83.

20 Silverstein J, Maclaren N, Riley W, Spillar R, Radjenovic D, Johnson S. Immunosuppression with azathioprine and prednisone in recent-onset insulin-dependent diabetes mellitus. *N Engl J Med* 1983; 319: 599–604.

21 Koivisto VA, Aro A, Cantell K, Haataja M, Huttunen J, Karonen S-L, Mustajoki P *et al.* Remissions in newly diagnosed type 1 (insulin-dependent) diabetes: influence of interferon as an adjunct to insulin therapy. *Diabetologia* 1984; 27: 193–7.

22 Feutren G, Mihatsch M. Risk factors for Cyclosporine-induced nephropathy in patients with autoimmune diseases. *N Engl J Med* 1992; 326: 1654–60.

23 Van Scoik KG, Johnson CA. The pharmacology and metabolism of the thiopurine drugs 6-mercaptopurine and azathioprine. *Drug Metab Rev* 1985; 142: 157–74.

24 Kinlen LJ. Immunosuppressive therapy and cancer. *Cancer Surveys* 1982; i: 566–83.

25 Sacks HS, Chalmers TC, Smith H. Randomized versus historical controls for clinical trials. *Am J Med* 1982; 72: 233–40.

26 Savilahati E, Tuomilehto J, Saukkonen TT, Akerblom HK, Virtala ET. Increased levels of cow's milk and beta-lactoglobulin antibodies in young children with newly diagnosed IDDM. *Diabetes Care* 1993; 16: 984–9.

27 Keller RJ, Eisenbarth GS, Jackson RA. Insulin prophylaxis in individuals at high risk of type 1 diabetes. *Lancet* 1993; 341: 927–8.

28 Erlanger BF. Do we know the site of action of cyclosporin? *Immunol Today* 1992; 13: 487–91.

29 Hawthorne AB, Hawkey CJ. Immunosuppressive drugs in inflammatory bowel disease: a review of their mechanisms of efficacy and place in therapy. *Drugs* 1989; 38: 267–88.

30 Mandrup-Poulsen T, Molvig J, Andersen HU, Helqvist S, Spinas GA, Munck M for the Canadian–European Randomized Control Trial Group. Lack of predictive value of islet cell antibodies, insulin antibodies and HLA-DR phenotype for remission in cyclosporine-treated IDDM patients. *Diabetes* 1990; 39: 204–10.

31 Petersen JS, Dyrberg T, Karlsen AE, Molvig J, Michelsen B, Nerup N, Mandrup-Poulsen T for the Canadian–European Randomized Control Trial Group. Glutamic acid decarboxylase autoantibodies in prediction of beta-cell function and remission in recent-onset IDDM after cyclosporine treatment. *Diabetes* 1994; 43: 1291–4.

32 The DCCT Research Group. Effects of age, duration and treatment of insulin-dependent diabetes mellitus on residual beta-cell function: observations during eligibility testing for the Diabetes Control and Complications Trial (DCCT). *J Clin Endocrinol Metab* 1987; 65: 30–6.

33 Hramiak IM, Dupre J, Finegood DT. Determinants of clinical remission in recent-onset IDDM. *Diabetes Care* 1993; 16: 125–32.

34 McCulloch DK, Klaff LJ, Kahn SE, Schoenfield SL, Greenbaum CJ, Mauseth RS,

Benson EA et al. A prospective study of subclinical beta-cell dysfunction among first-degree relatives of IDDM patients: 5 yr followup of the Seattle Family Study. Diabetes 1990; 39: 549–56.

35 Dahlqvist G, Blom L, Bolme P, Hagenfeldt L, Lindgren F, Persson B, Thalme B, Thoerell M, Westin S. Factors influencing the magnitude, duration, and rate of fall of B-cell function in type 1 diabetic children followed for two years from their clinical diagnosis. Diabetologia 1982; 31: 664–9.

36 Agner TP, Damm P, Binder C. Remission in IDDM: prospective study of basal C-peptide and insulin dose in 268 consecutively studied patients. Diabetes Care 1987; 10: 164–9.

37 Clarson C, Daneman D, Drash AL, Becker DJ, Ehrlich RM. Residual beta-cell function in children with IDDM: reproducibility of testing and factors influencing insulin secretory capacity. Diabetes Care 1987; 10: 33–8.

38 The Diabetes Control and Complications Trial Research Group. The effect of intensive treatment of diabetes on the development and progression of long-term complications in insulin-dependent diabetes mellitus. N Engl J Med 1993; 329: 977–86.

39 Eff C, Faber O, Deckert T. Persistent insulin secretion assessed by plasma C-peptide estimation in long-term juvenile diabetics with a low insulin requirement. Diabetologia 1979; 15: 169–72.

40 Sjoberg S, Gunnarsson R, Gjotterberg M, Lefvery AK, Persson A, Ostman J. Residual insulin production, glycemic control and prevalence of microvascular lesions and polyneuropathy in long-term type 1 diabetes mellitus. Diabetologia 1987; 30: 208–13.

41 The DCCT Research Group. Factors in the development of diabetic neuropathy. Diabetes 1988; 37: 476–81.

42 Madsbad S, Lauritzen E, Faber OK, Binder C. The effect of residual beta-cell function on the development of diabetic retinopathy. Diabetic Med 1986; 3: 42–5.

43 Bodansky HJ, Medbak S, Drury PL, Cudworth AG. Plasma C-peptide in long-standing type 1 diabetics with and without microvascular complications. Diabetic Med 1981; 7: 265–9.

44 Sberna P, Valentini U, Cimino A, Sabatti M, Rotundi A, Cristiq M, Spandrio S. Residual B-cell function in insulin dependent (type 1) diabetics with and without retinopathy. Acta Diab Lat 1986; 23: 339–44.

45 Bires B, Follansbee W, Orchard T. Does residual beta-cell function relate to the complications of IDDM? Diabetes 1989; 38 (supplement 1): 91A.

46 Smith RBW, Pyke DA, Watkins PJ, Binder C, Faber OK. C-peptide response to glucagon in diabetics with and without complications. N Zeal Med J 1979; 89: 304–6.

47 Haumant D, Borchy H, Toussaint D, Despontin M. Exogenous insulin needs. Relationship with duration of diabetes, C-peptidemia, insulin antibodies, and retinopathy. Helv Paed Acta 1982; 37: 143–50.

48 Eisenbarth GS. Type 1 diabetes mellitus. A chronic autoimmune disease. New Engl J Med 1986; 314: 1360–8.

49 Gorsuch AN, Spencer KM, Lister J, Mcnally JM, Dean BM, Bottazzo GF, Cudworth AG. Evidence for a long prediabetic period in type 1 (insulin dependent) diabetes mellitus. Lancet 1981; ii: 1363–5.

50 Millward BA, Alviggi L, Hoskins PJ, Johnston C, Heaton D, Botazzo GF, Vergani D et al. Immune changes associated with insulin dependent diabetes may remit without causing the disease: a study in identical twins. Br Med J 1986; 292: 793–6.

16

Insulin Treatment in Pre-diabetes

TIHAMER ORBAN and RICHARD JACKSON
Joslin Diabetes Center, Boston, Massachusetts, USA

BACKGROUND

Other chapters in this book document the abnormalities present in individuals before the onset of hyperglycemia and clinical diabetes. At the present time, the most effective way to identify high risk subjects is by screening first degree relatives, whose risk of developing diabetes is about 10 times that of the general population. Although a number of autoantibodies have now been identified, most of the clinical experience has been with islet cell antibodies (ICAs) and insulin autoantibodies (IAAs). These antibodies, combined with a measure of metabolic activity (the one plus three minute insulin values from an intravenous glucose tolerance test), can identify relatives at high risk for future development of Type 1 diabetes. Once such a group has been identified, the next question is "What treatment should we test as a possible intervention?" Data from three different sources provide support for intervention: (1) spontaneous animal models of autoimmune diabetes, currently the NOD mouse and the BB rat; (2) patients with new-onset Type 1 diabetes; and (3) other human autoimmune diseases, such as multiple sclerosis and rheumatoid arthritis.

INSULIN TREATMENT IN SPONTANEOUS ANIMAL MODELS

Many different therapies, detailed in previous chapters, have been successful in preventing hyperglycemia in the NOD mouse and the BB rat. There are

Prediction, Prevention and Genetic Counseling in IDDM. Edited by Jerry P. Palmer.
© 1996 John Wiley & Sons Ltd.

several interesting aspects of these studies, the most striking being the sheer number of methods which can successfully prevent diabetes in these models. Successful interventions also target a wide variety of pathways, from surgery to transfusion to diet to specific T-cell subset and lymphokine therapies. Many of these methods may not be applicable to human diabetes (neonatal thymectomy, whole body radiation, . . .), and others (high dose cyclosporin, lymphocyte transfusions, . . .) have worrisome side-effects. Of the several therapies which have been successful in the animal models and could be safely considered in humans, insulin is the one which has been best studied.

The BB rat develops a spontaneous autoimmune diabetes which becomes evident around 90 to 100 days of age. Insulin delivery to these animals starting at 35 to 40 days of age by either implantable insulinomas or Alzet mini pumps significantly reduced the incidence of diabetes (3 of 21 and 4 of 28 versus 14 of 16) as well as the incidence of insulitis[1]. The decrease in insulitis shows an effect on the basic disease process, separate from any simple metabolic effects. The insulin treatment was stopped at 120 days, and the rats were followed for another 50 days off insulin—no further diabetes developed. Another group similarly treated BB rats with ultralente insulin, beginning at 40 days and continuing to 142 days, again noting a reduction in diabetes (6 of 36 versus 15 of 36) and also in insulitis[2]. The same effect is seen with insulin given as a subcutaneous injection five times a week, from age 35 days to 120 days[3]. Again, no further diabetes was seen after the insulin injections were stopped, but there was an increase in insulitis during this time. In this same study a group of rats receiving insulin were transfused with Con-A activated splenocytes from diabetic rats. Rats which had received insulin injections for only 2 weeks developed diabetes after this splenocyte transfer, whereas rats which received at least 4 weeks of insulin injections were much less susceptible. Subcutaneous insulin protected 33-day-old rats which had just received Con-A activated lymphocytes from developing diabetes[4]. Although the insulin treatment seems to protect these rats from developing diabetes after adoptive transfer, the reverse does not hold true. BB rats (in this case RT6-depleted DR BB/Wor rats) which received insulin and sustained a reduction in diabetes and insulitis had their spleens harvested, and the splenocytes activated in culture with Con-A. These splenocytes were able to produce diabetes when transferred to other BB rats[5]. A Montreal group compared the effects of insulin with those of glyburide, an oral hypoglycemic agent, and diazoxide, which inhibits insulin secretion with resulting hyperglycemia[6]. Diazoxide had a diabetes-reducing effect similar to insulin, while glyburide had no effect on decreasing diabetes.

Similar results are reported in NOD mice, where daily protamine zinc insulin was given by injection to mice at weaning; diabetes was reduced to 3 of 34 versus 17 of 26 in the control group, and insulitis was also decreased[7]. As in the BB rat, insulin injections also protect NOD mice from adoptive transfer of diabetes[8]. Histologic examination found that the islets from insulin-treated mice had a higher insulin content than control NOD mice. The Gainesville group further analyzed the effects of parenteral insulin by using an "immunization" schedule, injecting insulin with incomplete Freund's adjuvant on an every four to eight week period for a total of four injections. Insulin given in this way would have very little metabolic effect, and was very effective in preventing diabetes and insulitis. Insulin B-chain given in this manner was also effective, while the insulin A-chain and insulin diluent were not effective. Splenocytes from NOD mice immunized with insulin or B-chain were also able to prevent diabetes when co-infused with diabetic splenocytes into a susceptible host[9].

Insulin has been effective in both spontaneous animal models of autoimmune diabetes in a variety of laboratories. The beneficial effect may be mediated through its metabolic actions, but part of the effect also appears to come from its immune modulating effects as an important beta-cell antigen, since immunizing doses and B-chain are also effective. The metabolic effects are probably also important, as interventions which limit endogenous insulin secretion (diazoxide) can decrease the incidence of disease.

INSULIN IN NEW-ONSET TYPE 1 DIABETES

One of the interesting results from the cyclosporin studies in new-onset patients with Type 1 diabetes was the chance to observe the placebo groups, and to document the degree of residual beta-cell function which exists at the onset of Type 1 diabetes. In the largest controlled study, a combination European and Canadian effort, the placebo group had a remission rate of 9.8% at the end of year[10]. Remission was defined as normal glycohemoglobin while off insulin treatment. At 6 months the remission rate in the control group was about 20%. Many more patients in the control group presumably had some residual beta cell function, but not enough to produce a full remission. This means that even at the onset of clinical diabetes, most patients still have islets capable of producing insulin, raising the possibility that this capability could be preserved, either by cyclosporin or by other means. Treatments which preserve some beta-cell function may be even more effective when applied to subjects who are much earlier in the disease process, and who still have normal glucose tolerance.

Many diabetes clinicians have felt that early treatment of type 1 diabetes with insulin was more likely to result in a honeymoon, an attitude typified by Robert Jackson's early studies in the 1940s[11]. In the 1970s a retrospective study in Sweden showed that patients who received higher insulin doses initially had better diabetes control 3 to 14 years later, and were also more likely to retain C-peptide[12]. Mirouze treated patients with Type 1 diabetes at onset with an "artificial pancreas" for 24 hours, and saw an increase in sustained remissions in this group[13]. Following this a number of studies looked at the effect of strict initial control on later residual beta cell function, and on ease of glucose control at later timepoints[14,15]. Positive effects were seen, but some studies found that the length of this positive effect was short-lived[16]. Then in 1989 Shah and Malone published a striking study in the *New England Journal of Medicine* in which they randomly assigned 26 adolescents with new-onset Type 1 diabetes into either a conventional group or a treatment group[17]. The treatment group received 14 days of in-patient intravenous (IV) insulin, and afterward received conventional insulin treatment identical to that of the conventional group. The two groups were then followed and treated in an identical manner, and evaluated after one year. The IV insulin group had significantly higher stimulated C-peptide secretion and markedly better glycohemoglobin values than the control group.

INTERVENTION THERAPY IN OTHER AUTOIMMUNE DISEASES

The area of oral tolerization is relatively new as applied to human disease, and is discussed in more detail in Chapter 18. The two animal models best studied are experimental autoimmune encephalitis (EAE), which is a model for human multiple sclerosis, and collagen-induced arthritis, a model for rheumatoid arthritis[18,19]. In each of these animals the antigen is specific for the involved tissue. Recently pilot trials in humans with multiple sclerosis and rheumatoid arthritis have shown positive results which have increased interest in this mode of therapy[20,21]. Oral administration of insulin can prevent diabetes in the NOD mouse, and this protection can be adoptively transferred with splenic T cells from an insulin-treated mouse[22,23]. The insulin B-chain is also effective orally, although the A-chain is not[24]. Thus insulin has a direct effect on the immune process, separate from any possible metabolically mediated effects.

HYPOTHESES FOR BENEFICIAL EFFECT

Why is subcutaneous insulin effective in the animal models? Hypotheses can be grouped under two main headings. One hypothesis is "beta cell rest", or perhaps better termed "beta cell assistance", and results from a metabolic effect of insulin on the beta cell. The insulin may cause a decrease in the density of beta-cell antigens which are involved in the ongoing immune-mediated destruction. If the metabolic activity of the beta cell is decreased, it may be less susceptible to damage from agents such as lymphokines or free radicals. Another group of hypotheses addresses a direct, non-metabolic effect of insulin. Support here comes from studies which use oral insulin, the B-chain of insulin, or insulin given in an immunizing schedule. Because of its long history as an essential metabolic hormone, the importance of insulin as one of the primary antigens involved in Type 1 diabetes is often overlooked. Insulin is beta-cell specific, appears on the cell surface, and in our family studies IAA is often the first autoantibody which appears. Wegman has shown that in the NOD, the earliest infiltrating T cells in the islets respond to insulin, and not to the other known autoantigens[25].

How do the islet cells change under the influence of insulin, or with changes in metabolic activity? A five day per week insulin injection regimen which was successful in decreasing diabetes and insulitis also produced smaller islets which had decreased insulin by immunocytochemistry[3]. The expression of beta cell antigens increases when beta cells are more active, and decreases when they are less active. These changes in antigen density are reflected by changes in antibody binding to these antigens. In vivo, feeding rats an insulin-stimulating diet high in sucrose and fat increases the binding of human islet cells antibody (ICA) positive serum to the rat islets, when these islets are used as the substrate in the standard ICA assays[26]. This same change in antigen expression also occurs for the two beta cell antigens recognized by monoclonal antibodies IC2 and A2B5. Culturing rat islets at increasing glucose concentrations, resulting in increasing beta cell metabolic activity, resulted in increasing expression of these two antigens[27]. Using the IC2 monoclonal, which binds to a beta cell specific antigen, these same investigators did in vivo experiments in mice and rats[28]. Fasted animals had decreased antigen expression compared to non-fasting animals, and animals treated with subcutaneous insulin for one week also showed decreased antigen expression. Insulin treatment of BB rats by means of transplantable RIN insulinomas causes a marked down-regulation of three different islet antigens recognized by monoclonal antibodies A2B5, R2D6 and 3G5[29]. The 64K-autoantigen, now known to be GAD, is also present in increasing amounts in rat islets and monkey islets exposed to increasing glucose concentrations[30,31], and this level of expression is linked to insulin secretion[32]. In fact, the increased expression associated with higher glucose values can be blocked by diazoxide[6], which inhibits glucose-stimulated insulin release, implying that the effect is related to decreased insulin production rather than hyperglycemia.

One of the prominent hypotheses explaining beta cell destruction is lysis by lymphokines[33]. Cultured rat islets are killed by both IL-1 and tumor necrosis factor (TNF), and beta cells may be more sensitive to these lymphokines than other islet cells[34]. This destruction is modulated by beta cell activity; islets cultured in increasing glucose concentrations are more susceptible to killing by both IL-1 and TNF[35]. "Resting" beta cells seem to be more resistant to the effects of IL-1 than beta cells which are active, that is, responding to glucose and secreting more insulin[36].

POSSIBLE SIDE-EFFECTS AND SAFETY ISSUES OF INSULIN TREATMENT

There is no evidence that insulin can precipitate hyperglycemia or glucose intolerance. Although one study in 1966, by Albert Renold, noted some lymphocytic islet infiltration in cows which received injections of bovine insulin in complete Freund's adjuvant (CFA), there was no diabetes or glucose intolerance in these animals, and no observable beta cell destruction[37]. Later studies using insulin alone or in combination with CFA showed neither insulitis nor diabetes[38]. In humans intramuscular insulin injections have frequently been used for treatment of various psychiatric disorders. A large retrospective study of 481 patients looked at subsequent development of diabetes[39]. These patients received an average of 59 injections each, with an average dose of 78 units. Over a mean follow-up time of 22 years, only one of these patients developed Type 1 diabetes, similar to the expected frequency in the general population.

The major side-effect of concern is hypoglycemia. In human pilot studies, described below, there has been minimal hypoglycemia. The risk of hypoglycemia can be controlled in several ways, the main method being the choice of a low insulin dosage. Also, since these subjects do not have diabetes, they have all of the compensatory systems intact, including the ability to suppress their own endogenous insulin secretion.

HUMAN STUDIES IN PRE-DIABETES

Family studies at the Joslin Clinic have provided a subject base for defining high risk relatives. We used a combination of IAA and IVGTT insulin values in ICA positive first degree relatives to select subjects who had a greater than 90% chance of developing diabetes within four years[40]. Based on the animal studies detailed above, we gave daily subcutaneous insulin to a small number of such high risk relatives. The aim of this pilot study was to assess the practicality and safety of this treatment, and to assess possible efficacy. At the time that the subcutaneous protocol was being developed, the report from Tampa on the positive effects of intravenous insulin in new-onset patients[17] appeared, and we added a once yearly intravenous insulin component to the protocol. All of the subjects were required to have a normal (by NDDG criteria) OGTT before starting treatment.

The dose of subcutaneous insulin was an important consideration, and could be approached in two ways. The first way involved giving as much insulin as possible, with the thought that this would maximize the chances of seeing a beneficial effect. This would involve taking insulin injections in much the same way as patients with diabetes; there would be multiple injections, frequent home glucose monitoring, restriction of diet and activity, and the unavoidable occurrence of hypoglycemia. Another approach would be to give a smaller dose of insulin, which could be given without diet or activity restrictions, without frequent monitoring, and with little or no risk of hypoglycemia. We chose the latter approach, with the goal of changing the subject's lifestyle as little as possible, with the exception of injections before breakfast and before bed.

Five subjects were treated and compared with two sets of controls; seven contemporary relatives who met the same high risk characteristics but declined treatment, and forty historical controls who met the same entry criteria[41]. The results showed that the insulin regimen was practical, and that there was minimal hypoglycemia—0 to 3 mild episodes per year, which either resolved spontaneously or were relieved by simple measures. The subjects received an average of 0.22 units of insulin per day. Two of the treated subjects developed diabetes, though at a delayed time compared to their predicted time for diabetes. These two had the highest diabetes risk, and in fact their "predicted time" to diabetes was negative with the model used. The seven subjects who declined treatment all developed diabetes within 2.2 years (Figure 16.1). Entry into the pilot study was stopped after the initial 12 subjects, and a randomized, controlled trial of parenteral insulin was begun. This study has since evolved into a multicenter NIH sponsored trial termed Diabetes Prevention Trial—Type 1, or DPT-1 which is ongoing.

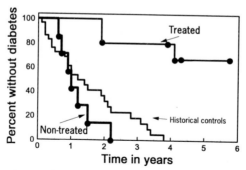

Figure 16.1. Progression to clinical IDDM in high risk subjects treated with parenteral insulin versus non-treated controls and historical controls

PRESENT AND FUTURE ACTIONS

The DPT-1 trial will screen 60 000 to 80 000 first degree relatives of patients with Type 1 diabetes. The initial screening will be done with ICA, and positive relatives will have subsequent IAA and IVGTT determinations to determine whether they are at high or medium risk for future development of diabetes. High risk relatives will be randomized to receive parenteral insulin versus no treatment (but close follow-up of their metabolic status), with a combination of subcutaneous and intravenous insulin. Subcutaneous insulin will be given in two doses of human ultralente insulin, 0.125 U/kg each, given before breakfast and before bed. Intravenous insulin will be given in an inpatient Clinical Research Center setting every 12 months, for a period of four days. Medium risk relatives will be randomized to receive oral insulin once a day or oral placebo. Entry into the intervention parts of the trial will begin in 1995, and subjects will be followed over a period of 5 to 6 years. This trial will serve as a prototype for any future intervention trials, whether refinements of insulin treatment are being investigated, or new therapies are being tried.

ACKNOWLEDGMENTS

The authors wish to express their thanks to Ruth Gerace and Terry Smith for their help with clinical material and to Ann Tolson for secretarial assistance.

REFERENCES

1 Appel MC, O'Neil JJ. Prevention of spontaneous diabetes in the bb/w rat by insulin treatment. *Pancreas* 1986; 1: 356.
2 Gotfredsen CF, Buschard K, Frandsen EK. Reduction of diabetes incidence of BB Wistar rats by early prophylactic insulin treatment of diabetes-prone animals. *Diabetologia* 1985; 28: 933–5.
3 Like AA. Insulin injections prevent diabetes (DB) in Bio-Breeding/Worcester (BB/Wor) rats. *Diabetes* 1986; 35 (Suppl 1): 74A.
4 Bertrand S, DePaepe M, Vigeant C, Yale JF. Prevention of adoptive transfer of BB rats by prophylactic insulin treatment. *Diabetes* 1992; 41: 1273–7.
5 Gottlieb PA, Handler ES, Appel MC, Greiner DL, Mordes JP, Rossini AA. Insulin treatment prevents diabetes mellitus but not thyroiditis in RT6-depleted diabetes resistant BB/Wor rats. *Diabetologia* 1991; 34: 296–300.
6 Vlahos WD, Seemayer TA, Yale JF. Diabetes prevention in BB rats by inhibition of endogenous insulin secretion. *Meab Clin Ex* 1991; 4018: 825–9.
7 Atkinson MA, Maclaren NK, Luchetta R. Insulitis and diabetes in NOD mice reduced by prophylactic insulin therapy. *Diabetes* 1990; 39: 933–7.
8 Thivolet CH, Goillot JE, Bedossa P, Durand A, Bonnard M, Orgiazzi J. Insulin

prevents adoptive cell transfer of diabetes in autoimmune non-obese diabetic mouse. *Diabetologia* 1991; **34**: 314–19.

9 Muir A, Peck A, Clare-Salzler M, Song Y-H, Cornelius J, Luchetta R, Krischer J, Maclaren N. Insulin immunization of NOD mice induces a protective insulitis characterized by diminished intra-islet interferon-γ transcription. *Diabetes* 1993; **42** (Suppl 1): 5A.

10 The Canadian–European Randomized Control Trial Group. Cyclosporin-induced remission of IDDM after early intervention: association of 1 year of cyclosporin treatment with enhanced insulin secretion. *Diabetes* 1988; **37**: 1574–82.

11 Jackson R, Boyd J, Smith T. Stabilization of the diabetic child. *Am J Dis Child* 1940; **59**: 332–41.

12 Ludvigsson J, Heding G, Larsson Y, Leander E. C-peptide in juvenile diabetics beyond the postinitial remission period. *Acta Paediatr Scand* 1977; **66**: 177–84.

13 Mirouze J, Selam JL, Pham TC, Mendoza E, Orsetti A. Sustained insulin-induced remissions of juvenile diabetes by means of an external artificial pancreas. *Diabetologia* 1978; **114**: 223–7.

14 Madsbad S, Krarup T, Regeur L, Faber OK, and Binder C. Effect of strict blood glucose control on residual B-cell function in insulin-dependent diabetics. *Diabetologia* 1981; **20**: 530–4.

15 Madsbad S, Krarup T, Faber OK, Binder C, Regeur L. The transient effect of strict glycaemic control on B cell function in newly diagnosed type I (insulin-dependent) diabetic patients. *Diabetologia* 1982; **22**: 16–20.

16 Perlman K, Ehrlich RM, Filler RM, Albisser AM. Sustained mormoglycemia in newly diagnosed type I diabetic subjects. *Diabetes* 1984; **33**: 995–1001.

17 Shah SC, Malone JI, Simpson NE. A randomized trial of intensive insulin therapy newly diagnosed insulin-dependent mellitus. *NEJM* 1989; March: 550–4.

18 Higgins PJ, Weiner HL. Suppression of experimental autoimmune encephalomyelitis by oral administration of myelin basic protein and its fragments. *J Immunol* 1988; **140**: 440–5.

19 Zhang J, Lee CSY, Lider O, Weiner H. Suppression of adjuvant arthritis in lewis rats by oral administration of Type II collagen. *J Immunol* 1990; **145**: 2489–93.

20 Trentham DE, Dynbesius-Trentham RA, Orav EJ, Combitchi D, Lorenzo C, Sewell KL, Hafler DA, Weiner HL. Effects of oral administration of Type II collagen on rheumatoid arthritis. *Science* 1993; **261**: 1727–30.

21 Weiner HL, Mackin GA, Matsui M, Orav EJ, Khoury SJ, Dawson DM, Hafler DA. Double-blind pilot trial of oral tolerization with myelin antigens in multiple sclerosis. *Science* 1993; **259**: 1321–4.

22 Zhang ZJ, Davidson L, Eisenbarth G, Weiner HL. Suppression of diabetes in nonobese diabetic mice by oral administration of porcine insulin. *Proc Natl Acad Sci USA* 1991; **88**: 10252–6.

23 Dong J, Muir A, Schatz D, Luchetta R, Hao W, Atkinson M, Maclaren N. Oral administration of insulin prevents diabetes in NOD mice. *Diabetes Res Clin Pract* 1991; **14**: S55.

24 Zhang J, Shoelson S, Miller A, Weiner HL. Insulitis is suppressed in NOD mice by oral administration of insulin peptides and glucagon. *FASEB (2)* 1992; **6**(5): abstract 4380.

25 Wegman DR, Gill RG, Norbury-Glaser M, Schlott N, Daniel D. Analysis of the spontaneous T cell response to insulin in NOD mice. *J Autoimmun* 1994; **7**: 833–43.

26 McCulloch DK, Barmeier H, Neifing JL, Palmer JP. Metabolic state of the pancreas affects end-point titre in the islet cell antibody assay. *Diabetologia* 1991; **34**: 622–5.

27 Aaen K, Rygaard J, Josefsen K, Petersen H, Brogren CH, Horn T, Buschard K.

Dependence of antigen expression on functional state of B-cells. *Diabetes* 1990; **39**: 697–701.

28 Buschard K, Brogren C-H, Ropke C, Rygaard J. Antigen expression of the pancreatic beta-cells is dependent on their functional state, as shown by a specific, BB rat monoclonal autoantibody IC2. *APMIS* 1988; **96**: 342–6.

29 Appel MC, Dotta F, O'Neil JJ, Eisenbarth GS. B-cell activity regulates the expression of islet antigenic determinants. *Diabetologia* 1989; **32**: 461.

30 Kampe O, Andersson A, Bjork E, Hallberg A, Karlsson FA. High-glucose stimulation of 64,000-Mr islet cell autoantigen expression. *Diabetes* 1989; **38**: 1326–8.

31 Hagopian WA, Karlsen AE, Petersen JS, Teague J, Gervassi A, Jiang J, Fujimotos W, Lernmark A. Regulation of glutamic acid decarboxylase diabetes autoantigen expression in highly purified isolated islets from *Macaca nemestrina*. *Endocrinology* 1993; **132**(6): 2647.

32 Bjork E, Kampe O, Andersson A, and Karlsson FA. Expression of the 64 kKa/glutamic acid decarboxlase rat islet cell autoantigen is influenced by the rate of insulin secretion. *Diabetologia* 1992; **32**: 490–3.

33 Mandrup-Poulsen T, Bendtzen K, Nerup J, Dinarello CA, Svenson M, Nielsen JH. Affinity-purified human interleukin 1 is cytotoxic to isolated islets of Langerhans. *Diabetologia* 1986; **29**: 63–7.

34 Nerup J, Mandrup-Poulsen T, Molvig J, Helquist S, Wogeusen L, Egeberg T. Mechanisms of pancretic beta cell destruction in Type 1 diabetes; an experimental model. *Diabetes Care* 1988; **11** (Suppl 1): 16–23.

35 Mehta VK, Hao W, Brooks-J, Worrell BM, Palmer JP. Low-dose interleukin 1 and tumor necrosis factor individually stimulate insulin release but in combination cause suppression. *Eur J Endocrinol* 1994; **130**: 208–14.

36 Palmer JP, Helzuist S, Spinas GA, Molvig J, Mandrup-Poulsen T, Anadersen HU, Newup J. Interaction of B-cell activity and IL-1 concentration and exposure time in isolated rat islets of langerhans. *Diabetes* 1989; **38**: 1211–16.

37 LeCompte PM, Steinke J, Soeldner JS, Renold AE. Changes in the islets of Langerhans in cows injected with heterologous and homologous insulin. *Diabetes* 1966; **15**(8): 586–96.

38 Augstein P, Kohnert K-D, Ziegler B, Furll B, Heinke P, Ziegler M. Induction of islet cell surface and insulin antibodies in balb/c mice by application of porcine insulin and Freund's adjuvant is not associated with insulitis. *Horm Metab Res* 1993; **25**: 344–7.

39 Bock T, Pedersen CR, Josefsen K, Bottazzo GF, Palmer JP, Buschard K. No risk of diabetes after insulin-shock treatment. *Lancet* 1992; **339**: 1504–6.

40 Jackson R, Vardi P, Herskowitz R, Eisenbarth G. Dual parameter linear model for prediction of onset of Type 1 diabetes in ICA positive relatives. *Clin Res* 1988; **36**: 585A.

41 Keller R, Eisenbarth G, Jackson R. Insulin prophylaxis in individuals at high risk of type 1 diabetes. *Lancet* 1993; **341**: 927–8.

17

The Use of Nicotinamide to Prevent Type 1 Diabetes

ROBERT B. ELLIOTT[1] and THOMAS MANDRUP-POULSEN[2]
[1]University of Auckland, New Zealand and [2]Steno Diabetes Centre, Denmark

INTRODUCTION

In designing strategies to prevent Type 1 diabetes, it is important to consider not only the biological plausibility of the agent used as the preventive, but also its safety and acceptability. None of the predictive tests used to define risk populations have 100% positive predictive value, so the safety and acceptability of an agent are as important as its potential biological activity when considering human preventive trials. High dose nicotinamide has been used successfully in the prevention of diabetes in the NOD mouse[1,2] and is an attractive agent as it has been in use clinically for a long time without apparent harmful effects.

The science of how nicotinamide exerts this protective effect has come a long way in the last decade, and its potential use in humans has gained some respectability. Nevertheless, the demonstration of protective function on β cells in vitro, and its successful use in an animal model—the NOD mouse—do not guarantee its usefulness in humans. Only clinical trials can establish this.

Not surprisingly, the first use of high dose nicotinamide in diabetes was in recently diagnosed humans. The effect on residual β-cell function has varied from small to non-existent[3-7]. Age at diagnosis seems to account for these different results[4,7], with younger children showing little if any response. This outcome is not surprising given the severe β-cell depletion which usually is present at the time of diagnosis—more so in the very young.

Prediction, Prevention and Genetic Counseling in IDDM. Edited by Jerry P. Palmer.
© 1996 John Wiley & Sons Ltd.

We will first present the evidence to date of the preventive effect of nicotinamide in humans as there would be little point in presenting the in vitro and animal model evidence of possible effectiveness if the human clinical trials showed no effect whatsoever.

EXPERIENCE IN HUMANS TO DATE

FIRST DEGREE RELATIVES OF TYPE 1 DIABETES

The trials so far reported either have been anecdotal or have used historical controls. In one such study 22 children aged less than 16 years old were drawn from two centers on the criteria of showing high levels of islet cell antibodies (80 or more units) and a degree of impairment of first phase insulin release in response to an infused bolus of glucose (less than 67 milliunits, sum of the 1' and 3' samples). Eight were not treated and all had developed diabetes within five years. The remainder were treated daily with 150–300 mg nicotinamide for every year of age. At a similar period of follow-up about half had the disease. The children were not randomly allocated to the two groups, and the treatment was not blind[8]. In an extension of this study, a much larger cohort of subjects who were relatives of all ages, with ICA of 20 or more JDF units, were also treated with nicotinamide. Their diabetes outcome was compared with two large untreated cohorts with similar characteristics[9]. Again a high degree of protection seemed apparent.

In another study three individuals, all of whom had high levels of islet and insulin autoantibodies and insulin release less than the third percentile, did not apparently benefit from treatment with nicotinamide compared with other individuals with the same characteristics[10].

Although none of these pilot trials demonstrates with any degree of certainty the effectiveness of nicotinamide, the discrepant results may be due to differences in selection criteria with the "unsuccessful" outcome being observed in individuals already very close to the onset of the disease.

GENERAL POPULATION STUDIES

Only one general population study has been reported in a preliminary fashion[9,11]. It involves a population of 80 000 children aged 5–7 at the time of admission to the trial. This was the entire available population of the city in which the trial was carried out. Some 33 000 of these children were randomly selected (by their school) to be tested for islet cell antibodies and of these some 20 000 accepted the offer of testing and 13 000 did not. The random remainder (48 000) were untested and constituted the control group. Those with persistent islet cell antibody levels of 20 or more JDF units plus those with 10 units of antibody and impaired first phase insulin release were offered treatment with nicotinamide.

After adjusting for the time it took to recruit the children, a mean follow-up time and subject/year exposure to diabetes risk could be calculated for the three groups and a diabetes incidence derived for the period of follow-up to date. The data are shown in Table 17.1. Some potential biases exist in the trial design, but most of these would mitigate against observing a protective effect. These potential biases include a possible lower ascertainment rate in the "control" group or the group who refused testing having a higher than expected diabetes incidence. The minor mean age difference in the three groups is very unlikely to have had any major effects on the results. It is implausible to attribute the high degree of significance of these results to these potential biases.

Table 17.1. Incidence of diabetes in school children (aged 5–7 at start of study)

Group	Subjects	Mean follow-up time (years)	Number developing diabetes	Diabetes incidence (per 100 000/year)
Control	48 335	5.2	55	21.0
Tested	20 195	4.2	6	7.1
Refused	13 463	4.2	10	17.7

A second trial involving 40 000 five-year-old children, avoiding age and possible microgeographical biases by better selection of the control group, is well past the recruiting stage and is yielding similar results to date.

The maximum follow-up time of these trial is six years, so it is far from certain that the effect observed will be maintained long term. However, an examination of the "failures" to date indicates that all have occurred in the first two years of follow-up and none in the third or subsequent years. This suggests that in some children the disease may have been too advanced at the time of recruitment to benefit from the treatment.

Large double-masked placebo-controlled studies of the preventive effect of nicotinamide in first degree relatives with ICA ≥ 20 units have been started in Europe and Canada. These will confirm these observations or otherwise, and possibly give a greater degree of quantitation to the short-term effect. They will be unable to provide information on the longer term effect as their design precludes this.

THE SCIENTIFIC RATIONALE OF THE USE OF NICOTINAMIDE

ANIMAL STUDIES

Streptozotocin-induced Diabetes in Rodents

The alkylating mutagen streptozotocin given intravenously to rodents causes swift destruction of the pancreatic β cells and in sufficient dose this leads to permanent diabetes. Large doses of nicotinamide given immediately before or within 1 hour of the intravenous or intraperitoneal injection of streptozotocin prevent the extremes of β-cell damage and diabetes[12-15].

Smaller doses of streptozotocin, individually insufficient to cause diabetes but given on five successive days, result in delayed appearance of diabetes (which may be immune mediated) and nicotinamide given after the completion of the course of the drug is ineffective in preventing the disease[16]. The putative mechanisms of the protective effect of nicotinamide are discussed below under the section on "in vitro" effects.

Effects in Rodent Models of Spontaneous Insulin-dependent Diabetes

The BB rat   Nicotinamide given to these animals even from weaning by intraperitoneal (i.p.) injection did not appear to have a protective effect against the spontaneous diabetes in these animals[17,18]. However, one author did note a protective effect of nicotinamide given in the drinking water[19].

The NOD mouse   Yamada et al.[1] were the first to show that nicotinamide given daily as a subcutaneous injection from the age of 80 days prevented the development of the disease. Subsequently the same effect could be obtained using a 1% solution of the vitamin in lieu of drinking water from weaning or 60 days of age. Thereafter this mode of administration was ineffective as were 0.1% solutions[2]. The protective effect appeared to wane after 230 days of age. Insulitis was present in all survivors at 250 days, but was of a lesser degree than controls[20]. Thus nicotinamide is ineffective if given too late or in insufficient doses.

EFFECTS OF NICOTINAMIDE ON β-CELL DESTRUCTION: BASIC STUDIES

Pathogenesis of β-Cell Destruction in IDDM

Recent studies point to the importance of free radicals as effectors of immune-mediated β-cell destruction. Thus, macrophages and endothelial cells activated by cytokines released in high local concentration in the inflammatory infiltrate in the islets synthesize nitric oxide radicals (NO) shown to be highly toxic to β cells in vitro[21]. Alternatively, cytokines, e.g. interleukin-1 (IL-1), tumor necrosis factor α (TNF) and interferon γ (IFN) produced by macrophages and T cells in synergy cause the synthesis of NO and free oxygen radicals (FOR) in the β cells[22]. Thus, cytokines induce the expression of the NO forming enzyme cytokine inducible nitric oxide synthase (iNOS) in rat and human islets. The intracellularly formed NO nitrosylates Fe-S groups in respiratory enzymes in mitochondria, especially aconitase, a key enzyme in the Krebs cycle[23]. When the activity of aconitase is inhibited, glucose oxidation is impaired leading to deficient ATP production and to functional inhibition of the β cell or cell death.

Depending upon the substrate concentration of L-arginine; iNOS activation may result in free oxygen radical production. Whether these radicals exert their action directly or interact with NO to form hydroxyl radicals (OH) is not clarified[24]. Both free oxygen derived radicals and NO cause DNA strand breaks, and cell death may be caused either from DNA damage directly if sufficiently massive, or from the process of repair of DNA damage. The repair process involves activation of the nuclear enzyme poly(adenosine diphosphate (ADP)-ribose) polymerase(P(ADPR)P)[25]. In the repair process the enzyme binds covalently to nucleic proteins to produce poly(ADP-ribose), using nicotinamide adenine dinucleotide (NAD) as a substrate. Thus, the cellular NAD pool may be depleted causing cell death or dysfunction, since NAD is also an essential co-factor in redox processes, including the mitochondrial electron transport chain.

Biochemical Mode of Action of Nicotinamide

Free oxygen derived radicals and NO radicals cause DNA strand breaks in islet cells which will activate P(ADPR)P and DNA repair[26], and the P(ADPR)P system has been shown to be activated in islets exposed to IL-1[27]. By inhibiting P(ADPR)P and the enzyme NADase that breaks down NAD and by repleting NAD stores, NA may prevent cellular NAD depletion and death.

NA also inhibits cytokine induced islet NO production[28–30] by inhibiting iNOS enzymatic activity and/or scavenging of NO radicals and at higher concentrations by inhibiting iNOS mRNA expression.

NA is known to be a weak scavenger of FOR and OH, but the chemistry of NA does not make a NO-scavenging action of NA likely, and preliminary studies in cell-free conditions support this notion[28].

NA prevents cytokine-induced MHC class II but not class I expression on cultured islet and thyroid cells[31,32]. The mechanism of action is unknown. The relevance of these findings is questionable, since class II expression on islet β cells in transgenic animals does not lead to autoimmune diabetes.

In summary, NA has several biochemical modes of action that are compatible with current concepts of the molecular mechanism leading to β-cell destruction in IDDM.

PHARMACOLOGY AND SAFETY OF NICOTAMIDE

NA is a white crystalline, odorless but bitter tasting, water-soluble power (MW 122.1 g mol^{-1}, melting point 128–131 °C). NA is derived from nicotinic acid (NI) by amidation of the carboxyl group of NI. NA exerts its most important biological functions by being converted into NAD$^+$ in the liver. NA is first deaminated to NI and then converted into NAD$^+$ which acts as a coenzyme for proteins involved in tissue respiration. When attached to these proteins NAD$^+$ functions as a dehydrogenase accepting hydrogen in the form of hybrid ions (H$^-$) from substrates and thereby being reduced to NADH.

NA is available in solution for injection and regular- or slow-release formulated tablets. It is readily absorbed from all sections of the intestine and is distributed in all tissues[33]. There is evidence that NA accumulates in the pancreatic islets. When injecting ^{14}C-labeled NA, NI or tryptophane to mice, a strong accumulation of labeling on whole body autoradiograms was found over islets in NA but not NI and tryptophane-injected animals, by far exceeding the intensity in blood[34]. The intensity was equal to that over kidney where the isotope is excreted. Although the accumulation was not precisely quantitated in this work, it suggests that islet concentrations of NA may be 100–1000-fold higher than in blood, accounting for the discrepancy between in vivo and in vitro findings in terms of effective concentrations.

NA is metabolized into N-methyl nicotinamide, which is further metabolized into N-methyl-2-pyridone-5-carboxamide and N-methyl-4-pyridone-3-car-boxamide[33]. These three metabolites are excreted in the urine, and N-methyl nicotinamide can be determined as a measure of drug compliance. When low doses of NA are given (50 mg day^{-1}) only very little unchanged NA appears in the urine. When high doses are administered the unchanged compound represents the major urinary component.

NA belongs to the family of B-vitamins. NA deficiency leads to pellagra which is characterized by abnormalities in the skin, gastrointestinal tract and CNS. The recommended daily intake is 0.30 mg kg^{-1} day^{-1}.

The following adverse effects in humans of NA doses from 3 to 12g day^{-1} have been reported[33,35]: rashes, facial erythema, hives, dry hair, soreness and tautness of the mouth, nausea and vomiting, heartburn, reversible elevation of liver function tests, dull headaches, fatigue, and inability to focus the eyes. Since some of these adverse effects are shared with nicotinic acid (rashes, dyspepsia, hepatotoxicity) they may be caused by the 4% contamination of the commercially available NA preparations with nicotinic acid.

When administered alone, NA has no carcinogenic potency[36], although the combination of NA and β-cell toxins causes islet cell tumors in rats and hamsters[37-39]. This oncogenicity is probably the result of an increased risk of mutation due to imbalance between the degree of DNA damage and the level of inhibition of DNA repair, i.e. P(ADPR)P activity. It is unknown whether NA alone has teratogenic effects. In rats 0.62–1 g kg^{-1} day^{-1} of NA in the drinking water or diet causes growth retardation, an effect that may be caused partly by a reduced water and food intake due to the foul taste of NA, and partly by deficiency of methionine, which is consumed during methylation of NA into its metabolites[40].

NA has by itself a bimodal time-dependent effect on β-cell function in vitro, short-term exposure leading to stimulation and long-term exposure to inhibition of glucose-stimulated insulin release[41-43]. In vivo, NI, but not NA, causes insulin resistance. NA does not acutely affect β-cell function in vivo[44].

CONCLUSIONS

Nicotinamide appears to be a relatively safe drug which is actively concentrated in the islets of Langerhans. It exerts a major protective effect against spontaneous diabetes in the NOD mouse if given in sufficient dose early enough. The protective effect appears to lie in the inhibition of the expression and enzymatic activity of cytokine-induced nitric oxide synthase, resulting in suppression of NO formation in the β cells and thereby resulting in less DNA damage and mitochondrial enzyme inactivation. Nicotinamide may further protect the β cells by inhibiting NAD depletion resulting from NO-induced DNA strand breaks and activation of an NAD-consuming DNA repair enzyme. Nicotinamide may have other helpful effects such as stimulating β-cell growth.

In humans nicotinamide appears to have a minor age-dependent β-cell sparing effect in newly diagnosed diabetics. In individuals considered at risk for developing the disease by reason of having islet cell antibodies with or without evidence of impaired insulin production, there is preliminary evidence that it exerts a protective effect against the development of diabetes. This evidence is strongest in a trial involving antibody positive school children, where the degree of protection over a four year period appears to be about 60–70%, with all of those not responding to treatment occurring in the first two years of follow-up. Large double-masked placebo-controlled trials in Europe and North America to confirm these results are well under way.

REFERENCES

1 Yamada K, Nonaka K, Hanfusa T, Miyazaki A, Toyoshima H, Tarui S. Preventive and therapeutic effects of large-dose nicotinamide injections on diabetes associated with insulitis. *Diabetes* 1982; **31**: 749–53.

2 Elliott RB, Reddy, S, Bibby NJ. Early nicotinamide treatment in the NOD mouse: effects on diabetes and insulitis suppression and autoantibody levels. *Diabetes Res* 1990; **15**: 95–102.
3 Pozzilli P, Visalli N, Ghirlanda G, Manna R, Andreani D. Nicotinamide increases C-peptide secretion in patients with recent onset type 1 diabetes. *Diabetic Med* 1989; **6**: 568–72.
4 Chase HP, Butler-Simon N, Garg S, McDuffie M, Hoops SL and O'Brien D. A trial of nicotinamide in newly diagnosed patients with Type 1 (insulin dependent) diabetes mellitus. *Diabetologia* 1990; **33**: 444–6.
5 Vialettes B, Picu R, Rostu MD, Charbonnel B, Rodier M, Mirouze J, Vexiau P, Passa P, Pehuet M, Elgrably F and Vague P. A preliminary multicentre study of the treatment of recently diagnosed Type 1 diabetes by combination nicotinamide-cyclosporin therapy. *Diabetes Care* 1990; **7**: 731–5.
6 Ilkova H, Görpe U, Kadioglu P, Ozyazar M and Bagriacik N. Nicotinamide in Type 1 diabetes mellitus of recent onset: a double blind placebo controlled trial. *Diabetologia* 1991; **34** (Suppl 2): A179.
7 Lewis CM, Canafax DM, Sprafka JM and Barbosa JJ. Double-blind randomised trial of nicotinamide on early-onset diabetes. *Diabetes Care* 1992; **15**: 121–3.
8 Elliott RB and Chase HP. Prevention or delay of type 1 (insulin dependent) diabetes mellitus in children using nicotinamide. *Diabetologia* 1991; **34**: 362–5.
9 Elliott RB, Pilcher CC, Stewart A, Fergusson D and McGregory MA. The use of nicotinamide in the prevention of Type 1 diabetes. *Immunosuppressive and Antiinflammatory Drugs, Ann NY Acad Sci* 1993; **696**: 333–41.
10 Herskowitz RD, Jackson RA, Soeldner JS, Eisenbarth GS. Pilot trial to prevent Type 1 diabetes: Progression to overt IDDM despite oral nicotinamide. *J Autoimmun* 1989; **2**: 733–7.
11 Elliott RB and Pilcher CC. Prevention of diabetes in normal school children. *Diabetes Res Clin Pract* 1991; **14**: S85.
12 Schein P, Cooney D and Vernon L. The use of nicotinamide to modify the toxicity of streptozotocin diabetes without loss of antitumour activity. *Cancer Res* 1967; **27**: 2324–32.
13 Dulin WE and Wyse BM. Studies of the ability of compounds to block the diabetogenic activity of streptozotocin. *Diabetes* 1969; **18**: 459–66.
14 Lazarus SS and Shapiro SH. Influence of nicotinamide and pyridine nucleotides on streptozotocin and alloxan induced pancreatic B cell cytotoxicity. *Diabetes* 1973; **22**: 499–506.
15 Schein PS, Rakieten N, Cooney DA, Davis R and Vernon ML. Streptozotocin diabetes in monkeys and dogs, and its prevention by nicotinamide. *Proc Soc Exp Biol Med* 1973; **143**: 514–18.
16 Rossini AA, Like AA, Chick WL, Appel MC and Cahill GF Jr. Studies of streptozotocin-induced insulitis and diabetes. *Proc Natl Acad Sci USA* 1977; **74**: 2485–9.
17 Rossini AA, Mordes JP, Gallina DL and Like AA. Hormonal and environmental factors in the pathogenesis of BB rat diabetes. *Metabolism* 1983; **32** (Suppl 1): 33–6.
18 Hermitte L, Vialettes B, Atlef N, Payan MJ, Doll N, Scheimann A and Vague P. High dose nicotinamide fails to prevent diabetes in BB rats. *Autoimmunity* 1989; **5**: 79–86.
19 Sarri Y, Mendola J, Ferrer J and Gomis R. Preventive effects of nicotinamide administration on spontaneous diabetes of BB rats. *Med Sci Res* 1989; **17**: 987–8.
20 Elliott RB, Bibby N and Reddy S. *Casein Peptide Precipitates Diabetes in the NOD Mouse and Possibly Humans. Genetic and Environmental Risk Factors for Type 1 Diabetes (IDDM) Including a Discussion on the Autoimmune Basis.* Laron Z and Karp M (eds).

Proceedings of the 8th International Beilinson Symposium on Prediabetes, Herzliya, Israel, October 1991: Karger Press 1992.

21 Kolb H, Kolb-Bachofen V. Type 1 (insulin-dependent) diabetes mellitus and nitric oxide. *Diabetologia* 1992; 35: 796–7.

22 Corbett JA, McDaniel ML. Does nitric oxide mediate autoimmune destruction of β cells? Possible therapeutic interventions in IDDM. *Diabetes* 1992; 41: 897–903.

23 Welsh N, Eizirik DL, Bendtzen K, Sandler S. Interleukin-1β-induced nitric oxide production in isolated rat pancreatic islets requires gene transcription and may lead to inhibition of the Krebs cycle enzymic aconitase. *Endocrinology* 1991; 129: 3167–73.

24 Beckman JS, Beckman TW, Chen J, Marshall PA, Freeman BA. Apparent hydroxyl radical production by peroxynitrite: implications for endothelial injury from nitric oxide and superoxide. *Proc Natl Acad Sci (USA)* 1990; 87: 1620–4.

25 Hayaishi O, Ueda K. Poly (ADP-ribose) and ADP-ribosylation of proteins. *Ann Rev Biochem* 1977; 46: 95–116.

26 Fehsel K, Jalowy A, Qi S, Burkart V, Hartmann B, Kolb H. Islet cell DNA is a target of inflammatory attack by nitric oxide. *Diabetes* 1993; 42: 496–500.

27 Fernandez-Alvarez J, Gomis R. Interleukin-1 induced activation of poly(ADP-ribose) synthease in pancreatic islets. *Diabetologia* 1990; 33: A19.

28 Andersen HU, Jrgensen KH, Egeberg J, Mandrup-Poulsen T, Nerua J. Nicotinamide prevents interleukin-1 effects on insulin release and nitric production in rat islets of Langerhans. *Diabetes* 1994; 43: 770–7.

29 Cetkovic-Cvrlje M, Sandler S, Eizirik DL. Nicotinamide and dexamethasone inhibit IL-1 induced nitric oxide production by RINm5F cells without decreasing mRNA expression for nitric oxide synthase. *Endocrinology* 1993 (in press).

30 Buscema M, Vinci C, Gatta C, Rabuazzo MA, Vignen R, Purrello F. Nicotinamide partially reverses the interleukin-1β inhibition of glucose-induced insulin release in pancreatic islets. *Metabolism* 1992; 41: 296–300.

31 Yamada K, Miyajima E, Nonaka K. Inhibition of cytokine-induced MHC class II but not class I molecule expression on mouse islets cells by niacinamide and 3-aminobenzamide. *Diabetes* 1990; 39: 1125–30.

32 Hiromatsu Y, Sato M, Yamada K, Nonaka K. Nicotinamide and 3-aminobenzamide inhibit recombinant human interferon gamma induced HLA-DR antigen expression, but not HLA-A,B,C antigen expression, on cultured human thyroid cells. *Clin Endocrinol* 1992; 36: 91–5.

33 Goodman LS, Gilman A. *The Pharmacological Basis of Therapeutics*. New York: Macmillan, 1975, pp 1554–6.

34 Tjälve, Wilander E. The uptake in the pancreatic islets of nicotinamide, nicotinic acid and tryptophane and their ability to prevent streptozotocin diabetes in mice. *Acta Endocrinol* 1976; 83: 357–64.

35 Zakheim HS, Vasily DB, Westphal ML, Hastings CW. Reactions to niacinamide. *J Am Acad Dermatol* 1981; 4: 736–7.

36 Toth B. Lack of carcinogenicity of nicotinamide and isonicotinamide following lifelong administration to mice. *Oncology* 1983; 40: 72–5.

37 Rakieten ML, Gordon BS, Beaty A, Cooney DA, Schein PS. Pancreatic islet cell tumours produced by the combined action of streptozotocin and nicotinamide. *Proc Soc Exp Biol Med* 1971; 137: 280–3.

38 Kazumi T, Yoshino G, Baba S. Pancreatic islet cells tumours found in rats given alloxan and nicotinamide. *Endocrinol Japan* 1980; 27: 387–93.

39 Bell RH, McCullough PJ, Pour PM. Influence of diabetes on susceptibility to experimental pancreatic cancer. *Am J Surg* 1988; 155: 159–64.

40 Petley AM, Wilkin TJ. Oral nicotinamide impairs growth in young rats. *Diabetologia* 1992; **35**: A202.
41 Golden P, Baird L, Malaisse WJ, Malaisse-Lagae F, Walker MM. Effect of streptozotocin on glucose-induced insulin secretion by isolated islets of Langerhans. *Diabetes* 1971; **20**: 513–18.
42 Zawalich WS, Dye ES, Matschinsky FM. Nicotinamide modulation of rat pancreatic islet cell responsiveness in vitro. *Horm Metabol Res* 1979; **11**: 469–71.
43 Sandler S, Andersson A. Long-term effects of exposure of pancreatic islets to nicotinamide in vitro on DNA synthesis, metabolism and β-cell function. *Diabetologia* 1986; **29**: 199–202.
44 Visalli N, Boccuni ML, Pozzilli P. Acute administration of nicotinamide does not modify C-peptide and insulin secretion in normal subjects. *Diab Nutr Metab* 1993; **6**: 159–61.

18

Oral Tolerance

HOWARD L. WEINER
Center for Neurologic Diseases, Brigham and Women's Hospital and Harvard
Medical School, Boston, Massachusetts, USA

INTRODUCTION

The goal of treatment for autoimmune diseases is to specifically suppress the autoreactive immune processes without affecting the remainder of the immune system. This is especially important in juvenile diabetes in which a non-toxic therapy that can be administered in a clinically appropriate fashion to children is most desirable. We have been studying oral tolerance as a means to suppress autoimmune diseases in both animals and man[1]. Oral tolerance represents the exogenous administration of antigen to the peripheral immune system via the gut. As such, it is a form of antigen-driven peripheral immune tolerance. Immunologic tolerance is not programmed into the germ-line but is acquired during maturation of the immune system by mechanisms that delete or inactivate antigen-reactive clones. There are three basic mechanisms to explain antigen-driven tolerance: clonal deletion, clonal anergy, and active suppression. A large number of studies have shown that one of the primary mechanisms associated with oral tolerance is the generation of active suppression[2]. More recently, clonal anergy has been demonstrated[3,4] and in some instances clonal deletion may occur[95]. The type of tolerance generated is dependent on dose[5].

GUT-ASSOCIATED LYMPHOID TISSUE (GALT)

The gut-associated lymphoid tissue consists of lymphoid nodules termed Peyer's patches, villi containing epithelial cells and intraepithelial lymphocytes

Prediction, Prevention and Genetic Counseling in IDDM. Edited by Jerry P. Palmer.
© 1996 John Wiley & Sons Ltd.

and lymphocytes scattered throughout the lamina propria (reviewed in reference 6)[6].

Peyer's patches are well-organized lymphoid nodules containing T and B lymphocytes, macrophages, dendritic cells and a germinal center with B lymphocytes. They are overlaid by M cells which function for antigen uptake and transfer. The distal surface of M cells has a dendritic morphology which may function to directly transfer antigen to underlying macrophages and dendritic cells. T lymphocytes present in the dome are predominantly CD4+ cells of both Th1 and Th2 phenotypes, whereas parafollicular T cells are both CD4+ and CD8+. Peyer's patches are one of the primary areas in the GALT where specific immune responses are generated. Peyer's patches are a major source of IgA producing B cells and T cells from the Peyer's patches have been reported to preferentially induce sIgA+B cells to differentiate into plasma cells. Peyer's patches have also been shown to be a site where regulatory cells are generated which mediate the active suppression component of oral tolerance[7-9]. Recent studies have suggested that Th2 type responses may be preferentially generated in Peyer's patches. Investigators have shown separation of Peyer's patch T cells into IL-5 and IL-2 producing subsets[10]. Daynes *et al.* have reported that the lymphoid tissue microenvironment can determine the pattern of T-cell responses in different lymphoid organs[11]. T cells in lymphoid organs drained by non-mucosal sites such as axillary or inguinal lymph nodes secreted IL-2 as the primary T-cell growth factor after activation, whereas T cells from mucosal sites such as Peyer's patch produced IL-4. Xu-Amano *et al.*, have reported the selective induction of Th2 cells (IL-5 secreting cells as measured by elispot) in murine Peyer's patches following oral immunization with sheep red blood cells as compared to systemic immunization in which IFN-γ producing cells predominated[12]. We have found that antigen-specific TGF-β producing cells appear in Peyer's patches after orally administered myelin basic protein and that these cells can adoptively transfer protection against EAE[8]. In addition, mesenteric lymph node cells from fed animals secrete TGF-β, IL-4 and IL-10 but little IFN-γ when restimulated in vitro with fed antigen[13]. TGF-β and IL-4 regulate the adhesiveness of Peyer's patch high endothelial venule cells for lymphocytes[14]. As discussed below, cells secreting these cytokines are preferentially generated in the gut associated lymphocyte tissue.

Intraepithelial lymphocytes (IEL) are adjacent to the columnar epithelial layer of small intestinal villi and possess a number of unique features that are distinct from lymphocytes in other lymphoid tissues[15]. IEL have been shown to be oligoclonal, activated and cytolytic but proliferate poorly. These properties may be secondary to their anatomic location and constant exposure to bacterial antigens; they may play a role in the cellular immune defense of the intestinal epithelial barrier. There is no evidence that they play a role in mediating oral tolerance as they apparently do not migrate in vivo and attempts to transfer oral tolerance with IEL were unsuccessful as opposed to Peyer's patch lymphocytes. However, they have been reported to abrogate oral tolerance (discussed below). Lamina propria lymphocytes are found diffusely interspersed in the lamina propria with a ratio of CD4+/CD8+ cells more closely resembling the Peyer's patch and peripheral blood[6]. Epithelial cells of the small intestine express class II on their surface and can present antigen in vitro—they are discussed below.

MECHANISM OF ORAL TOLERANCE

The primary factor which determines which form of peripheral tolerance develops following oral administration of antigen is the dose of antigen fed. Low doses of antigen favor the generation of active suppression or regulatory-cell-driven tolerance whereas high doses of antigen favor anergy-driven tolerance (Figure 18.1). Although these forms of oral tolerance are not mutually exclusive and may occur simultaneously, they are distinct and the use of oral tolerance to treat autoimmune diseases such as IDDM is critically dependent on which of these two mechanisms is triggered.

The delineation of these two mechanisms of oral tolerance was based on the following: (1) investigations in our laboratory in which low doses of orally administered autoantigens were shown to suppress experimental autoimmune diseases via the generation of regulatory cells that suppressed in vitro and in vivo via the secretion of down-regulatory cytokines such as TGF-β[16]; (2) investigations from other laboratories which demonstrated clonal anergy following oral administration of large doses of antigen with no evidence of active suppression[3,4]; (3) a large series of investigations demonstrating transferable suppression following oral tolerance (reviewed in reference 2) including work which showed two components of oral tolerance, one that was abrogated by treatment with low dose cyclophosphamide and one that was not, a difference that was dose dependent[17]; and (4) direct comparison in our laboratory demonstrating that the two mechanisms depend on the dose[5].

As shown in Figure 18.1, low doses of antigen result in the generation of antigen-specific regulatory cells and as such involve presentation of antigen by gut-associated antigen presenting cells. Such presentation preferentially induces regulatory cells which upon subsequent recognition of antigen in vivo or in vitro, secrete the suppressive cytokine TGF-β. In addition, Th2 responses are preferentially generated in the gut, resulting in cells which secrete IL-4 and IL-10. These antigen-specific regulatory cells migrate to lymphoid organs and suppress immune responses by inhibiting the generation of effector cells and to the target organ and suppress disease by releasing antigen non-specific cytokines (bystander suppression). Certain factors can

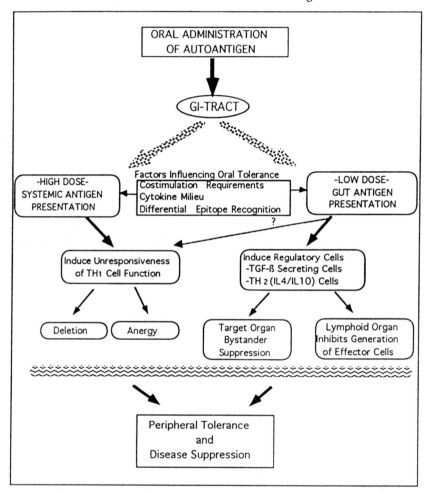

Figure 18.1. Effect of antigen dosage on peripheral tolerance

affect the generation of regulatory cells including costimulation requirements and the cytokine milieu in which the immune response is generated.

High doses of orally administered antigen result in systemic antigen presentation after the antigen passes through the gut and enters the systemic circulation either as intact protein or antigen fragments. High doses of antigen induce unresponsiveness of Th1 cell function, primarily via clonal anergy. The degree to which clonal anergy following high doses of antigen merely represents the direct passage of small amounts of antigen into the systemic or portal circulation or is dependent on filtration by the gut is unknown. Why there is reduced active suppression with high doses of orally administered antigen is unclear, but could relate to anergizing or deleting cells involved in the generation of active suppression.

FATE OF ORALLY ADMINISTERED ANTIGEN

Although dietary antigens are degraded by the time they reach the small intestine, studies in humans and rodents have indicated that degradation is partial and that some intact antigen is absorbed as well[18,19]. Absorbed antigen, either undegraded or partially degraded, might have an important role in the generation of oral tolerance, since serum containing antigen absorbed from the gut 1 hour after feeding transfers tolerance as measured by suppression of systemic DTH responses. Serum from animals injected systemically with ovalbumin (OVA) or to which OVA was added directly did not suppress, suggesting there may be unique tolerogenic properties of antigen that passes through the gut[19,20]. These studies involved administration of large doses of antigen (25 mg OVA). Depending on the antigen, the amount fed, and the nature of the fragments generated, absorbed antigen could induce active suppression and/or clonal anergy after being processed by the gut and absorbed into the circulation. Some authors have suggested that digestion of antigen is required for the generation of oral tolerance[21,22]. Further studies using different doses of peptide fragments of an antigen will help clarify these issues.

ACTIVE SUPPRESSION

Many studies demonstrate that active suppression is an important mechanism for oral tolerance (reviewed in reference 2). After feeding antigens such as ovalbumin or sheep red blood cells, transferable suppression mediated by T cells from Peyer's patches, mesenteric lymph node and spleen has been demonstrated. Investigators have also reported initial sensitization prior to the appearance of suppression[23]. Of note are the studies of Mowat *et al.*[17] who reported that high doses of ovalbumin induced tolerance not abrogated by cyclophosphamide and such tolerance affected antibody responses. Low doses of ovalbumin induced a state of tolerance that could be reversed by cyclophosphamide and primarily affected cell-mediated responses. Cyclophosphamide is believed to abrogate active suppression. It appears that these studies were delineating components of active suppression versus anergy depending on dose. In addition, Hanson and Miller[24] reported two components of oral tolerance following oral administration of ovalbumin. They found tolerance was observed both in cyclophosphamide treated and untreated animals but they were unable to transfer tolerance from cyclophosphamide treated animals.

Our studies of oral tolerance in autoimmune models have found active suppression to be a primary mechanism and have identified regulatory cells generated following oral tolerance which act via the secretion of antigen-nonspecific down-regulatory cytokines following triggering by the fed antigen (reviewed in reference 1). In the SJL mouse both CD4+ and CD8+ regulatory cells are generated which act via the secretion of TGF-β or IL-4/IL-10. We have successfully cloned CD4+T cells from the mesenteric lymph nodes of SJL mice that had been orally tolerized to MBP[13]. These clones were structurally identical to Th1 type encephalitogenic CD4+ clones in TCR usage, MHC restriction and epitope recognition. However, they produced TGF-β with varying amounts of IL-4 and IL-10 and no IFN-γ and suppressed EAE induced with either myelin basic protein (MBP) or proteolipid protein. These results suggest that cells capable of regulating immune responses are not a unique type of suppressor cell but conventional T cells whose major down-regulatory activity is mediated by their cytokines. The cytokine profile appears stable and depends on the microenvironment in which they are induced. Oral tolerance can be induced in CD8-depleted mice, and in the NOD mouse orally tolerized with insulin, protection may be more easily transferred with CD4+ than CD8+ cells (unpublished observations). In the Lewis rat fed guinea pig MBP, these regulatory cells are predominantly CD8+[25] and act via the secretion of TGF-β following antigen-specific triggering[16]. In addition, TGF-β-secreting regulatory cells can be found in Peyer's patches 24–48 hours after one feeding of MBP[8]. Of note is that cells from Peyer's patches removed after one feeding of MBP do not proliferate in response to MBP even though they release TGF-β upon in vitro stimulation.

ANTIGEN-DRIVEN BYSTANDER SUPPRESSION

It has become clear that in human autoimmune diseases such as multiple sclerosis and IDDM there are, most probably, reactivities to multiple autoantigens from the target organ, even if the disease was initiated by a single antigen. The mechanism of bystander suppression following oral tolerance obviates this major conceptual problem. Bystander suppression was first demonstrated in vitro when it was shown that cells from MBP-fed animals could suppress proliferation of an ovalbumin line across a transwell[26]. The cells from MBP-fed animals suppressed across the transwell only when triggered by the fed antigen. In an analogous fashion, cells from OVA-fed animals suppressed a MBP line across the transwell when stimulated with OVA. The soluble factor shown to be responsible for the suppression was TGF-β. Bystander suppression was then demonstrated in vivo. Feeding ovalbumin has no effect on MBP-induced EAE in the Lewis rat. However, if animals are fed ovalbumin and then given aqueous ovalbumin in the footpad following immunization in the footpad with MBP/CFA, EAE is suppressed. Suppression is mediated by OVA-specific regulatory cells which migrate to the draining lymph node and secrete TGF-β upon encountering OVA and thus inhibit the generation of the MBP-specific immune response being generated in the lymph node. Bystander suppression is specific to the fed antigen and is transferable. Further demonstration of bystander or tissue-specific suppression in vivo was obtained using MBP peptides. In the Lewis rat, MBP peptide 21–40 is a non-encephalitogenic epitope whereas 71–90 is the encephalitogenic epitope[27]. Peptide 21–40 triggers TGF-β release following oral tolerization and orally administered 21–40 suppresses 71–90 induced EAE in the Lewis rat. Furthermore, in 71–90 immunized animals protected by oral administration of peptide 21–40, DTH responses in the ear to peptide 71–90 are not suppressed whereas DTH responses to whole MBP are suppressed and suppression occurs because the 21–40 epitope is present in whole MBP to trigger TGF-β-secreting cells. Other examples of tissue-specific bystander suppression are the suppression of PLP-peptide-induced disease in the SJL mouse by feeding myelin basic protein or MBP peptides[28].

NEONATAL TOLERANCE

Although neonatally administered antigens have been shown to induce tolerance, studies have demonstrated that feeding ovalbumin or human gammaglobulin to newborn animals may result in immune priming for both humoral and cell-mediated immune responses whereas tolerance occurs when the same antigens are fed to adult animals[29,30]. We have found that orally administered MBP to neonatal rats did not result in tolerization to MBP but instead primed for immunologic responses[31]. Proliferative responses to MBP and its encephalitogenic epitope were present in animals fed MBP. Furthermore, neonates fed MBP and immunized 6–8 weeks later with MBP and adjuvant had enhanced disease severity and were not protected from a second attack upon active reinduction of EAE. Suppression of EAE began to appear in animals fed MBP at 4 weeks of age and was similar to oral tolerance in adult animals when animals were fed at 6 weeks of age. These results suggest that immaturity of the immunoregulatory network associated with oral tolerance and sensitization to autoantigens via the gut in the neonatal period may contribute to the pathogenesis of autoimmune diseases. This hypothesis is consistent with a recent report demonstrating that following exposure to cow's milk during early infancy, individuals genetically susceptible to insulin-dependent diabetes developed anti-BSA antibodies that cross-react with a pancreatic beta cell surface protein[32] (see Chapter 11).

MODULATION OF ORAL TOLERANCE

Treatment of animals with INF-γ abrogated oral tolerance as measured by antibody responses to orally administered BSA[33]. Gamma interferon was shown to enhance class II expression in the gut and the authors postulate that poor expression of class II MHC on epithelial cells of the small intestine contribute to the induction of oral tolerance. An alternative explanation is that the active suppression component of oral tolerance is dependent on the induction of Th2 responses and administration of gamma interferon favors Th1 responses. We have found that orally administered bacterial lipopolysaccharide (LPS) enhances protection by orally administered MBP. This is not seen when LPS is given systematically[34]. The LPS synergistic effect is associated with the expression of IL-4 in the brain of orally tolerized animals[35] suggesting that LPS may act by affecting presentation of antigen in the gut in a manner that induces Th2-type responses. Consistent with this is the observation that LPS plus MBP had no effect on antibody responses when LPS was given orally. Experimental graft versus host disease[36], which increased class II MHC expression in gut epithelium, was also reported to abrogate oral tolerance as was stimulation of the reticuloendothelial system with oestradiol[37]. Other studies have suggested an immunoregulatory role for murine intraepithelial lymphocytes which are $\gamma\delta$ positive. When transferred into animals, these cells abrogate oral tolerance to red blood cells as measured by antibody production[38]. IELs that are $\alpha\beta$ had no effect. The mechanism of action of these cells is unknown.

ANTIGEN PRESENTATION IN THE GUT

There are several cells capable of antigen presentation in the gut-associated lymphoid tissue[39-41]. These include macrophages and dendritic cells in Peyer's patches and lamina propria, B lymphocytes and epithelial cells. MHC class II is constitutively expressed on the small intestinal epithelium. These are expressed at low density and the intensity of expression is increased during inflammation, graft versus host disease or following the injection of gamma interferon[41]. Macrophage-enriched cells obtained from mice fed OVA are able to stimulate antigen-primed lymph node T cells in vitro in an antigen-specific fashion without further exposure to antigen[42]. Dendritic cells also appear to acquire antigen fragments following oral or intraintestinal injection[43]. Epithelial cells may preferentially trigger the activation of CD8+ suppressor T cells. In the rat, these epithelial-cell-induced CD8+ T lymphocytes are antigen-specific[44] whereas in the human they were found to be antigen-nonspecific[45]. Initial experiments from our laboratory suggest that oral antigen associates with both class I and class II MHC in gut epithelial cells (Gonnella and Weiner, unpublished). The mechanism of antigen presentation within the gut is crucial for the generation of active suppression. It is possible that such cells preferentially stimulate Th2-type responses because of the gut environment, specific properties of the antigen-presenting cells, or different costimulatory signals. There does not appear to be a difference of acquisition of antigen by dendritic cells as compared to dendritic cells from other parts of the body.

IMMUNIZATION VIA THE GUT

Oral tolerance has been an impediment in developing orally administered synthetic vaccines[46]. Since the oral route can generate an immune response as well as tolerance, vaccine efficacy depends upon its capacity to override tolerogenic stimuli. The expression of a dietary protein in *Escherichia coli* renders it strongly antigenic to gut lymphoid tissue as measured by biliary IgA antibodies, suggesting that mucosal immunogenicity may depend on how the protein is presented to gut-associated lymphoid tissue[47]. Cholera toxin has been studied as a strong mucosal adjuvant[48] and recently it has been shown that coupling a protein or cells to the cholera B toxin can enhance oral tolerance[49].

TREATMENT OF ORGAN-SPECIFIC AUTOIMMUNE DISEASES IN ANIMALS

A large series of studies have demonstrated that orally administered autoantigens can suppress experimental models of autoimmunity (Table 18.1) including diabetes in the NOD mouse. Features of each of these models are discussed below.

Table 18.1. Suppression of animal models of autoimmunity by oral tolerance

Animal model	Antigen fed
EAE (MS)	MBP, PLP
Arthritis (CII, AA)	Type II collagen
Uveitis	S-antigen, IRBP
Diabetes (NOD mouse)	Insulin, GAD
Myasthenia gravis	AChR
Thyroiditis	Thyroglobulin
Transplantation	Alloantigen, MHC peptide

EAE

Orally administered guinea pig MBP to suppress EAE was first shown in the Lewis rat model[50,51]. In a series of experiments we have shown this to be mediated by antigen-specific CD8+T cells that act via the secretion of TGF-β[16,26,27]. Whitacre *et al.* have also shown suppression of EAE in the Lewis rat with guinea pig MBP but have found clonal anergy to be the primary mechanism[3,51,52]. As discussed previously, it appears that the dosage of antigen fed accounts for the differences. In our experiments, a total of 3–5 mg was fed in 1 mg doses whereas Whitacre *et al.* fed 20 mg given in 5 mg doses plus soybean trypsin inhibitor (STI) which prevented degradation of antigen in the gut. Of note is that Whitacre *et al.* also used male rats which have a more severe form of EAE and thus may be more difficult to tolerize orally. Although mechanisms of tolerization may have been different, both groups find suppression of disease, decreased proliferative responses, and decreased inflammatory responses in the brain.

Chronic relapsing EAE in the Lewis rat and strain 13 guinea pig was also suppressed by oral administration of MBP or a bovine myelin preparation that is also being administered in human clinical trials.[53] There was no exacerbation of disease in these animals demonstrating that orally administered antigens do not appear to prime but rather suppress an already immunized animal. In the guinea pig model 10 mg of bovine myelin fed three times per week over a 3 month period suppressed disease and histologic manifestations whereas feeding 50 mg of bovine myelin did not. This may indicate that bystander suppression was responsible for the effect on chronic disease and that in some instances the oral administration of too high a dose will not suppress autoimmune models. As discussed later, loss of protection by orally administered antigen at higher doses was also seen with orally administered collagen to suppress adjuvant arthritis and orally administered insulin to suppress diabetes in the NOD mouse.

Detailed immunohistology was performed in animals orally tolerized with MBP and in animals naturally recovering from EAE[35]. Brains from OVA fed animals at the peak of disease showed perivascular infiltration with activated mononuclear cells which secreted the inflammatory cytokines IL-1, IL-2, TNF-α, IFN-γ, IL-6 and IL-8. Inhibitory cytokines TGF-β and IL-4 and prostaglandin E2 (PGE$_2$) were absent. In MBP orally tolerized animals there was a marked reduction of the perivascular infiltrate and down-regulation of all inflammatory cytokines. In addition, there was up-regulation of the inhibitory cytokine TGF-β. When bacterial lipopolysaccharide (LPS) was fed in addition to MBP, protection against EAE was enhanced and was associated with elevated IL-4 and PGE$_2$ in the brain[34,35]. In control recovering animals (day 18) staining for inflammatory cytokines was diminished and there was up-regulation of TGF-β and IL-4. These results suggest that the suppression of EAE, by oral tolerization and natural recovery, is related to regulatory cells that secrete inhibitory cytokines at the target organ. As discussed below, oral administration of insulin is associated with increased IL-4 expression in pancreatic islets.

Prior feeding of MBP protects against actively induced EAE in the Lewis rat although it does not protect from adoptively transferred EAE[3,54]. Nonetheless, spleen cells from orally tolerized animals will suppress adoptively transferred EAE when co-transferred with encephalitiogenic cells or when injected into recipient animals at a different site at the time encephalitogenic cells are transferred[54]. This suppression was mediated by CD8+T cells. Presumably, prior oral tolerization does not prevent adoptively transferred disease as the adoptively transferred cells migrate rapidly to the brain and initiate the inflammatory response before sufficient numbers of orally induced regulatory cells appear in the brain to down-regulate the response. However, if regulatory cells from orally tolerated animals are transferred into the animal at the same as the encephalitogenic cells, they migrate to the brain simultaneously and are activated by MBP to release factors such as TGF-β to prevent encephalitogenic cells from initiating the inflammatory response.

In studies of a variety of species, it was found that suppression of EAE was most effective when MBP from the homologous species was orally administered[55]. This has important implications for treatment of human autoimmune diseases. Human recombinant MBP has been cloned and expressed and is effective in suppressing EAE in the SJL mouse model[56] and plans for oral tolerance therapy IDDM will involve human recombinant insulin.

As described previously, in the SJL model of EAE, we have found suppression of MBP and PLP induced disease by orally administered MBP or PLP and have also found suppression by the administration of MBP peptides[28]. Both CD4+ and CD8+ regulatory cells are generated following oral tolerance in the murine model and we have recently cloned CD4+ mucosally derived regulatory cells that suppress EAE[13].

Inhaled antigen also induces antigen specific suppression and investigators have reported suppression by nasally administered antigens[57]. Aerosolization of MBP to Lewis rats suppressed acute EAE and relapsing EAE when given after recovery from the first attack[58].

ARTHRITIS

Previous investigators have demonstrated suppression of collagen-induced arthritis by feeding collagen type II[59,60]. We have studied adjuvant arthritis (AA) in the rat, a well-characterized and more fulminant form of experimental arthritis[61]. Oral administration of chicken collagen type II (CII), given at a dose of 3 μg per feeding consistently suppressed the development of AA. A decrease in DTH responses to CII was observed that correlated with suppression to AA. Suppression was antigen specific in that feeding collagen type II did not suppress EAE, and feeding MBP did not suppress AA. Suppression of AA could be adoptively transferred by T cells from CII-fed animals and was observed when CII was fed after disease onset. Of note is that suppression was observed at doses of 3 and 30 μg, but not at 300 or 1000 μg. These results suggest that oral collagen is suppressing AA via bystander suppression rather than clonal anergy since active suppression may be lost at higher doses. The effectiveness of such small amounts of oral collagen may be related to the fact that collagen has repeating amino acid subunits. To test further the bystander suppression concept, we fed type II collagen to animals with antigen-induced arthritis in which animals are immunized with BSA and then BSA injected into the joint. There was a reduction of arthritis in Lewis rats fed 3 or 30 μg of collagen but not 300 μg[96]. Oral type II collagen has also been shown to suppress pristane-induced arthritis[62] and more recent studies have shown suppression of collagen-induced arthritis by active suppression[63].

UVEITIS

Oral administration of S-antigen (S-Ag), a retinal autoantigen that induces experimental allergic uveitis (EAU), prevented or markedly diminished the clinical appearance of S-Ag-induced disease as measured by ocular inflammation[64] [66]. Furthermore, oral administration of S-Ag also markedly diminished uveitis induced by the uveitogenic M and N fragments of the S-Ag. Oral administration of S-Ag did not prevent MBP-induced EAE. In vitro studies demonstrated a significant decrease in proliferative responses to the S-Ag in lymph node cells draining the site of immunization from fed versus nonfed animals. Furthermore, the addition of splenocytes from S-Ag-fed animals to cultures of a CD4+ S-Ag-specific lymphocyte line profoundly suppressed the line's response to the S-Ag, whereas these splenocytes had no effect on a PPD-specific lymphocyte line. The antigen-specific in vitro suppression was blocked by anti-CD8 antibody, demonstrating that suppression was dependent on CD8+T lymphocytes. As in EAE, EAU was also suppressed by feeding S-Ag-related peptides that were either uveitogenic, cross-reactive or synthetic [65–68]. Gregerson et al., using high and low doses of S-Ag peptides, also found that low doses of antigen favor suppression whereas high doses induce unresponsiveness or anergy[66].

DIABETES

To test oral tolerance in the NOD model, we first initiated a series of experiments in which animals were administered a pancreatic extract from neonatal rats, rich in islets. We observed a delay in the onset of diabetes in these animals. We then initiated studies using defined antigens and chose insulin for two reasons. First, it is uniquely localized to the pancreatic islets and, second, it is a candidate autoantigen as a target for the autoimmune response in NOD mice. We administered porcine insulin at a dose of 1 mg orally twice a week for five weeks and then weekly until one year of age[69]. The severity of lymphocytic infiltration of pancreatic islets was reduced by oral administration of insulin and there was a delay in the onset of diabetes. A decreased incidence of diabetes was seen in animals followed for one year. As expected, orally administered insulin had no metabolic effect on blood glucose levels. Suppression of insulitis was observed at a dose of 1 mg but not 5 mg. These findings suggest that oral insulin is acting by the induction of regulatory cells that are suppressing by the bystander suppression mechanism as higher doses were not effective against insulitis. Splenic T cells from animals orally treated with insulin adoptively transferred protection against diabetes, whereas cells from MBP-fed animals did not, demonstrating that oral insulin generates active cellular mechanisms that suppress disease. Initial characterization of those cells in our laboratory suggests that they are CD4+ as opposed to CD8+, a finding recently reported by Thivolet as well[70]. Ongoing studies in our laboratory have demonstrated the ability to suppress insulitis by administering the B chain of insulin, peptides of the B chain, or GAD. Immunohistochemical studies were performed on animals fed porcine insulin over a 5 week period. As shown in Table 18.2, there is an increase of IL-4, IL-10, PGE and TGF-β in the islets of insulin-fed animals and a decrease of IFN-γ, TNF-α and IL-2[97]. These results suggest that a Th2 type response is being generated in association with the ameliorating effects of oral insulin. Our results are analogous to a recent report of cytokine patterns in NOD mice treated with adjuvant to suppress autoimmune diabetes[71]. These investigators reported that CFA decreased the frequency of INF-γ producing cells and increased the number of IL-4 secreting cells. Given the mechanism of antigendriven bystander suppression, our results do not implicate autoreactivity to insulin as a pathogenic mechanism in the NOD mouse. Indeed, initially experiments suggest that orally administered glucagon can suppress insulitis.

Table 18.2. Histology of cells and cytokines at week 10 in pancreas of NOD mice fed insulin or ovalburmin*[97]

Feature	Insulin-fed	Ovalbumin-fed
Histology	Mild to moderate peri-islet MNC	Dense peri and intra-islet MNC infiltrates
T cells	>75% MNC+ve	>75% MNC+ve
CD4+ subset	>75% MNC+ve	>75% MNC+ve
CD8+ subset	Few cells/section	~5% peri-islet cells
Macrophages	Few adventitial and peri-islet MNC	5 to 10% of MNC (intra- and peri-islet cells)
IL-2R	Few cells/section	5 to 10% MNC+ve
IL-2	Negative	5 to 10% MNC+ve
IFN-γ	Negative	>50% intra- and peri-islet MNC
TNF-α	Negative	>50% intra- and peri-islet MNC
IL-4	5 to 10% intra- and peri-islet MNC	Negative
IL-10	5 to 10% intra- and peri-islet MNC	Negative
TGF-β	10 to 20% intra- and peri-islet MNC	Negative
PGE	10 to 20% intra- and peri-islet MNC	Negative

*n=3 animals/group.

EAMG

The oral administration of Torpedo acetylcholine receptor (AChR) to Lewis rats prior to immunization with AChR and Freund's adjuvant prevented or delayed the onset of experimental autoimmune myasthenia gravis (EAMG)[72]. The levels of anti-acetylcholine receptor antibodies in the serum were lower in orally tolerized animals as compared to control animals. This response was dose-dependent, requiring a minimum of 5 mg of AChR plus STI to prevent breakdown in the stomach. Thus it appears that these results may relate to the induction of anergy given the relatively large doses fed (up to 20 mg).

TRANSPLANTATION

Oral tolerance to allogenic spleen cells prevents sensitization by skin grafts and transforms accelerated rejection of vascularized cardiac allografts to an acute form typical of unsensitized recipients[73]. In addition, the mixed lymphocyte response in vitro and DTH responses were suppressed following oral administration of antigen. In a second series of experiments we found induction of immunity and oral tolerance with polymorphic class II major histocompatibility complex allopeptides in the rat[74]. Inbred Lewis rats were immunized or fed class II synthetic MHC allopeptides. In vivo these animals developed DTH responses. Furthermore, oral administration of the allopeptide mixture daily for 5 days before immunization reduced DTH responses both to the allopeptide mixture and to allogenic splenocytes and this reduction was antigen specific. Orally administered alloantigen was accompanied by elevation of intragraft IL-4[75]. The prevention of accelerated graft rejection by alloantigens administered intravenously was not associated with increased intragraft IL-4. In the pig, islet allograft survival was reported to be prolonged by oral tolerization with islet tissue[76]. Thus, oral tolerance may be of benefit in down-regulating alloreactivity associated with transplantation.

TREATMENT OF AUTOIMMUNE DISEASES IN HUMANS

The first attempts of oral tolerization may have been utilized by native Americans who were thought to have fed their children *Rhus* leaves to prevent them from becoming sensitized to poison ivy[77]. Investigators have shown that exposure of a contact-sensitizing agent via the mucosa prior to subsequent skin challenge led to unresponsiveness in a portion of the subjects studied[78]. In another study on human volunteers, serum antibodies to bovine serum albumin (BSA) were measured before and after feeding large amounts of this antigen (0.1–1.5 mg of BSA per pound per day). Those subjects that had anti-BSA antibodies prior to eating BSA showed a rise in their serum anti-BSA titers. A similar response was observed when some subjects were given an injection of BSA. Subjects who did not have anti-BSA antibodies before or after the test did not respond to subsequent intradermal immunization[79]. Oral desensitization has also been attempted in Rh disease[80]. In an attempt at oral immunization, human volunteers were given capsules containing killed *Streptococcus mutans* and circulating IgA-producing cells were found in some subjects[81]. This suggests that some generation of a secretory immune response can occur following oral ingestion of microbial antigens. Orally administered KLH, 50 mg given daily for two weeks over a three week period, has been reported to decrease subsequent cell-mediated immune responses although antibody responses were not affected[82].

MULTIPLE SCLEROSIS

In order to determine whether orally ingested autoantigens could affect the clinical course and immune responses in patients with an autoimmune disease, 15 patients with relapsing remitting multiple sclerosis were fed a capsule containing 300 mg of bovine myelin or placebo daily for one year[83]. Results demonstrated a decrease in myelin basic protein reactive cells in the bloodstream of MS patients as compared to controls. There was no evidence of sensitization either as measured by antibody levels to MBP or PLP or by increased proliferation responses to the fed antigens at a one year period. Clinical responses demonstrated that 12 of 15 placebo-fed patients had major MS attacks whereas only 6 of 15 in the control group had attacks ($p = 0.06$). It appeared that a subgroup of patients that were either males or DR2– preferentially responded to the oral tolerization. However, the sample size was small and the degree to which this subgroup response will occur in future studies is unknown. Based on these observations, a multicenter 500 patient phase III double-blind placebo-controlled trial of bovine myelin in DR2– and DR2+ relapsing remitting MS patients, both males and females, is in progress. Some patients have received oral myelin for up to 5 years with no apparent toxicity. In contrast, myelin basic protein given by multiple subcutaneous injections results in prominent immune responses to the antigen[84].

RHEUMATOID ARTHRITIS

A 60-patient double-blind trial of oral collagen administration to patients with rheumatoid arthritis demonstrated a decrease in joint swelling and disease index in patients fed collagen compared to placebo controls[85]. Patients were those previously or currently on immunosuppressant drugs such as methotrexate that had failed such therapy. Patients were taken off these medications and treated for a 3 month period. In the first month they received

100 µg of oral collagen per day and in the second and third month 500 µg per day. These doses were extrapolated from the small amounts of collagen used to suppress adjuvant arthritis in the Lewis rat. There were no toxicities or evidence of sensitization to type II collagen in fed patients as measured by anti-collagen antibodies. There was no linkage to either DR type or sex in the patients that responded. In patients treated with the collagen there was less need for narcotic use during the course of the study and four patients in the collagen-treated group apparently had complete remission of their rheumatoid arthritis. A multicenter and double-blind placebo-controlled phase II dosing trial of oral collagen was recently finished. Patients had a washout period from their drugs and then received 6 months of oral collagen at daily doses of 20, 100, 500, or 2500 µg. Statistically significant improvement was observed in the 20 µg collagen-treated group compared to placebo. Given what is known of the mechanism of oral tolerization, these studies do not establish that type II collagen is a target autoantigen in the disease. Indeed, given the low doses fed, it is possible that the effect may have been mediated by regulatory cells that migrated to the joint and released anti-inflammatory cytokines such as TGFβ or IL-4. Whether patients that went into complete remission represent a separate category remains to be determined.

UVEITIS

An open-label pilot study has been performed on two patients with uveitis, one with Behcet's disease[86] and the second with pars planitis. In this open label trial, patients had required steroids and/or cyclosporin to maintain visual function. Patients were started on 30 mg of bovine S-antigen three times a week and then tapered from steroids and immunosuppressive medication. A positive therapeutic response was observed in both patients over a two year period. They were able to reduce their previous medication without worsening vision and with decrease in S-antigen responsiveness. A double-masked placebo-controlled trial of 45 patients is currently in progress.

DIABETES

Based on the current understanding of mechanisms of oral tolerance and IDDM and animals' studies showing that oral insulin can affect the development of diabetes in the NOD mouse, a trial of oral insulin in IDDM is being planned. The ease of administration and apparent lack of toxicity make oral insulin an attractive approach for prevention of diabetes. The diabetes prevention trial (DPT-1) will involve two intervention protocols, first parenteral insulin subjects with a 5 year risk of IDDM greater than 50% and oral insulin or potentially another islet-specific antigen in subjects with a 5 year risk of IDDM of 25–50%. The objective of the trial is to determine whether antigen-based therapies of non-diabetic relatives can delay development of clinical IDDM. Relatives less than age 45 will be screened for ICA and then staged with tissue-typing, IAA and IVGTT. For eligibility in the oral antigen protocol, subjects must be positive ICA and IAA in two samples and must not have protective HLA types. The outcome measure will be the development of IDDM. The details of the oral antigen protocol are currently being decided in terms of the antigen to be fed, the dosage and specific outcome measures. The two major candidate antigens are insulin and GAD. Proinsulin may also be considered for this protocol. In addition, plans are being formulated to treat new-onset diabetics with oral insulin or an insulin derivative. The purpose of the trial in new-onset IDDM will be to determine whether oral insulin alters the need for subsequent insulin therapy and/or makes subsequent insulin therapy easier to maintain. A "honeymoon" or clinical remission of IDDM occurs in many patients and is characterized by a partial or temporary return of insulin secretion and sensitivity to insulin. Immunomodulatory treatment with cyclosporin A and nicotinamide has been associated with phases of enhanced insulin secretion as well as insulin sensitivity. It will be determined whether oral insulin has similar effects. Patients will begin oral insulin a short time after diagnosis and will be followed by C-peptide levels and glycohemo-globulin.

FUTURE DIRECTIONS

Given the results in animal models of autoimmunity and initial studies in human disease states it appears that orally administered autoantigens may find a place in the treatment of human organ-specific inflammatory autoimmune diseases. Such therapy would have the advantages of being orally administered, non-toxic and antigen specific. The mechanism of bystander suppression solves a major problem related to designing antigen or T-cell specific therapy of inflammatory autoimmune diseases since one need not necessarily identify the target autoantigen for oral tolerance to be effective. In animal models of autoimmunity, during the course of a chronic inflammatory autoimmune process, there is intra- and interantigenic spreading of autoreactivity at the target organ[87-91]. It is likely that in human autoimmune disease states such as IDDM there are reactivities to multiple autoantigens from the target organ and multiple epitopes given that humans are an outbred population. In multiple sclerosis there is immune reactivity to three myelin antigens, MBP, PLP and MOG[92,93]. Similarly, in IDDM there are multiple islet cell autoantigens that could be the target of autoreactivity[94]. Dosing appears to be important for stimulating the active suppression component of oral tolerance and identification of regulatory cells in humans following oral tolerization is critical for demonstrating the immunologic effects of oral tolerization. Given the results in animal studies, one would predict that homologous protein and the use of synergists or enhancers would increase the biologic efficiency of oral tolerance. In this regard, recombinant human proteins and the concomitant administration of immune adjuvants to enhance generation of regulatory cells would be required.

ACKNOWLEDGMENT

The author wishes to thank Patricia Nelson for editorial review. This work was supported by National Institutes of Health grants N529352 and NDDK 45078 and a grant from AutoImmune, Inc. In accordance with disclosure guidelines of the Harvard Medical School, H.L.W. has a financial interest in AutoImmune.

REFERENCES

1 Weiner HL, Friedman A, Miller A, Khoury SJ, Al-Sabbagh A, Santos LMB, Sayegh M, Nussenblatt RB, Trentham DE, Hafler DA. Oral tolerance: immunologic mechanisms and treatment of murine and human organ specific autoimmune diseases by oral administration of autoantigens. *Ann Rev Immunol* 1994; **12**: 809–37.
2 Mowat AM. The regulation of immune responses to dietary protein antigens. *Immunol Today* 1987; **8**: 93–8.
3 Whitacre CC, Gienapp IE, Orosz CG, Bitar D. Oral tolerance in experimental autoimmune encephalomyelitis. III. Evidence for clonal anergy. *J Immunol* 1991; **147**: 2155–63.
4 Melamed D, Friedman A. Direct evidence for anergy in T lymphocytes tolerized by oral administration of ovalbumin. *Eur J Immunol* 1993; **23**: 935–42.
5 Friedman A, Weiner HL. Induction of anergy or active suppression following oral tolerance is determined by antigen dosage. *PNAS* 1994; **191**: 6688–92.
6 Brandtzaeg P. Overview of the mucosal immune system. *Curr Topics Microbiol Immunol* 1989; **146**: 13–28.
7 MacDonald TT. Immunosuppression caused by antigen feeding. II. Suppressor T cells mask Peyer's patches B cell priming to orally administered antigen. *Eur J Immunol* 1983; **13**: 138–42.
8 Santos LMB, Al-Sabbagh A, Londono A, Weiner HL. Oral tolerance to myelin basic proteins induces regulatory TGF-β secreting T cells in Peyer's patches of SJL mice. *Cell Immunol* 1994; **157**: 439–47.
9 Mattingly JA. Immunological suppression after oral administration of antigen. III. Activation of suppressor-inducer cells in the Peyer's patches. *Cell Immunol* 1984; **86**: 46–52.
10 Schoenbeck S, Hammen MJ, Kagnoff MF. Vicia villosa agglutinin separates freshly isolated Peyer's patch T cells into interleukin 5- or interleukin 2- producing subsets. *J Exp Med* 1989; **169**: 1491–6.
11 Daynes RA, Araneo BA, Dowell TA, Huang K, Dudley D. Regulation of murine lymphokine production in vivo. III. The lymphoid tissue microenvironment exerts regulatory influences over T helper cell function. *J Exp Med* 1990; **171**: 979–96.

12 Xu-Amano J, Aicher WK, Taguchi T, Kiyono H, McGhee JR. Selective induction of Th₂ cells in murine Peyer's patches by oral immunization. *Internat Immunol* 1992; 4: 433-45.

13 Chen Y, Kuchroo VK, Inobe J-I, Hafler DA, Weiner HL. Regulatory T cell clones induced by oral tolerance: suppression of autoimmune encephalomyelitis. *Science* 1994; 265: 1237-40.

14 Chin YH, Cai JP, Xu XM. Transforming growth factor-β1 and IL-4 regulate the adhesiveness of Peyer's patch high endothelial venule cells for lymphocytes. *J Immunol* 1992; 148: 1106-12.

15 Lefrancois L. Intraepithelial lymphocytes of the intestinal mucosa: curiouser and curiouser. *Seminars in Immunol* 1991; 3: 99-108.

16 Miller A, Lider O, Roberts AB, Sporn M, Weiner HL. Suppressor T cells generated by oral tolerization to myelin basic protein suppress both in vitro and in vivo immune responses by the release of TGF-β following antigen specific triggering. *Proc Natl Acad Sci USA* 1992; 89: 421-5.

17 Mowat AM, Strobel S, Drummond HE, Ferguson A. Immunological responses to fed protein antigens in mice. I. Reversal of oral tolerance to ovalbumin by cyclophosphamide. *Immunology* 1982; 45: 105-13.

18 Husby S, Jensenius JC, Svehag S-E. Passage of undegraded dietary antigen into the blood of healthy adults. Further characterization of the kinetics of uptake and the size distribution of the antigen. *Scand J Immunol* 1986; 24: 447-52.

19 Bruce MG, Ferguson A. The influence of intestinal processing on the immunogenicity and molecular size of absorbed, circulating ovalbumin in mice. *Immunology* 1986; 59: 295-300.

20 Peng HJ, Turner MW, Strobel S. The generation of a "tolerogen" after the ingestion of ovalbumin is time-dependent and unrelated to serum levels of immunoreactive antigen. *Clin Exp Immunol* 1990; 81: 510-15.

21 Michael JG. The role of digestive enzymes in orally induced immune tolerance. *Immunol Invest* 1989; 18(9&10): 1049-54.

22 Hanson DG, Roy MJ, Green GM, Miller SD. Inhibition of orally-induced immune tolerance in mice by prefeeding an endopeptidase inhibitor. *Reg Immunol* 1993, 5: 94-102.

23 Gautam SC, Chikkala NF, Battisto JR. Oral administration of the contact sensitizer trinitrochlorobenzene: initial sensitization and subsequent appearance of a suppressor population. *Cell Immunol* 1990; 125: 437-48.

24 Hanson DG, Miller SD. Inhibition of specific immune responses by feeding protein antigens. V. Induction of the tolerant state in the absence of specific suppressor T cells. *J Immunol* 1982; 128: 2378-81.

25 Lider O, Santos LMB, Lee, CSY, Higgins PJ, Weiner HL. Suppression of experimental autoimmune encephalomyelitis by oral administration of myelin basic protein II. Suppression of disease and in vitro immune responses is mediated by antigen-specific CD8⁺ T lymphocytes. *J Immunol* 1989; 142: 748-52.

26 Miller A, Lider O, Weiner HL. Antigen-driven bystander suppression following oral administration of antigens. *J Exp Med* 1991; 174: 791-8.

27 Miller A, Al-Sabbagh A, Santos LMB, Prabhu-Das M, Weiner HL. Epitopes of myelin basic protein (MBP) that trigger TGF-β release following oral tolerization to MBP are different from encephalitogenic epitopes. *J Immunol* 1993; 151: 7307-15.

28 Al-Sabbagh A, Miller A, Santos LMB, Weiner HL. Antigen-driven tissue-specific suppression following oral tolerance: orally administered myelin basic protein suppresses proteolipid induced experimental autoimmune encephalomyelitis in the SJL mouse. *Eur J Immunol* 1994; 24: 2104-9.

29 Hanson DG. Ontogeny of orally induced tolerance to soluble proteins in mice. *J Immunol* 1981; **127**: 1518–24.
30 Strobel S, Ferguson A. Immune responses to fed protein antigens in mice. 3. Systemic tolerance or priming is related to age at which antigen is first encountered. *Ped. Res* 1984; **18**: 588–93.
31 Miller A, Lider O, Abramsky O, Weiner HL. Orally administered myelin basic protein in neonates primes for immune responses and enhances experimental autoimmune encephalomyelitis in adult animals. *Eur J Immunol* 1994; **24**: 1026–32.
32 Karjalainen J, Martin JM, Knip M, Ilonen J, Robinson BH, Savilahti E, Akerblom HK, Dosch H-M. A bovine albumin peptide as a possible trigger of insulin-dependent diabetes mellitus. *New Engl J Med* 1992; **327**: 302–7.
33 Zhang Z, Michael JG. Orally inducible immune unresponsiveness is abrogated by IFN-γ treatment. *J Immunol* 1990; **144**: 4163–5.
34 Khoury SJ, Lider O, Al-Sabbagh A, Weiner HL. Suppression of experimental autoimmune encephalomyelitis by oral administration of myelin basic protein. III. Synergistic effect of lipopolysaccharide. *Cell Immunol* 1990; **131**: 302–10.
35 Khoury SJ, Hancock WW, Weiner HL. Oral tolerance to myelin basic protein and natural recovery from experimental autoimmune encephalomyelitis are associated with downregulation of inflammatory cytokines and differential upregulation of transforming growth factor β, interleukin 4, and prostaglandin E expression in the brain. *J Exp Med* 1992; **176**: 1355–64.
36 Strobel S, Mowat AM, Ferguson A. Prevention of oral tolerance induction to ovalbumin and enhanced antigen presentation during a graft-versus-host reaction in mice. *Immunology* 1985; **56**: 57–64.
37 Mowat AM, Parrot DM. Immunological responses to fed protein antigens in mice. IV. Effects of stimulating the reticuloendothelial system on oral tolerance and intestinal immunity to ovalbumin. *Immunology* 50: 547–54.
38 Fujihashi K, Taguchi T, Aicher WK, McGhee JR, Bluestone JA, Eldridge JH, Kiyono H. Immunoregulatory functions for murine intraepithelial lymphocytes: γ/δ T cell receptor-positive (TCR⁺) T cells abrogate oral tolerance while α/β TCR⁺ T cells provide B cell help. *J Exp Med* 1992; **175**: 695–707.
39 Bland P. MHC class II expression by the gut epithelium. *Immunol Today* 1988; **9**(6): 174–8.
40 Mayrhofer G, Pugh CW, Barclay AN. The distribution, ontogeny and origin in the rat of Ia-positive cells with dendritic morphology and of Ia antigen in epithelia, with special reference to the intestine. *Eur J Immunol* 1983; **13**: 112–22.
41 Steiniger B, Falk P, Lohmüller M, Van Der Meide PH. Class II MHC antigens in the rat digestive system. Normal distribution and induced expression after interferon-gamma treatment in vivo. *Immunology* 1989; **68**: 507–13.
42 Richman LK, Graeff AS, Strober W. Antigen presentation by macrophage-enriched cells from the mouse Peyer's patch. *Cell. Immunology* **62**: 110–18.
43 Liu LM, MacPherson GG. Antigen acquisition by dendritic cells: intestinal dendritic cells acquire antigen administered orally and can prime naive T cells in vivo. *J Exp Med* 1993; **177**: 1299–307.
44 Bland PW, Warren LG. Antigen presentation by epithelial cells of the rat small intestine. II. Selective induction of suppressor T cells. *Immunology* 1986; **58**: 9–14.
45 Mayer L, Shlien R. Evidence for function of Ia molecules on gut epithelial cells in man. *J Exp Med* 1987; **166**: 1471–83.
46 Mowat AM, Thomas MJ, MacKenzie S, Parrott DM. Divergent effects of bacterial lipopolysaccharide on immunity to orally administered protein and particulate antigens in mice. *Immunology* 1986; **58**: 677–83.

47 Dahlgren UIH, Wold AE, Hanson LA, Midtvedt T. Expression of a dietary protein in *E. coli* renders it strongly antigenic to gut lymphoid tissue. *Immunology* 1991; 73: 394–7.

48 Elson CO. Cholera toxin and its subunits as potential oral adjuvants. *Curr Topics Microbiol Immunol* 1989; 146: 29–34.

49 Sun J-B, Holmgren J, Czerkinsky C. Cholera toxin B subunit: an efficient transmucosal carrier-delivery system for induction of peripheral immunological tolerance. *PNAS* 1994; 91: 10795–9.

50 Higgins P, Weiner HL. Suppression of experimental autoimmune encephalomyelitis by oral administration of myelin basic protein and its fragments. *J. Immunol.* 1988; 140: 440–5.

51 Bitar DM, Whitacre CC. Suppression of experimental autoimmune encephalomyelitis by the oral administration of myelin basic protein. *Cell Immunol.* 1988; 112: 364–70.

52 Fuller KA, Pearl D, Whitacre CC. Oral tolerance in experimental autoimmune encephalomyelitis: Serum and salivary antibody responses. *J. Neuroimmunol* 1990; 28: 15–26.

53 Brod SA, Al-Sabbagh, A, Sobel RA, Hafler DA, Weiner HL. Suppression of experimental autoimmune encephalomyelitis by oral administration of myelin antigens. IV. Suppression of chronic relapsing disease in the Lewis rat and strain 13 guinea pig. *Ann. Neurol.* 1992; 29: 615–22.

54 Miller A, Zhang ZJ, Sobel RA, Al-Sabbagh A, Weiner HL. Suppression of experimental autoimmune encephalomyelitis by oral administration of myelin basic protein. VI. Suppression of adoptively transferred disease and differential effects of oral vs. intravenous tolerization. *J. Neuroimmunol.* 1993; 46: 73–82.

55 Miller A, Lider O, Al-Sabbagh A, Weiner HL. Suppression of experimental autoimmune encephalomyelitis by oral administration of myelin basic protein. V. Hierarchy of suppression by myelin basic protein from different species. *J. Neuroimmunol.* 1992; 39: 243–50.

56 Oettinger HF, Al-Sabbagh A, Zhang J, LaSalle JM, Weiner HL, Hafler DA. Biological activity of recombinant human myelin basic protein. *J Neuroimmunol* 1993; 44: 157–62.

57 Hoyne GF, O'Hehir RE, Wraith DC, Thomas WR, Lamb JR. Inhibition of T cell and antibody responses to house dust mite allergen by inhalation of the dominant T cell epitope in naive and sensitized mice. *J. Exp. Med.* 1993; 178: 1783–8.

58 Weiner HL, Al-Sabbagh A, Sobel R. Antigen driven peripheral immune tolerance: suppression of experimental autoimmune encephalomyelitis (EAE) by aerosol administration of myelin protein. *FASEB J* 1990; 4: 2102 (Abstract).

59 Thompson HSG, Staines NA. Gastric administration of type II collagen delays the onset and severity of collagen-induced arthritis in rats. *Clin Exp Immunol* 1986; 64: 581–6.

60 Nagler-Anderson C, Bober LA, Robinson ME, Siskind GW, Thorbecke FJ. Suppression of type II collagen-induced arthritis by intragastric administration of soluble type II collagen. *Proc Natl Acad Sci USA* 1986; 83: 7443–6.

61 Zhang JZ, Lee CSY, Lider O, Weiner HL. Suppression of adjuvant arthritis in Lewis rats by oral administration of type II collagen. *J. Immunol.* 1990; 145: 2489–93.

62 Thompson SJ, Thompson HSG, Harper N, Day MJ, Coad AJ, Elson CJ, Staines NA. Prevention of pristane-induced arthritis by the oral administration of type II collagen. *Immunology* 1993; 79: 152–7.

63 Thompson HSG, Harper N, Bevan DJ, Staines NA. Suppression of collagen induced arthritis by oral administration of type II collagen: changes in immune

and arthritic responses mediated by active peripheral suppression. *Autoimmunity* 1993; **16**: 189–99.

64 Nussenblatt RB, Caspi RR, Mahdi R, Chan CC, Roberge F, Lider O, Weiner HL. Inhibition of S-antigen induced experimental autoimmune uveoretinitis by oral induction of tolerance with S-antigen. *J Immunol* 1990; **144**: 1689–95.

65 Singh VK, Kalra HK, Yamaki K, Shinohara T. Suppression of experimental autoimmune uveitis in rats by the oral administration of the uveitopathogenic S-antigen fragment or a cross-reactive homologous peptide. *Cell Immunol* 1992; **139**: 81–90.

66 Gregerson DS, Obritsch WF, Donoso LA. Oral tolerance in experimental autoimmune uveoretinitis: distinct mechanisms of resistance are induced by low versus high dose feeding protocols. *J Immunol* 1993; **151**: 5751–61.

67 Thurau SR, Chan C-C, Suh E, Nussenblatt RB. Induction of oral tolerance to S-antigen induced experimental autoimmune uveitis by a uveitogenic 20mer peptide. *J Autoimmun* 1991; **4**: 507–16.

68 Vrabec TR, Gregerson DS, Dua HS, Donoso LA. Inhibition of experimental autoimmune uveoretinitis by oral administration of S-antigen and synthetic peptides. *Autoimmunity* 1992; **12**: 175–84.

69 Zhang JA, Davidson L, Eisenbarth G, Weiner HL. Suppression of diabetes in NOD mice by oral administration of porcine insulin. *Proc Natl Acad Sci USA* 1991; **88**: 10252–6.

70 Bergerot I, Fabien N, Maguer V, Thivolet C. Oral administration of human insulin to NOD mice generates CD4+T cells that suppress adoptive transfer of diabetes. *J Autoimmunity* 1994; **7**: 655–63.

71 Shehadeh NN, LaRosa F, Lafferty KJ. Altered cytokine activity in adjuvant inhibition of autoimmune diabetes. *J Autoimmun* 1993; **6**: 291–300.

72 Wang Z-Y, Qiao J, Link H. Suppression of experimental, autoimmune myasthenia gravis by oral administration of acetylcholine receptor. *J Neuroimmunol* 1993; **44**: 209–14.

73 Sayegh MH, Zhang ZJ, Hancock WW, Kwok CA, Carpenter CB, Weiner HL. Down-regulation of the immune response to histocompatibility antigen and prevention of sensitization by skin allografts by orally administered alloantigen. *Transplantation* 1992; **53**: 163–6.

74 Sayegh MH, Khoury SJ, Hancock WH, Weiner HL, Carpenter CB. Induction of immunity and oral tolerance with polymorphic class II major histocompatibility complex allopeptides in the rat. *Proc Natl Acad Sci USA* 1992; **89**: 7762–6.

75 Hancock WW, Sayegh MH, Kwok CA, Weiner HL, Carpenter CB. Oral but not intravenous alloantigen prevents accelerated allograft rejection by selective intragraft Th2 cell activation. *Transplantation* 1993; **55**: 1112–18.

76 Hrstka J, Hesse UJ, Hrstka V, Danis J, Schmitz-Rode M, Tunggal B, Hordegen P, Peters S. Prolongation of islet allograft survival following immunologic conditioning by antigen feeding in the pig. *Transplant Proc* 1992; **24**: 663–4.

77 Dakin R. Remarks on a cutaneous affection produced by certain poisonous vegetables. *Am J Med Sci* 1829; **4**: 98–100.

78 Lowney ED. Immunologic unresponsiveness to a contact sensitizer in man. *J Investig Derma* 1968; **51**(6): 411–17.

79 Korenblatt PE, Rothberg RM, Minden P, Farr RS. Immune responses of human adults after oral and parenteral exposure to bovine serum albumin. *J Allergy* 1968; **41**: 226–35.

80 Gold WR Jr, Queenan FT, Woody J, Sacher RA. *Am J Obstet Gynecol* 1983; **146**: 980.

81 Czerkinsky C, Prince SJ, Michalek SM, Jackson S, Russell MW, Moldoveanu Z,

McGhee JR, Mestecky J. IgA antibody-producing cells in peripheral blood after antigen ingestion: Evidence for a common mucosal immune system in humans. *Proc Natl Acad Sci* 1987; **84**: 2449–53.

82 Husby S, Mestecky J, Moldoveanu Z, Holland S, Elson CO. Oral tolerance in humans: T cell but not B cell tolerance after antigen feeding. *J Immunol* 1994; **152**: 4663–70.

83 Weiner HL, Mackin GA, Matsui M, Orav EJ, Khoury SJ, Dawson DM, Hafler DA. Double-blind pilot trial of oral tolerization with myelin antigens in multiple sclerosis. *Science* 1993; **259**: 1321–4.

84 Salk RJS. A study of myelin basic protein as a therapeutic probe in patients with multiple sclerosis. In Hallpike JF, Adams CWM, Toutellotte WW (eds), *Multiple Sclerosis*. University Press, pp 621–30.

85 Trentham DE, Dynesius-Trentham RA, Orav EJ, Combitchi D, Lorenzo C, Sewell KL, Hafler DA, Weiner HL. Effects of oral administration of collagen on rheumatoid arthritis. *Science* 1993; **261**: 1727–30.

86 Nusenblatt RB, de Smet MD, Weiner HL, Gery I. *The Treatment of the Ocular Complications of Behcet's Disease with Oral Toleration*. 6th International Conference on Behcet's disease. Amsterdam: Elsevier, 1993; 641–6.

87 McCarron R, Fallis R, McFarlin D. Alterations in T cell antigen specificity and class II restriction during the course of chronic relapsing experimental allergic encephalomyelitis. *J Neuroimmunol* 1990; **29**: 73–80.

88 Lehmann PV, Forsthuber T, Miller A, Sercarz EE. Spreading of T cell autoimmunity to cryptic determinants of an autoantigen. *Nature* 1992; **358**: 155–8.

89 Cross AH, Tuohy VK, Raine CS. Development of reactivity to new myelin antigens during chronic relapsing autoimmune demyelination. *Cell Immunol* 1993; **146**: 261–7.

90 Kaufman DL, Clare-Salzier M, Tian J, Forsthuber T, Ting GSP, Robinson P, Atkinson MA, Sercarz EE, Tobin AJ, Lehmann PV. Spontaneous loss of T cell tolerance to glutamate decarboxylase in murine insulin-dependent diabetes. *Nature* 1993; **366**: 72–5.

91 Tisch R, Yang X-D, Singer SM, Liblau RS, Fugger L, McDevitt HO. Immune response to glutamic acid decarboxylase correlates with insulitis in non-obese diabetic mice. *Nature* 1993; **366**: 72–5.

92 Zhang J, Markovic S, Raus J, Lacet B, Weiner HL, Hafler DA. Increased frequency of IL-2 responsive T cells specific for myelin basic protein and proteolipid protein in peripheral blood and cerebrospinal fluid of patients with multiple sclerosis. *J Exp Med* 1993; **179**: 973–84.

93 Kerlero de Rosbo N, Milo R, Lees MB, Burger D, Bernard CCA, Ben-Nun A. Reactivity to myelin antigens in multiple sclerosis: peripheral blood lymphocytes respond predominantly to myelin oligodendrocyte glycoprotein. *J Clin Invest* 1993; **92**: 2602–8.

94 Harrison LC. Islet cell antigens in insulin-dependent diabetes: Pandora's box revisited. *Immunol Today* 1992; **13**: 348–52.

95 Chen Y, Inobe J-i, Marks R, Gonnella P, Kuchroo VK, Weiner HL. Peripheral deletion of antigen-reactive T cells in oral tolerance. *Nature* 1995; **376**: 177–80

96 Yoshino S, Quattrocchi E, Weiner HL. Supression of antigen-induced arthritis in Lewis rats by oral administration of type II collagen. *Arthritis and Rheumatism* 1995; **38**: 1092–6.

97 Hancock WW, Polanski M, Zhang J, Blogg N, Weiner HL. Suppression of insulitis in Non-Obese Diabetic (NOD) mice by oral insulin administration is associated with selective expression of Interleukin-4 and -10, transforming growth factor-β, and prostaglandin-E. *Am. J. Path.* 1995; **147**: 1193–9.

19

Lessons from the Animal Models: BB Rat

JEAN-FRANÇOIS YALE[1], FRASER W. SCOTT[2] and ERROL B. MARLISS[1]

[1]McGill Nutrition and Food Science Center, Royal Victoria Hospital, Montreal, Canada and [2]Nutrition Research Division, Banting Research Centre, Ottawa, Canada

INTRODUCTION

The prevention of the spontaneous autoimmune diabetes syndrome in the BB rat by cyclosporine[1] was one of the strongest arguments put forward to justify human trials in newly diagnosed subjects (reviewed elsewhere in this volume). Much was learnt in this sequence of studies about both the rat and human syndromes. This is perhaps the most tangible example to date of the comparisons and contrasts between the two diabetes "models", and of the advantages—and limitations—of such a comparison. As BB rat investigators with a combined experience beginning with the original description of the syndrome[2], we have argued for the utility and have warned of the potential limitations of studies in the rat being relevant to the human[3,4].

The BB rat was discovered in 1974 in a Wistar-derived commercial breeding colony (in Ottawa, Ontario, Canada) from which its name is derived. The first publication on it appeared in 1977[2], and since then over 1000 published articles have defined the genetics, etiology and pathogenesis, metabolic consequences, diabetes-related complications, therapy and strategies for prediction, reversal and prevention. Certain features of the BB rat syndrome must be borne in mind in interpreting the published data. Incidence, severity, immunologic features, and other aspects do vary among colonies and sub-lines from a given colony. The principal sources of rats for

Prediction, Prevention and Genetic Counseling in IDDM. Edited by Jerry P. Palmer.
© 1996 John Wiley & Sons Ltd.

study have been Ottawa, Ontario and Worcester, Massachusetts, as well as colonies in Denmark, Germany, Japan, and several other countries. They are usually designated by the colony of origin, with BB alone referring to Ottawa, BB/Wor to Worcester, BB/OK from Karlsburg, Germany, etc. Additional designations are: *BBdp* or *DP-BB*, referring to diabetes-prone lines; *BBn* to lines derived from the original Ottawa colony that never develop diabetes and may be considered to be "normal"; *BBd* to overtly diabetic rats; and *DR-BB* to a line that is ordinarily diabetes-resistant but becomes diabetic very rapidly after administration of antibody against the RT6[a] T cell alloantigen[5]. Studies of diabetes prevention have been performed in BBdp rats, in RT6 depleted DR-BB, and in a variety of derivative models, such as adoptive transfer and disease recurrence/occurrence in islets transplanted into susceptible animals.

The genetic susceptibility appears to reside in at least two, and probably more than three loci, including MHC (the RT1[u] haplotype or gene(s) in tight linkage disequilibrium with it, is required), an autosomal recessive gene responsible for the lymphopenia, and others yet to be defined (see Chapter 12). The usual onset of diabetes is peri- and postpubertal, both sexes are affected equally, with variable numbers in different litters (and also of sequential litters from the same breeding pair), after a very short period of demonstrable abnormalities of insulin secretion and glucose tolerance. The disease is truly insulin dependent. Incidence in different lines may vary from 25% to close to 100%, but it typically 40–70%.

The islets show variable degrees of intensity of insulitis in early stages, but with extensive mononuclear cell infiltration at the onset of hyperglycemia. The earliest infiltrating cells into the islets are dendritic cells or macrophages. The islets of insulin-treated rats show only residual inflammation, fibrosis, and persistence of non-beta cells. Autoimmune thyroiditis also occurs. Multi-organ antibodies have been found, not only anti-islet (but *not* anti-insulin) but also thyroid, gastric parietal cell, smooth muscle, and anti-lymphocyte as well. There is typically a severe lymphopenia affecting all lymphatic tissues except the thymus and the intraepithelial lymphocytes in the intestine. The most affected subsets are virtual absence of CD8+T lymphocytes, marked reduction of CD4+T cells, with absence of expression of the differentiation alloantigen RT6. A relative increase in B cells and NK cells is found, as are activated T cells expressing MHC class II antigen. Altered energy substrate metabolism in all immunocytes except thymocytes has been documented[6].

Marked immunocyte functional alterations have been described, including impaired proliferative responses to mitogens in vitro, decreased responsiveness in mixed lymphocyte reactions, impaired lymphokine production, the absence of functional cytotoxic T cells, yet with presence of beta cytotoxic lymphocytes. Certain of these decreased responses can be restored by removal of macrophages. The presence of (or the ability to generate) beta cytotoxic cells has been demonstrated in part by the adoptive transfer of the pathogenic process to susceptible recipient animals using a variety of activated immunocyte preparations originating from BBd spleens. Adoptive transfer very reliably induces diabetes usually in less than 2 weeks.

A delicate balance appears to exist among those factors leading to beta cell destruction, and factors conferring protection/resistance to the process. The presence of environmental (and other) triggers/amplifiers or inhibitory factors of the process is clear, in part from the variable disease expression despite the fact that the rats are genetically homogeneous and are raised in an (apparently) identical environment. It has been suggested that there may be a "protective" islet mononuclear cell infiltration as well as one that is destructive. This is consistent with current hypotheses regarding the presence of natural autoimmunity that remains suppressed permanently in nonsusceptible individuals, but whose expression in susceptible individuals is dependent upon a critical balance between autoaggressive and protective mechanisms. One such effector pathway appears to relate to the dynamic equilibrium between Th1 and Th2 cells and their cytokine products. It is perhaps because of a multifactorial etiopathogenesis in the BB rat that an extremely wide variety of interventions appear capable of altering the balance between autoaggressive and protective factors, with resultant prevention of overt expression of the disease.

One must be cautious in interpreting the catalog of interventions that follows. It should not be presumed that the suppression of overt Type 1 diabetes necessarily interrupts the pathogenic process. Many studies do not include data on the presence of milder forms of the syndrome that are demonstrable only by glucose tolerance testing and study of pancreatic islet pathology. This is one very important lesson to carry from animal to human studies, namely, that the absence of overt insulin dependence may only mean attenuation of the process, or "delaying the inevitable", rather than total arrest of the process which is the ultimate goal of preventive strategies. For reasons of space restriction, we cannot cite all reported studies. Results of studies that did not report diabetes prevention, or are abstracts, as well as other key references are referred to in the text by the first author of the reports and the year of publication.

IMMUNOSUPPRESSION

The autoimmune nature of the diabetes syndrome of the BB rat has prompted the investigation of numerous immunosuppressive approaches for its prevention and treatment. The results of certain of these trials are summarized below.

CYCLOSPORINE A

The immunosuppressive agent cyclosporine has been very successful in organ transplantation and is now routinely used clinically. The group of Stiller et al.[1,7] was the first to show prevention of diabetes in diabetes-prone BB rats by cyclosporine administration started at a young age and continued throughout the susceptibility period, and their findings have been amply confirmed (Table 19.1)[1,7–18]. The best results were obtained with uninterrupted administration of cyclosporine using therapeutic dosage schedules that resulted in trough plasma levels between 100 and 300 ng ml^{-1}. Similarly, starting the treatment later or interrupting it before the end of the usual susceptibility period led to lesser efficacy in prevention of diabetes. Treatment for a very limited duration (60–70 days)[16] did decrease the incidence of diabetes, suggesting that short-term treatment led to a persistent protection in *some* rats. It is possible that such a limited treatment, started at a critical point in the evolution of the pathophysiologic process, could result in long-term prevention in all rats. The data available suggest variability in the age at

Table 19.1. Diabetes prevention studies with cyclosporine A in BB rats

| Ref. | Treatment | | Diabetes incidence | | | |
	Dose	Duration Age (days)	Experimental %	n	Control %	n
1, 7	10 mg kg^{-1} day^{-1} po	34–55				
	8 mg kg^{-1} day^{-1} po	56–120	0	0/40	75	30/40
8	10–20 mg kg^{-1} day^{-1} po	40–165	0	0/58	47	29/62
9	10 mg kg^{-1} day^{-1} po	30–100	0	0/38	34	13/38
10	10 mg kg^{-1} day^{-1} po	30–150	22	5/23	32	6/19
11	10 mg kg^{-1} day^{-1} po	40–105	0	0/12	45	9/20
12	10 mg kg^{-1} day^{-1} po	42–120	0	0/30	49	45/92
13, 14	15 mg kg^{-1} day^{-1} SC	50–65				
	followed by 15 mg kg^{-1} Q2 wks	65–160	11	4/38	59	26/44
	15 mg kg^{-1} day^{-1} SC	30–50				
	followed by 15 mg kg^{-1} Q2 wks	50–160	10	5/48	42	20/48
15	10 mg kg^{-1} day^{-1} po	42–147	0	0/25	46	11/24
		42–119	20	3/15	50	7/14
		56–161	25	5/20	60	12/20
16	10 mg kg^{-1} day^{-1} po	30–40	20	2/20	30	3/10
		40–50	50	7/14	43	6/14
		50–60	67	10/15	67	10/15
		60–70	23	7/30	73	22/30
		70–80	37	11/30	45	13/29
17	5 mg kg^{-1} day^{-1} po	42–137	25	3/12	75	9/12
21	5 mg kg^{-1} day^{-1} po	30–125	35	6/17	88	15/17

po = oral or by gavage; SC = subcutaneous injection.

which the process begins as well as in its rate of progression between rats. Therefore there would be difficulty in defining this critical "window of opportunity" in individual rats.

Cyclosporine prevented the normal increase with age in numbers of T cells, resulting in lower numbers in the treated rats compared with their untreated littermates[10]. Its disease prevention efficacy was therefore associated with a worsening of the immunosuppression. When started at diabetes onset, cyclosporine had no effects on the evolution of diabetes in at least three studies[19,20]. Likewise, it was unable to prevent the adoptive transfer of diabetes from recent-onset BBd rats to young diabetes-prone BB rats by Con-A stimulated splenocytes[20]. That is, once cells that are activated to destroy the beta cells are present or introduced exogenously, the drug appears unable to arrest the process. However, it can prevent recurrence of diabetes after islet transplantation if started either before or at the time of the transplant into BBd rats (Konigsberger *et al.* 1987). Furthermore, when BB rats were treated at the diagnosis of glucose intolerance, one-third remained intolerant without evolving to overt diabetes for more than 60 days, in contrast to the untreated rats that all became diabetic within 8 days[20]. The prevention studies also revealed that cyclosporine treatment of BBn or other normal rats at therapeutic dosage *itself* led to glucose intolerance, through a decrease in insulin secretion and peripheral insulin resistance[21,22]. Thus, in addition to its nephrotoxic effects, this agent is a "double-edged sword" in relation to the beta cell itself. The effects of cyclosporine in BB and normal rats has been reviewed in more detail in reference 20.

In summary, the potent protective effect of cyclosporine against diabetes in BB rats was a prototype in the testing of an agent first in the rat, followed directly by human clinical trials. Because of the difficulty in predicting disease susceptibility in the human at the time of these studies, it was tried first in new-onset patients. Though the effects were tantalizing in a proportion of the patients, they were of short duration and accompanied in many with undesirable side-effects. The detailed BB rat studies would have clearly predicted that this drug is likely to be most potent when started early, whereas late introduction after the destructive process had destroyed sufficient beta cells to have caused hyperglycemia is much less efficacious. It also appeared unable to protect "normal" beta cells from pre-activated immune cells.

OTHER IMMUNOSUPPRESSIVE AGENTS

A wide variety of approaches has been used, almost uniquely with individual drugs. It is noteworthy that certain agents appear not to have been used or more probably have not been reported because of lack of efficacy. Among these are the "classical" immunosuppressants, azathioprine and cyclophosphamide. The absence of data on these and other agents in the present review therefore should not be construed as evidence for absence of trials being conducted, but that the authors are unaware of them. An additional cautionary note must be sounded about the interpretation of published studies on immunosuppressants. Many studies did not include follow-up off the drug for a sufficient period to know whether prevention had the potential for permanence or not. Few studies tested "successful" BBdp recipients for glucose intolerance; more studies did include islet pathology. Finally, we also do not present details of side-effects of certain of the agents tested; these are presented in some but not all published papers.

FK-506 is a macrolide that suppresses T-cell activation by inhibiting the transcription of mRNA for early phase lymphokines, and has been shown to prevent transplant rejection. FK-506 was shown to be very potent in preventing diabetes in BB rats[23-25] (Table 19.2) and furthermore, the absence of insulitis in treated animals was demonstrated. Ciamexone, an immunomodulatory drug derived from the immunostimulant group of 2-cyanaziridines, showed a beneficial effect on adjuvant arthritis, and suppressed local graft versus host reaction. Its use in young BBdp rats resulted in a mild protective effect[12] (Table 19.2).

Fusidic acid, an antibiotic used for staphylococcus infections, exhibits in vitro and in vivo immunosuppressive properties. Its use for prevention of

Table 19.2. Diabetes prevention studies with other immunosuppressive drugs

| Ref. | Treatment (dose and duration) | Diabetes incidence | | | |
| | | Experimental | | Control | |
		%	n	%	n
23, 24	FK-506 1 mg kg^{-1} po 30–120 days	16	3/19	75	15/20
	FK-506 2 mg kg^{-1} po 30–120 days	0	0/20	75	15/20
25	FK-506 25 μg 6 days/wk IM 27–120 days	0	0/10	68	34/50
12	Ciamexone 1 mg kg^{-1} po 42–120 days	27	9/33	39	13/33
	Ciamexone 10 mg kg^{-1} po 42–120 days	34	32/93	49	45/92
	Fusidic acid 2 mg IM 6 days/wk 30–120 days	45	9/20	75	15/20
	4 mg IM 6 days/wk 30–120 days	50	10/20	75	15/20
	8 mg IM 6 days/wk 30–120 days	80	12/15	75	15/20
	Cortisone acetate 250 μg kg^{-1} day^{-1} po 21–120 days	45	18/40	53	21/40
26	Mycophenolate mofetil 20 mg^{-1} day^{-1} 40–140 day po	0	0/24	55	10/18
	40–70 days po	40	6/15		
	60–90 days po	47	8/17		

IM = intramuscular; po=oral or by gavage.

diabetes in BB rats by Nicoletti *et al.* (1994) resulted in only modest effects (Table 19.2). Cortisone acetate, 250 μg kg^{-1} day^{-1} from 21 to 120 days, did not influence the frequency of diabetes nor the appearance of islet cell antibodies (Dyrberg *et al.* 1985). Mycophenolate mofetil is able to inhibit lymphocyte proliferation, presumably by an inhibitory effect on enzymes in the purine nucleotide synthetic pathway[26]. It prevented diabetes if treatment was prolonged, and was less effective if stopped at 70 or 90 days. Short-term treatment with 15-deoxyspergualin at 2 mg kg^{-1} pre- and post-islet transplantation into BBd rats was reported by von Specht *et al.* to markedly prolong graft survival[27].

IRRADIATION

Total lymphoid irradiation to BBdp rats was among the earlier interventions that prevented diabetes in surviving rats[28]. A subsequent study with gamma irradiation in single low doses to 30-day-old rats did not show such an effect in BBdp rats[29], interpreted by the authors to suggest that the cytotoxic effector cells are relatively radioresistant. In contrast, DR-BB rats showed a dose-related increase in diabetes frequency with irradiation, consistent with removal of a more radiosensitive regulatory cell population that inhibits the beta-cell destructive process. A further amplification of the latter effect occurred in adoptive transfer of activated BBd cells to DR-BB recipients. The same study showed no effect of ultraviolet (UVB) irradiation on diabetes frequency. This would appear to be a line of investigation worth pursuing for the present only in animal models.

IMMUNOTHERAPY

This section groups a wide variety of interventions aimed at producing major alterations in the immune system, by eliminating or altering differing populations of cells defined according to the specificity of the interventions. They include administration of cytokines, monoclonal (and a few polyclonal) antibodies to immune cell subsets, cytokines or cytokine receptors, agents to disable/destroy macrophages, removal of lymphatic tissues, and interventions aimed at altering immunocyte activation by altering their metabolic state. These interventions are difficult to classify strictly according to mechanism of effect.

INTERVENTIONS DIRECTED AT IMMUNOCYTE SUBSETS

Following the initial demonstration that antilymphocyte serum[30] with or without other immunosuppressant drugs[31] was able to arrest or even reverse diabetes, a wide variety of monoclonal antibodies have been found to be equally or more effective (Table 19.3(a)). The latter added a variable degree of

Table 19.3. Immunotherapeutic interventions in BB rats

Ref.	Intervention	Model			Monoclonal antibody	Diabetes incidence						P <
		BBdp	DR-BB	Islet Tx		Experimental			Control			
						%	n	Days to DM*	%	n	Days to DM*	
(a) Antibodies to immune cells												
30	Antilymphocyte serum	✓				0	0/27		33	8/24		0.05
31	Antilymphocyte serum (×1)+glucocorticoids +cyclosporine	✓				29	14/48†		46	23/50		0.004
32	Anti-CD5	✓			OX19	0	0/49		61	43/70		0.001
	Anti CD8+NK	✓			OX8	12	11/90		61	43/70		0.001
	Anti CD4 (+	✓			W3/25	34	12/35		61	43/70		0.02
	variables other subsets)	✓			OX38	55	11/20		61	43/70		NS
		✓			OX35	39	14/36		61	43/70		0.05
	Anti "Ia - A"	✓			OX6	50	28/56		61	43/70		NS
	"Ia - E"	✓			OX17	32	7/22		61	43/70		0.03
	"Ia - A"	✓			3JP	63	10/16		61	43/70		NS
33	Anti CD2 (T+NK cells)	✓			(OX34,OX53, OX54,OX55 OX54+55)	0 to 34	0/66 to 11/32		77	23/30		0.01
34	Anti-NK	✓			3.2.3	73	19/26		84	27/32		NS
	Anti-CD8+NK	✓			OX8	16	3/19		84	27/32		0.01
	Anti-MHC Class II											
	"I-E"	✓			GY 15/195	14	2/14		43	6/14		NS
	"I-A"	✓			GY 15/361	65	11/17		43	6/14		NS

				%	Incidence	Days to DM*	Incidence	Days to DM*	p
35	Anti-CD4(+macrophages)	W3/25	✓		5	24.6	10	21.5	NS
	Anti-CD5	OX19	✓		5	16	10	21.5	NS
	Anti-CD8+NK	OX8	✓		5	>100	10	21.5	0.05
	Anti-NK	αAsialoGM$_1$	✓		5	>100	10	21.5	0.05
36	Anti-NK	αAsialoGM$_1$	✓		5	82	10	22	0.01
(b) Antibodies to cytokines, receptors or adhesion molecules									
37	Anti-interferon-γ		✓ (BBd)	14	2/14	75	15/20		0.001
38	Anti IL-2 receptor antibody (+low-dose cyclosporine A)		(BBd)	67	8/12‡				
	Anti IL-2 receptor antibody (+low-dose cyclosporine A)		(BBd)	63	7/11‡				
	Anti IL-2 receptor antibody (ART-18)		✓		10	>120	12	30	0.01
39	Anti IL-2 receptor antibody (ART-18)		✓		13	>42	12	11	0.01
	Anti leukocyte-function associated antigen-1 (LFA-1)		✓	58	7/12	100	12/12		0.05
	Anti intercellular adhesion molecule-1 (ICAM-1)		✓	82	9/11	100	10/10		NS

* Days to DM refers to absence of diabetes in BBd transplant recipients.
† Also effective in reversing diabetes if given at onset.
‡ This number of diabetic rats became normoglycemic with treatment.

specificity in terms of targeting phenotypically defined populations, depending upon how restricted the antigen(s) recognized are, and the capacity of the antibody to delete the targeted population. Further, the dose(s) selected, age at onset of treatment, treatment schedule, duration of treatment, and development of antibodies to the monoclonal preparation are variables in determining outcome.

In the BBdp rat, the following findings have been reported. An anti-CD5 antibody (OX19) was capable of total abrogation of overt diabetes, markedly decreased insulitis, and likewise decreased the intensity of thyroiditis[32]. A variety of other antibodies, to CD8+ and NK cells (OX8) and to CD4+ cells were variably effective, and most but not all anti-class II antibodies were ineffective[32]. A range of anti-CD2 antibodies all caused significant decreases in diabetes incidence[33], interpreted as due to CD4+T-cell depletion, prevention of effector cell activation, or blocking the CD2–ligand interaction between effector and target cells. To define further whether the OX8 effect was due to the CD8+T cells and/or NK cells, a more specific anti-NK antibody, 3.2.3, was used, which appeared ineffective itself[34]. Whereas an anti I-E antibody, OX17, was effective in one study[32], another antibody (GY 15/195) showed a nonsignificant trend toward a decrease, and another anti I-A antibody (GY 15/361) was not effective (Boitard et al. 1985). The latter study was among those whose power to show effects was limited by small numbers of rats studied and a rather low "control" incidence. A study of prevention of insulitis in normal islets transplanted into BBd rats confirmed the effectiveness of the OX8 antibody but not of OX19 or W3/25[35]. Marked prolongation of graft survival was found with an anti-NK antibody, anti-asialo GM_1[36]. The latter antibody alone prevented diabetes in BBdp rats[36], but did not prevent diabetes in the RT6-depleted DR rat either alone or combined with OX8[5] (Woda et al. 1987). The foregoing studies are consistent with a key role for T lymphocytes, especially those identified by OX8, though this subset is numerically markedly reduced in peripheral lymphoid tissues in BBdp rats. A role for NK cells is suggested by the OX8 and anti-asialo GM_1 results, but not by the antibody 3.2.3 results. There is less certainty about this in the DR-BB model, but this is only one of several lines of evidence that suggest that the effector mechanisms are different in these rats than in BBdp rats.

Table 19.3(b) lists three other effective interventions. These include anti-interferon-γ[37], anti-IL-2 receptor antibody in recent-onset diabetes[38] (Hahn et al. 1988) and in the islet transplant model[39] (Hahn et al. 1990). A study by Kitagawa et al. (1994) with anti-leukocyte-function associated antigen (LFA-1), an adhesion molecule, showed modest but significant effects, though anti-ICAM-1 was without effect. Interpretations of these studies are complex and thus far have provided interesting probes more than detailed insights into disease mechanisms. For example, since IL-2 receptors can be expressed on activated T, B, NK cells and macrophages, the effect of

Table 19.4. Effects of cytokine administration

Reference	Intervention	Model BBdp	DR-BB	Experimental %	n	%	Control n	$P<$
				Diabetes incidence				
40	*Interleukin-1β*							
	High dose	✓		95	21/22*	83	20/24	NS
	Low dose	✓		50	11/22	83	20/24	0.05
	High dose		✓	5	1/21	<3		
41	Interleukin-2	✓		53	17/32	23	8/35	0.025
42	Interleukin-2							
	"Low-incidence"	✓		53	17/32	23	8/35	0.01
	"Hi-incidence"	✓		32	6/19	73	19/26	0.01
	Interleukin-2							
	Low dose	✓		50	7/14	64	9/14	NS
	High dose	✓		70	7/10	60	6/10	NS
	High dose		✓	0	0/10			
43	Tumor necrosis factor α	✓		0	0/21	36	8/22	0.001
44	Tumor necrosis factor β (lymphotoxin)	✓						
	Low dose			38	10/26	80	24/30	0.01
	High dose			14	4/29	80	24/30	0.0001

*Age of onset was lower with high dose (9/22 developed DM before the first control rat).

anti-receptor antibody, though impressively potent, requires further study to establish why it works.

CYTOKINE ADMINISTRATION

Table 19.4 summarizes studies of effects of interleukins 1 and 2 and tumor necrosis factors γ and β. In one study of IL-1β in BBdp rats, both acceleration of the onset with high doses (without altering incidence) and decreased incidence with low doses were found[40]. Higher incidence was found after IL-2 in a line of BBdp rats with a rather low (23%) incidence[41]. The same group showed decrease in incidence in another line with higher control incidence (73%)[42]. They postulated the differences to be due to different settings of the "cytokine network" controlling the disease process, or possibly to different levels of inhibitors of IL-2. Another study showed no effect of IL-2 (Burstein *et al.* 1987).

Satoh *et al.* showed total prevention of diabetes with tumor necrosis factor α (TNFα)[43]. The mechanism of this effect is also unknown, but is not thought to be correction of low endogenous TNFα production, as is the case in the NOD mouse. Many possibilities exist, including decreased NK cell activity, increased superoxide dismutase activity in beta cells, induction of production of other cytokines, and others. It is noteworthy that the insulitis was not prevented by TNFα. The same group showed prevention with TNFβ (lymphotoxin)[44]. Low production of endogenous TNF was also found, as shown in other in vivo and in vitro studies by Lapchak et al. (1992). The immunostimulatory effect of streptococcal preparation OK-432 that also leads to lowered diabetes incidence (see below) is postulated to be due at least in part to stimulation of TNF production.

INTERVENTIONS DIRECTED AT MACROPHAGES

Since the first cells to appear in the insulitis are macrophages, as documented by several authors, to target these cells specifically has been an interesting preventive strategy. Kolb et al. (1990) showed that macrophages bearing the ED1 marker are capable of lysing islet cells in vitro. His group first showed that intraperitoneal silica injection to impair macrophage function prevented BBdp rats from becoming diabetic[45,46]. Only 4 of 111 treated (4%), compared with 38 of 121 (32%) of control rats developed diabetes. The group of Yoon confirmed these findings[47], and extended them with an adoptive transfer paradigm and suggested the mechanism to be a decrease in macrophage-dependent T-lymphocyte and NK cell cytotoxicity. The same intervention, silica injections in DR-BB rats depleted of RT6+T cells, did *not* prevent them from developing diabetes (Cormier et al. 1989). Nor did this treatment of either donors or recipients prevent adoptive transfer of diabetes, suggesting a different pathogenic role for macrophages in this model.

THYMECTOMY

Neonatal thymectomy, if complete, results in the systemic elimination of mature thymus-derived T cells. In an early experiment, this intervention was successful in preventing diabetes[48]. However, it is a rather nonspecific intervention, and can only be interpreted as showing that pathophysiologic process requires such cells to be present, rather like prevention with antilymphocyte serum. Adult thymectomy is less effective at preventing diabetes, and correspondingly less effective in extensively depleting T cells (Like et al. 1986).

INTERVENTIONS DIRECTED AT THE METABOLIC ACTIVITY OF IMMUNOCYTES

Cells of the immune system are metabolically very active, and when functionally stimulated, require increased uptake and metabolism of energy and biosynthetic substrates to sustain their activities[6]. The carbon flux from the quantitatively most important energy substrates, glucose and glutamine, is primarily via glycolysis (the principal product being lactate) and glutaminolysis (with principal products being glutamate and aspartate), respectively. Newsholme (1989) postulated that this provides for a very rapid and precise "buffering mechanism" of availability of other intermediates for biosynthetic pathways. Since glutamine is a precursor for purine and pyrimidine nucleotide as well as protein synthesis, it is not surprising that immunocytes with the greatest capacity for proliferation are those that have the greatest rates of glutamine utilization, with relatively less glucose utilization[6]. The highest rates of substrate oxidation are in macrophages, followed by blood mononuclear cells, splenocytes, then lymph node lymphocytes, and with thymocytes the least active. Macrophages are notable in respect to glucose metabolism in that a larger proportion is directed via the pentose phosphate pathway. This is relevant to their production of oxygen free radicals (see below).

Of note is the marked increase in energy metabolism of immunocytes of the BBd rat, that to some extent is also found in BBdp rats[6]. The fact that it is present in BBdp rats as early as 50 days old suggested to one of us (EBM), that attenuation of this increase in metabolism (without damaging the integrity of the immunocytes) could be a useful strategy to prevent diabetes. We addressed ourselves first to glutamine, using the antimetabolite acivicin in doses considerably less than for chemotherapy. It was very effective at suppressing disease expression at the level of insulitis, glucose intolerance and overt diabetes[49]. The success of this approach suggests that other agents that are not directed at interrupting immunologic functional activation, but rather at immunocyte metabolism, are worth exploring. One such approach is directed toward adenosine deaminase activity, shown to be elevated in peripheral sites in BBd rats. The adenosine deaminase inhibitor 2'-deoxycoformycin decreased diabetes incidence from 78 to 32% in BBdp rats[50]. Though such agents have cytotoxic actions, this is not the goal of their deployment in preventing the autoimmune process, so lower doses and/or combinations of agents (each used at doses without demonstrable toxicity) may be effective.

IMMUNOMODULATION AND/OR TOLERANCE INDUCTION

Several lines of evidence confirm the ability of restoration of immune regulation in BBdp rats to prevent diabetes, with or without prevention of insulitis. These outcomes have been achieved by transfer of cell populations (either mixtures or relatively purified) from a variety of donor animal types. The mechanism(s) responsible for such prevention have been difficult to define. Other means of influencing the balance between autoaggressive and protective actions of the immune system, including induction of tolerance to islet cells, and treatment with agents with "immunomodulating" activity are also reviewed in this section.

BONE MARROW TRANSPLANTATION

Naji *et al.* were the first to show that bone marrow cells from Wistar–Furth rats injected neonatally into BBdp rats prevent diabetes[51,52]. They documented that such inoculations restored certain aspects of lymphocyte function and numbers toward normal[53], results consistent with the preventive outcome being due to the introduction of a missing cell population capable of suppressing the beta-cytotoxic process. Similar findings were subsequently obtained by bone marrow transplantation from non-diabetes-prone rats into irradiated adult BBdp recipients[54,55]. These studies pointed to cells derived from bone marrow stem cells being responsible, but could not exclude the possibility that protection was from T cells in the inoculum.

TRANSFERS OF INDIVIDUAL AND MIXED-CELL POPULATIONS

Following the initial demonstration that whole blood transfusions[56], then buffy-coat transfusions[57], were able to prevent diabetes and attenuate insulitis, it was shown that this effect resided in the T cells transferred[57]. A single injection of MHC-compatible spleen cells from either Wistar–Furth or DR-BB rats was also found to prevent diabetes[58] if given early in life. The requirement for transferred cells persisting in the recipient has likewise been demonstrated, as has the efficacy of a T-helper (W3/25+) enriched (but not an OX-8+ enriched) population of cells[59]. In the BB/hooded (BB/h) hybrid, both splenocytes and concanavalin-A activated blasts were able to prevent diabetes[60].

The studies involving transfers from DR-BB donors, that were effective at preventing diabetes in association with long-term engraftment of RT6+ cells were interpreted as consistent with cells co-expressing other T-cell markers (e.g. W3/25+) with RT6 as responsible[5]. A more recent study of transfer of cells from BBdp rats beyond the usual age of diabetes occurrence (232 days) to 92-day-old BBdp recipients was designed to determine whether the "resistance" of the donors could be transferred[61]. These cells were all RT6−, yet were able both to prevent diabetes after a single injection into BBdp rats and to prevent recurrence of diabetes after syngeneic islet grafts into BBd rats. Thus, though the identity of these cells remains unknown, there exists in some BBdp rats a population capable of suppressing the ability to other cells in the same rats to destroy the beta cells. Whether this regulatory action is a direct cell–cell interaction or mediated via cytokine release at key sites remains to be determined. One study of transplantation of diabetes-resistant rat thymus suggested that bone-marrow-derived antigen-presenting cells within the thymus not only permitted restoration of T-cell function in the BBdp recipients, but completely prevented diabetes and decreased both the incidence and severity of the insulitis[62]. If the preventive mechanism(s) were established in the animal model, it could lead to a more specific cell population to isolate for use in future human trials.

INTRATHYMIC ISLET TRANSPLANTATION

Having demonstrated prolonged islet graft survival and function in BBd rats receiving intrathymic transplants (Posselt *et al.* 1991, 1992), the group of Naji and colleagues went on to show complete prevention of diabetes in BBdp rats neonatally injected with small numbers of islets from adult Wistar–Furth rats, into the thymus[63,64]. The mechanism implicated was of tolerance induction to beta cells, since both pancreatic and intrathymic islets remained normal, since the systemic lymphopenia and immunodeficiency in the recipients was unaltered, and since diabetes did not develop after adult thymectomy in the protected rats. Another study produced protection from diabetes with irradiated adult DR-BB islets injected intrathymically to 32-day-old BBdp recipients: incidence was 8 of 23 (35%) compared to 22 of 25 (88%) in control rats[65]. Similar findings were reported using MHC-incompatible (Lewis) islets introduced into the thymus of BBdp rats at 28–42 days of age, with 0 of 13 (0%) developing diabetes, compared with 13 of 13 (100%) of controls[66]. Interestingly, the same group (Brayman *et al.* 1993) found partial protection from subsequent diabetes using MHC-compatible Wistar–Furth islets (6 of 10 or 60%). In contrast, in the RT6-depleted DR-BB model, neither iso- nor allografted islets into the thymus prevented diabetes, nor reversed existing diabetes[67]. This again demonstrates the different disease mechanism(s) of the latter model. However, because of the rapid development of the beta cell destructive process in these rats, it could be that the age of transplantation (30 days) was too late for tolerance induction. Another possibility is that the ability to develop tolerance is interfered with by depletion of RT6+ cells. Thus, this approach needs much further investigation before it may be considered for human studies.

OTHERS

Anti-inflammatory Agents

Given the presence of inflammatory cells in the insulitis in BBdp and BBd rats, the induction by cytokines of eicosanoids with deleterious effects on islet integrity, the in vitro protection from such effects by some anti-inflammatory agents (Rabinovitch *et al.* 1990), and the acceleration of diabetes in BBdp rats by derivatives of prostoglandin E_1[68], it is surprising that more studies on anti-inflammatory agents have not been reported. One study of a novel anti-inflammatory agent tetrandrine, a bisbenzylisoquinoline alkaloid, showed decrease in diabetes incidence from 76 to 11% when begun at 35 days of age, and from 63 to 29% when started at age 70 days[69]. A corresponding decrease in insulitis intensity was reported. The precise mechanism was not identified.

Platelet activating factor (PAF) is a phospholipid mediator in a variety of inflammatory conditions, whose activity is antagonized by Ginkgolide B (BN 52021). This agent can abolish alloxan-induced diabetes in the rat and can protect islets in vitro from toxicity mediated by splenocytes. Although it reduced the severity of insulitis when given from age 25 to 105 days to BBdp rats, there was a rather puzzling absence of effect on overall incidence of diabetes (Beck *et al.* 1991). Such a divergent effect on insulitis compared with diabetes occurrence has not been reported with other interventions.

Other Immunomodulating Drugs

The "immunopotentiator", B-1,6; 1,3 D-glucan (a 500 kDa polysaccharide) prevents diabetes and insulitis in BBdp rats[70]. When given intravenously beginning at 28 days it decreased diabetes incidence from 13 of 30 (43%) to 2 of 30 (7%) and insulitis from 82 to 26% by 140 days. An agent that appears to be able to induce antigen non-specific "suppressor cell" activity, the azaspirane compound SK&F 106610, decreased diabetes incidence in BBdp rats from 24 of 30 (80%) to 10 of 31 (32%), accompanied by decreased insulitis[71]. Prevention by the immunomodulating maneuvers, injection of complete Freund's adjuvant and the streptococcal preparation OK-432 are reviewed below.

"PROTECTION" OF THE BETA CELL FROM AUTOIMMUNE ATTACK

AGENTS AFFECTING BETA CELL SECRETORY ACTIVITY

The observation of Gotfredsen *et al.*[72] that exogenous insulin administered from a young age markedly reduced diabetes incidence in BBdp rats supported the hypothesis that beta cell rest could result in decreased antigen expression at the surface of beta cells, thereby protecting them from the immune attack. This finding was subsequently confirmed by numerous reports (Table 19.5)[72-75] (see also Like 1986). In an attempt to differentiate whether this protective effect was related to the hypoglycemia or to an inhibition of insulin secretion, one of us (JFY) administered diazoxide to inhibit beta cell secretion and to cause mild hyperglycemia. To test for the possibility of increased diabetes susceptibility due to increased secretion, and corresponding hypoglycemia, we gave the sulfonylurea glyburide. While

Table 19.5. Prevention of diabetes by prophylactic insulin in BBDP rats

Reference	Insulin dose	Plasma glucose (mmol/l)	Diabetes incidence Experimental		Controls	
			%	n	%	n
72	15 units/kg daily 10–25 units/kg for	?	17%	6/36	42%	15/36
	5–7 d	Lower	2%	1/65	56%	24/43
73	2 units per day	1.4–3.6	14%	3/21	88%	14/16
74	15 units/kg/d	3.0–3.6	20%	4/20	42%	8/19
75	15–20/units/kg/d	4.7	10%	1/10	25%	1/4

glyburide had no effect, diazoxide was as potent as insulin in preventing the appearance of diabetes[74]. We also showed that insulin treatment of young diabetes-prone recipients greatly reduced the rate of adoptive transfer of diabetes (from 95 to 29%) from acutely diabetic rats[76], revealing that insulin treatment (in contrast to cyclosporine) could prevent the destruction of pancreatic β cells by previously activated immune cells. In the RT6-depleted DR-BB/Wor rat model of diabetes, Gottlieb *et al.* showed that prophylactic insulin greatly reduced the frequency of diabetes and insulitis[75]. However, spleen cells from the protected rats were still capable of inducing adoptive transfer of diabetes. This extremely potent effect in three settings in which it is certain that autoreactive cells are present, yet diabetes expression is attenuated or delayed, has considerable importance in relation to the human interventions that have been designed as a result of the animal data.

Buschard *et al.* reported that neonatal stimulation of β cells in BBdp rats with glucagon or arginine reduced the subsequent onset of diabetes from 65 to 20–23%[77]. They argued that this stimulation may have accelerated β-cell maturation, and thereby induced antigen expression on these cells, resulting in tolerance that would not have occurred in the normal course of maturation. The inhibition of β-cell insulin secretory activity has been shown in vitro to decrease the expression of autoantigens at the surface of the β cells, an effect that could explain the reduced β-cell destruction observed in vivo. However, inhibition of insulin secretion has also been shown to reduce the susceptibility of islet cells to the cytotoxic effects of IL-1β, suggesting that the resting β cells may be more resistant to cytotoxic insults through other mechanisms as well. The relationship between beta cell function and diabetes occurrence has been reviewed in greater detail in reference 78.[78]

OXYGEN FREE RADICALS

A role has been proposed for oxygen free radicals in beta cytotoxicity, generated both within beta cells themselves and by infiltrating macrophages and other immunocytes, under the influence of cytokines (reviewed in reference 79).[79] Islets have low superoxide dismutase (SOD) and glutathione peroxidase activity, which would tend to make them more susceptible to damage. BBdp rat islets have even lower SOD levels, possibly making them even more prone to oxidative damage (Pisanti *et al.* 1988). Given the clear role of macrophages and their capacity for oxygen free radical production, the increased activity of macrophage pentose phosphate pathway we showed in BBd cells[6], and the NADPH this would provide for forming O_2^- and its derivatives, they could well contribute to the cytotoxicity. Once attracted to the islet, activated BBd macrophages could release large amounts of superoxide anion, hydrogen peroxide (Wu *et al.* 1993) and hydroxyl radical. It is noteworthy that cyclosporine has been shown to inhibit the oxidative burst in macrophages (Goldin and Keisary 1989). Many lines of evidence have been adduced to implicate the involvement of these molecular species in vitro and in vivo systems (Mandrup-Poulsen *et al.* 1990). Within the beta cells themselves, the effects of tumor necrosis factor (TNF) and interferon-gamma (IFNγ) have been suggested to act via free radical generation (Pukel *et al.* 1988). Sumoski *et al.* (1989) have attributed the functional and cytotoxic effects of mixtures of cytokines (IL1, TNF, IFNγ) incubated with normal islet cells to free radicals based on similar effects of known free-radical generators, and on protection by the combination of dimethylthiourea and citiolone. They have implicated lipid peroxidation as a mechanism by use of a potent inhibitor (U78518E) of this process (Rabinovitch *et al.* 1992).

In the BB rat, several antioxidant interventions have decreased diabetes incidence, via probable antioxidant effects. Behrens *et al.* showed decreased diabetes incidence with α-tocopherol administration[80], following which they have demonstrated an alteration in not only vitamin E but also in ascorbic acid and dehydroascorbic acid metabolism in BBdp rats, possible contributing factors to susceptibility to diabetes. Probucol both decreased the incidence and delayed the onset of diabetes[81]. Of interest is the decreased susceptibility of BB rats with essential fatty acid deficiency (especially of *n*-6 polyunsaturated fatty acids) to diabetes[82].

Nicotinamide is effective in preventing diabetes in NOD mice, and is currently being used in human trials. In the BB rat, it did not prevent diabetes[83]. In combination with vitamin E and Max EPA (a source of *n*-3 fatty acids), nicotinamide negated an otherwise significant effect (diabetes occurred in 14 of 17 rats). The combination of ebselen, vitamin E and Max EPA was effective in lowering incidence (to 7 of 17 compared with 12 of 16 controls) and delaying onset age (in females) in this study[84]. Another study of an oral mixture of four free-radical scavengers added to feed had modest effects in delaying onset and decreasing diabetes incidence[85]. The mixture included allopurinol, mercaptoproprionyl-glycine, dimethylthiourea and vitamin E. These investigators (Murthy *et al.* 1990) also reported failure of injections of superoxide dismutase and catalase to prevent diabetes in BB rats. The iron chelator desferoxamine was studied using a high molecular weight hydroxyethyl starch (HES) conjugate and HES as the control[86]. It was partially effective, but an effect was also seen with HES compared to untreated rats. These antioxidant studies taken together suggest that there may be an agent or combination of agents that may be of interest in prevention of diabetes. It would require an extraordinarily nontoxic agent or mixture however, as many of the individual compounds in this category have a significant incidence of side-effects.

NITRIC OXIDE

There has been a virtual explosion of interest in the role of nitric oxide (NO) as a mediator of beta cell damage. NO is the product of two different forms of NO synthase, with arginine as substrate, citrulline as product and requiring NADPH. The constitutive form (calcium and calmodulin dependent) is widely distributed in endothelium, brain, platelets and islets. The inducible form is stimulated by endotoxin, IFNγ and IL-1 and is found in smooth muscle, microglial cells, hepatocytes, macrophages and beta cells. Considerably larger amounts of NO are produced by the latter form, and have inhibitory effects on cell function as well as cytolytic effects. Some NO effects are guanylate-cyclase mediated and the cytotoxic effects may be via destruction of iron-sulfur centers of iron-containing enzymes, leading to altered mitochondrial function and DNA synthesis. Furthermore, NO appears to be able to react with superoxide anion to form hydroxyl radicals, themselves capable of damaging mitochondria and impairing DNA synthesis.

Several lines of evidence support the relevance of NO to Type 1 diabetes[79]. As with free radicals, NO can be released by infiltrating immune cells in the islet and generated within the beta cell itself. Wu and Flynn (1993) have found marked increases in NO production by BBd peritoneal macrophages. The inhibition of insulin secretion by NO can be blocked in vitro by inhibitors of the constitutive NO synthase, the arginine analogs, L-N^G-monomethyl-L-arginine (L-NMMA) and L-N^G-nitro-L-arginine (L-NAME). Activated macrophage-mediated islet cell cytotoxity is also inhibited in vitro by these agents. Aminoguanidine, a protein-glycosylation inhibitor, is also a potent and selective inhibitor of inducible NO synthase. Wu found a delay in onset of diabetes of 13–15 days with subcutaneous injection of L-NMMA and oral aminoguanidine, but no effect on overall diabetes incidence[87]. A decrease in diabetes incidence was shown with oral L-NAME, without effect on age of onset[88]. The interpretation of the decrease in incidence was complex, however, in that a number of the treated rats died without diabetes prior to ending the study at 150 days of age. Possible explanations for failure to show greater effects are that NO synthesis within the islets was incompletely inhibited, or that there may be NO-sensitive and NO-insensitive phases in the β-cytotoxic process[87]. This promises to be a productive area for ongoing work, but the results are too preliminary to allow for extrapolation to the human syndrome.

AGENTS IN THE ENVIRONMENT

Many kinds of data point to involvement of environmental factors in diabetes pathogenesis in both persons and BB rats, the most studied being foods and infectious agents, and to a lesser extent, stress.

DIET

It will be almost impossible to determine the diabetes-including potential of individual foods from epidemiological data. The identity of food diabetogens, the mechanisms by which they act and when and how long the susceptible host must be exposed to these agents can be defined from studies in animals. The chances of designing successful diet interventions in humans will be enhanced if the food diabetogens can be characterized at the molecular level in diabetes-prone animals.

Protein

Several lines of evidence now strongly suggest that semi-purified diets containing non-diabetogenic protein sources inhibit diabetes development. In the first study of long-term effects of defined diets in BBdp rats, two diets were fed, one a mainly plant-based diet and the other, a modified, AIN-76A semi-purified diet consisting of casein (20% w/w) as the sole protein source, with 15% corn oil, 55% corn starch plus micronutrients and cellulose fiber[89]. The diabetes incidence was 11 out of 40 and 0 out of 40 respectively, whereas usual diabetes frequency was 68±7% in BBdp rats fed standard, mainly plant-based diets such as Purina 5001 or NIH-07. In contrast, casein (10±6% diabetes incidence) or hydrolyzed casein (HC, 14±7%) diets prevent or delay onset of diabetes, dampen insulitis and preserve greater islet mass (HC versus NIH, 0.88±0.41 versus 0.45±0.41 mm^2, $p = 0.007$ Scott *et al.* unpublished). Others have confirmed this finding[90,91] and Elliott and Martin found that feeding a diet with an amino acid mixture in place of protein was also protective[92]. Thus, more than 85% of BBdp rat diabetes may be food-induced[93].

Issa-Chergui *et al.*[90] fed a semi-purified casein-based diet to low incidence (20–25%) hybrid BBdp rats and found that the diet had to be fed before 30 days of age to be protective. Another study by Daneman *et al.*[94] used two mainly plant-based Purina Chow® diets, one with 1.0% cow's milk protein (CMP) and the other without CMP. Both plant-based diets with and without CMP, when fed post-weaning, produced a high incidence of diabetes in rats exposed to CMP between days 14 and 24. Avoiding exposure to CMP between days 14 and 24 inhibited appearance of diabetes. One of us (FWS) reported that a beneficial effect is still apparent when the pups are weaned at 23 days on to the protective casein-based diet despite being exposed orally from day 14 to plant-based diets fed to the dam[95]. Even when first exposure to NIH-07 occurred as late as 50 days of age, diabetes incidence was still 66% and only age at onset was delayed by 3–4 weeks. Thus, food diabetogens do not act only as "triggers" of the diabetes process but require a certain susceptibility, dose, and duration of exposure to induce diabetes.

Further indirect evidence suggests that the protein source is important. Add-back studies aimed at identifying which diet modifications increased the diabetes incidence of the protective diets indicated the following modifications of carbohydrate, fat and fiber composition did not increase diabetes frequency: corn starch changed to lactose[95], sucrose[95] or fructose, increasing the amount of corn oil from 5 to 15% or changing the fat source altogether from corn oil to 15% lard, 15% menhaden fish oil[90] or 15% safflower oil,[90] or increasing the amount of fiber from 5 to 19% by adding wheat bran[96].

Further extensive add-back studies suggested that modification of the protein source (many with heterogeneous protein) was the key to the dietary modification of diabetes in the BB rat[89,95–98]. When all the major components of the NIH-07 diet were assayed for diabetes-inducing potential, wheat gluten and various soy preparations were found to be major diabetogens (45–50% incidence individually, but not additive) and skim milk powder was a mild and highly variable diabetogen[94]. More recent studies used large amounts of wheat and soy fractions either as sole sources, supplemented with amino acids or as add-backs to casein or hydrolyzed casein diets. These indicate the wheat diabetogen(s) may be a low molecular weight glutenin protein whose diabetogenic activity is changed depending on reducing or oxidizing treatments. The soy diabetogenic activity is decreased by papain hydrolysis, only marginally affected by ethanol extraction, generally heat stable, and seems *not* to be related to the Kunitz protease inhibitor and therefore could be a heat stable protein unrelated to ethanol-extractable phytoestrogens.

A diet high in alfalfa seeds, which contain the systemic lupus erythematosus (SLE)-linked amino acid canavanine, resulted in a diabetes incidence of 33%. Certain other protein sources are non-diabetogenic when fed in semi-purified diets: fish meal, rapeseed flour, lactalbumin, hydrolyzed lactalbumin, kidney beans, peanut meal, ground corn[93]. Thus, the focus in studies of the BBdp rat has been mainly on food protein sources and chemically treated food fractions.

Fish Oil and Essential Fatty Acid (EFA) Deficiency

Others have tried to decrease the diabetogenic effect of plant-based laboratory diets by treating BBdp rats with fish oil. In one report (Paul *et al.* 1990), there was no effect of oral dosing with fish oil on diabetes incidence. Another group reported a significantly lower diabetes incidence (17%) in animals fed a supplemented diet between 50 and 120 days where 15% of calories were from fish oil (Woehrle *et al.* 1989). The dose of fish oil was ~30 mg day^{-1} in the former and ~900 mg day^{-1} in the latter study. These studies suggest that to have an effect, fish oil *n*-3 fatty acids must be ingested in large amounts not usually taken in the diet.

In another study[82], where a casein-based semi-purified diet deficient in essential fatty acids (EFA) was fed to BBdp rats, a protective effect was observed with only 12 of 41 rats becoming diabetic compared to 29 of 40 fed a Purina Chow®5001 diet. Repletion with linoleate three times per week, resulted in diabetes incidence that was intermediate and not significantly different from either the EFA-deficient (casein-fed) group or the Purina Chow®-fed group.

Cow's Milk Proteins

Considerable interest has been raised by the suggestion that human Type 1 diabetes is related to components of bovine milk. The incidence of diabetes associated with cow's milk whey protein sources is variable in the BB rat. Casein is the major protein fraction of cow's milk, making up ~80% of total protein and consisting mainly of α_{s1}, κ, β, γ-caseins. A recent preliminary report from Bibby and Elliott (1993) and colleagues indicated that a β-casein fraction, fed in a basal diet of soy protein isolate-containing infant formula increased diabetes incidence in a low incidence line of NOD mouse. As noted, casein is not diabetogenic in the BBdp rat. One current controversial hypothesis that bovine serum albumin (BSA) causes diabetes was based in part on the early studies of Elliott and Martin[92] and Daneman *et al.*[94]. Dosch and colleagues (1992) have suggested that a 17 amino acid portion of the BSA molecule, ABBOS, was similar to a β-cell molecule, ICA69. It was postulated that this similarity might permit cross-reactive BSA antibodies to interact in some way with the target β cell. However, we have found that the diabetogenicity of different whey protein materials varies considerably and there was no relationship between daily dose of BSA in the diet and BB rat diabetes frequency[93]. Although there were BSA antibodies present in some BBdp rats fed large amounts of milk proteins, their presence or level did not predict which animals became diabetic. This is similar to earlier findings in the NOD mouse (Leiter, 1990) and is supported by another study in the NOD mouse showing no correlation between disease onset and BSA antibody level (Petersen *et al.* 1994). Previous studies also indicated that a lactalbumin diet was not diabetogenic when fed to BBdp rats[95]. Therefore, it appears that cow's milk preparations such as skim milk powder are *sometimes* mildly diabetogenic but there is great variation from batch to batch and the diabetogenicity is unlikely to be associated with commercial casein, lactalbumin or bovine serum albumin.

INFECTIOUS AGENTS

The idea that infectious agents, particularly viruses, might *cause* diabetes has been a focus of much speculation and research. There is evidence that congenital rubella syndrome is associated with diabetes in humans and coxsackie B4 virus injection into susceptible SJL/J mice and Patas monkeys can result in diabetes. Rossini and colleagues (1979) first looked at infectious agents in BBdp rat diabetes by raising 12 germ-free BB rats, 3 of which became diabetic. Like *et al.* (1991) reported that cesarean derivation of BBdp rats into an environment free of selected viruses, *increased* the rate of appearance and frequency of diabetes, further suggesting that infectious agents are not a prerequisite. Vertical transmission of virus is thought not to occur in rats although this may be the case in NOD mice (Suenaga and Yoon, 1988). Virus infection of DR-BB but not BBdp rats causes diabetes. This was one outcome of investigation of epidemics in the diabetes-resistant BB rat line in the colony at Worcester, Massachusetts (Thomas *et al.* 1991; Like *et al.* 1991; Guberski *et al.* 1991). Injection of young DR-BB rats with a parvovirus, Kilham's rat virus (KRV), produced diabetes and insulitis in 61% of animals without affecting the levels of CD4+ and CD8+ lymphocytes (Guberski *et al.* 1991). This effect appears to be specific to KRV and involves infection of lymphoid tissues but not the target β cells (as in previous models of virus-induced diabetes). The mechanism of KRV-induced DR-BB diabetes is not clear but several have been suggested: antigen mimicry involving cross-reactivity between KRV and β cells, compromised immunoregulation, altered vascular permeability in the pancreas, or an increased anti-viral response producing cytokines that might trigger resident autoreactive cells. In BBdp rats, diabetes is not normally induced by KRV unless the animals are reconstituted with concanavalin-A-activated spleen cells from DR-BB rats. Polyinosinic poly-cytidilic acid (poly I:C), which induces IFN-α similar to viral infections, rapidly induces diabetes in young BBdp and DR-BB rats in a dose-dependent manner (Sobel *et al.* 1994). The fact that this occurs in both BBdp and DR-BB rats suggests that the KRV infection may act in a different manner.

Diabetes expression is not only increased by viruses and poly I:C; prevention of diabetes by viruses or bacterial products has also been reported. Raising BBdp rats and NOD mice in an ultra-clean environment increases diabetes incidence (Leiter 1990; Singh and Rabinovitch 1993; Rabinovitch 1994). This is consistent with the finding that injection with a lymphocytic choriomeningitis virus (LCMV), clone 13, prevented insulitis and diabetes in BBdp rats[99] and NOD mice (Oldstone 1988). This virus infects a subpopulation of lymphocytes and may enhance production of suppressor cells or inhibit lymphocytes required for the β-cell destructive process. Thus, infection of lymphocytes can both protect from or promote development of diabetes depending on the strain of virus (e.g. LCMV compared with KRV) and the status of the immune system of the susceptible host (e.g. DR-BB compared with BBdp). Injection of other viruses such as encephalomyocarditis virus, lactate dehydrogenase virus and mouse hepatitis virus also protects NOD mice from developing diabetes.

Complete Freund's adjuvant[100] (containing *Mycobacterium tuberculosis*), given as one injection before age 28 days, and OK432[101] (a *Streptococcus pyogenes* A3 preparation), injected weekly from 5 to 20 weeks of age inhibit insulitis and diabetes development in BB rats. Similar effects are seen in the NOD mouse, in which other agents such as the fungal polypeptide, LZ-8, and BCG (containing *Mycobacterium bovis*) also prevent or delay insulitis and diabetes (Singh and Rabinovitch 1993; Rabinovitch 1994). These microbial agents are immunostimulants and may be promoting expansion of natural suppressor T cells, or affecting the distribution of Th1/Th2 lymphocytes, as well as cytokine secretion and action. The fact that an ultra-clean environment actually increases diabetes frequency suggests that environmental immuno-stimulation is required for normal immune function. This apparent contra-diction, that both immunosuppressive and immunostimulatory regimes can inhibit diabetes was addressed recently by Rabinovitch (1994). He proposed that microbial extracts as well as relevant autoantigens such as GAD up-regulate a Th2 lymphocyte subset and secretion of associated cytokines, IL-4 and IL-10. These cytokines would in turn down-regulate diabetes-including Th1 subsets of lymphocytes and their associated cytokine products, IFN-γ and IL-2. This hypothesis is based mainly on data from the NOD mouse and although some evidence supports a similar concept, it is not clear yet if such a mechanism will apply in the BBdp and DR-BB rats.

STRESS

The role of stress was investigated by Carter *et al.* (1987), who found that various combined stressors such as immobilization for 1 hour three times per week, physically rotating the cage, crowding or randomly reassigning animals to different groups significantly decreased the age of onset but had no effect on final diabetes incidence. As the relationship between neurochemical, endocrine and immune networks becomes better understood, the role of stress in diabetes pathogenesis may yet be found to be important, and may have preventive implications as well.

CONCLUSION

The BB rat literature has a very substantial proportion of its content addressed to trials of prevention of the diabetic syndrome. At least two approaches used first in the BB rat have been tested or are currently undergoing trials in human subjects—cyclosporine at onset of diabetes and prophylactic insulin given to high risk individuals. Many of the other successful interventions reported in the rat cannot be tested in the human for the present. Others lack specificity, or would require drugs (such as antibodies) that would have to be appropriate to accommodate to the species differences. The other major problem in carrying animal findings forward to clinical trials is that certain interventions are already known to work either in the BBdp or DR-BB rat or in the NOD mouse or the BB rat, but not in both. An example of the latter is nicotinamide. For the present, one cannot rely on there being a greater likelihood of analogies between one or other BB model or species of rodent, and the human.

There is no simple unifying message that can be derived from the study of successful and unsuccessful animal trials, except that they underscore the multifactorial nature of the syndromes. This was very nicely summarized, albeit in a broader context, in the report of a recent meeting that addressed the fundamental question of whether Type 1 diabetes is caused by an autoimmune and/or an inflammatory process[102]. There is a huge advantage to animal studies in that large numbers of whole litters of animals can be studied and thoroughly "dissected" at the end, to unravel the effects of the primary process and the interventions. Clearly a dynamic equilibrium between the "beta-cytotoxic" and "protective" forces exists, that has yet to be well characterized in terms of what causes it to tilt in the direction of producing disease versus remaining quiescent or subclinical. What is impressive is the vast array of interventions that alters this balance in the BB rat. What remains for future investigations is the challenge of determining the key element of each intervention that tips the balance. In so doing, not only can single-drug treatments be refined, but ingenious combinations can be tested in a setting in which each is given at dose levels shown to be as safe as can be determined experimentally (and without interactions). This approach could well lead to clinical trials that can be applied to large groups of persons at risk for the disease.

REFERENCES

1 Laupacis A, Gardell C, Dupre J, Stiller CR, Keown P, Wallace AC, Thibert P. Cyclosporin prevents diabetes in BB Wistar rats. *Lancet* 1983; **1:** 10–12.
2 Nakhooda AF, Like AA, Chappel CI, Murray FT, Marliss EB. The spontaneously diabetic Wistar rat. Metabolic and morphologic studies. *Diabetes* 1977; **26:** 100–12
3 Marliss EB, Nakhooda AF, Poussier P, Sima AAF. The diabetic syndrome of the 'BB' Wistar rat: possible relevance to type I (insulin-dependent) diabetes in man. *Diabetologia* 1982; **22:** 225–32.
4 Marliss EB, Yale J-F. Immunomodulatory interventions in spontaneous rodent Type I diabetes mellitus. Relevance to the human. In Proceedings of the 13th Congress of the International Diabetes Federation. Excerpta Medica International Congress Series No. 800, 1989, pp 427–30.

5 Mordes J, Handler ES, Burstein D *et al*. Immunotherapy of the BB rat. In Eisenbarth GS (ed), *Immunotherapy of Diabetes and Selected Autoimmune Diseases*. Boca Raton: CRC Press, Inc, 1989, pp 36–52.

6 Wu G, Field CJ, Marliss EB. Immunocyte metabolism and its alterations in the spontaneous autoimmune diabetes syndrome of the BB rat. In Shafrir E (ed), *Lessons from Animal Diabetes*, Vol V. London: Smith Gordon, 1994, pp 49–58.

7 Stiller CR, Laupacis A, Keown PA, Gardell C, Dupre J, Thibert P, Wall W. Cyclosporine: action, pharmacokinetics, and effect in the BB rat model. *Metab Clin Exp* 1983; 32(Suppl 1): 69–72.

8 Jaworski MA, Honore L, Jewell LD, Mehta JG, McGuire-Clark P, Schouls JJ, Yap WJ. Cyclosporin prophylaxis induces long-term prevention of diabetes and inhibits lymphocytic infiltration in multiple target tissues in high-risk BB rat. *Diabetes Res* 1986; 3: 1–6.

9 Bone AJ, Walker R, Varey AM, Cooke A, Baird J. Effect of cyclosporin on pancreatic events and development of diabetes in BB/Edinburgh rats. *Diabetes* 1990; 39: 508–14.

10 Yale J-F, Grose M, Seemayer TA, Marliss EB. Immunological and metabolic concomitants of cyclosporin prevention of diabetes in BB rats. *Diabetes* 1987; 36: 749–57.

11 Baquerizo H, Leone J, Perkel C, Wood P, Rabinovitch D. Mechanisms of cyclosporine protection against spontaneous diabetes mellitus in the BB/WOR rat. *J Autoimmun* 1989; 2: 133–50.

12 Kiesel U, Maruta K, Treichel U, Bicker U, Kolb H. Suppression of spontaneous insulin-dependent diabetes in BB rats by administration of Ciamexone. *J Immunopharmacol* 1986; 8(3): 393–406.

13 Brayman KL, Armstrong J, Barker CF, Naji A. Intermittent cyclosporine administration and prevention of diabetes in the BB rat. *Transpl Proc* 1986; 18: 1545–7.

14 Brayman KL, Armstrong J, Shaw LM, Rosano TG, Tomaswewski JE, Barker CF, Naji A. Prevention of diabetes in BB rats by intermittent administration of cyclosporine. *Surgery* 1987; 102: 235–41.

15 Jaworski MA, Jewell LD, Honore L, Mehta JG, Bayens-Simmonds J, McGuire-Clark P, Schouls JJ, Yap WY. Immunosuppression in autoimmune disease: the double-edged sword. *Clin & Invest Med* 1987; 10: 488–95.

16 Like AA, Dirodi V, Thomas S, Guberski DL, Rossini AA. Prevention of diabetes mellitus in the BB/W rat with cyclosporine-A. *Am J Pathol* 1984; 117: 92–7.

17 Mahon JL, Gunn HC, Stobie K, Gibson C, Garcia B, Dupre J, Stiller CR. The effect of bromocriptine and cyclosporine on spontaneous diabetes in BB rats. *Transpl Proc* 1988; 20: 197–200.

18 Rabinovitch A, Sumoski WL. Theophylline protects against diabetes in BB rats and potentiates cyclosporine protection. *Diabetologia* 1990; 33: 506–8.

19 Yale J-F, Grose M, Roy RD, Seemayer TA, Marliss EB. Response to cyclosporine administration at onset of diabetes in BB rats. *Diabetes Res* 1987; 5: 129–33.

20 Yale JF. Cyclosporine A for prevention and therapy of Type I diabetes in the BB rat. In Shafir E, Renolds AE (ed), *Frontiers in Diabetes Research. Lessons from Animal Diabetes II*, 1988, pp 145–8.

21 Yale J-F, Roy D, Grose M, Seemayer TA, Murphy GF, Marliss EB. Effects of cyclosporine on glucose tolerance in the rat. *Diabetes* 1985; 34: 1309–13.

22 Yale J-F, Chamelian M, Courchesne S, Vigeant C. Peripheral resistance and decreased insulin secretion after Cyclosporine A treatment. *Transpl Proc* 1988; 20: 985–8.

23 Murase N, Lieberman I, Nalesnik MA, Mintz DH, Todo S, Drash AL, Starzl TE. Effect of FK 506 on spontaneous diabetes in BB rats. *Diabetes* 1990; 39: 1584–6.

24 Murase N, Lieberman I, Nalesnik M, Todo S, Drash AL, Starzi TE. FK 506 prevents spontaneous diabetes in the BB rat. *Transpl Proc* 1991; **23**(1): 551–5.

25 Nicoletti F, Meroni PL, Barcellini W, Grasso S, Borghi MO, Lunetta M, Di Marco R, Stepani S, Mughini L. FK-506 prevents diabetes in diabetes-prone BB/Wor rats. *Int J Immunopharmac* 1991; **13**: 1027–30.

26 Hao L, Wang Y, Chan SM, Lafferty KJ. Effect of mycophenolate mofetil on islet allografting to chemically induced or spontaneously diabetic animals. *Transpl Proc* 1992; **24**: 2843–4.

27 Von Specht BU, Debelius A, Konigsberger H, Lodde G, Roth H, Permanetter W. Prolongation of islet and pancreas graft survival in spontaneous diabetic BB/W rats by perioperative cyclosporin or 15-deoxyspergualin therapy. *Transpl Proc* 1989; **21**: 965–7.

28 Rossini AA, Slavin S, Woda BA, Geisberg M, Like AA, Mordes JP. Total lymphoid irradiation prevents diabetes mellitus in the Bio-Breeding/Worcester (BB/W) rat. *Diabetes* 1984 **36**: 543–7.

29 Handler ES, Mordes JP, McKeever U *et al*. Effects of irradiation on diabetes in the BB/Wor rat. *Autoimmunity* 1989; **4**: 21–30.

30 Like AA, Rossini AA, Guberski DL, Appel MC. Spontaneous diabetes mellitus reversal and prevention in the BB/W rat with antiserum to rat lymphocytes. *Science* 1979; **206**: 1421–3.

31 Like AA, Anthony M, Guberski DL, Rossini AA. Spontaneous diabetes mellitus in the BB/W rat. Effects of glucocorticoids, cyclosporin-A, and antiserum to rat lymphocytes. *Diabetes* 1983; **32**: 326–30.

32 Like AA, Biron CA, Weringer EJ, Byman K, Sroczynski E, Guberski L. Prevention of diabetes in Biobreeding/Worcester rats with monoclonal antibodies that recognize T lymphocytes or natural killer cells. *J Exp Med* 1986; **164**: 1145–59.

33 Barlow AK, Like AA. Anti-CD2 monoclonal antibodies prevent spontaneous and adoptive transfer of diabetes in the BB/Wor rat. *Am J Pathol* 1992; **141**: 1043–51.

34 Ellerman K, Wrobleski M, Rabinovitch A, Like A. Natural killer cell depletion and diabetes mellitus in the BB/Wor rat (revisited). *Diabetologia* 1993; **36**: 596–601.

35 Markmann JF, Jacobson JD, Kimura H, Brayman KL, Barker CF, Naji A. Prevention of autoimmune damage to islet grafts in BB rats by antibody therapy. *Transpl. Proc.* 1989; **21**: 2703.

36 Jacobson JD, Markmann JF, Brayman KL, Barker CF, Naji A. Prevention of recurrent autoimmune diabetes in BB rats by anti- asialo-GM$_1$ antibody. *Diabetes* 1988; **37**: 838–41.

37 Nicoletti F, Meroni PL, Landolfo S, Gariglio M, Guzzardi S, Barcellini W, Lunetta M, Mughini L, Zanussi C. Prevention of diabetes in BB/Wor rats treated with monoclonal antibodies to interferon-gamma. *Lancet* 1990; **336**: 319.

38 Hahn HJ, Lucke S, Kloting I, Volk HD, Baehr RV, Diamanstein T. Curing BB rats of freshly manifested diabetes by short-term treatment with a combination of a monoclonal anti-interleukin 2 receptor antibody and a subtherapeutic dose of cyclosporin A. *Eur J Immunol* 1987; **17**: 1075–8.

39 Hahn HJ, Kuttler B, Kloting I, Dunger A, Besch W, Diamanstein T. Extended survival of MHC-identical allogeneic islet grafts in diabetic BB rats—the effect of an interleukin 2 receptor-targeted immunotherapy. *Transplantation* 1992; **54**: 555–8.

40 Vertrees S, Wilson CA, Ubungen R, Wilson D, Baskin DG, Toivola B, Jacobs C, Boiani N, Baker P, Lernmark A. Interleukin-1β regulation of islet and thyroid autoimmunity in the BB rat. *J Autoimmun* 1991; **4**: 717–32.

41 Kolb H, Zielasek J, Treichel V, Freytag G, Wrann M, Kiesel U. Recombinant

interleukin 2 enhances spontaneous insulin- dependent diabetes in BB rats. *Eur J Immunol* 1986; **16**: 209–12.

42 Zielasek J, Burkart VS, Naylor P, Goldstein A, Kiesal U, Kolb H. Interleukin-2-dependent control of disease development in spontaneously diabetic BB rats. *Immunology* 1990; **69**: 209–14.

43 Satoh J, Seino H, Shintani S, Tanaka S, Ohteki T, Masuda T, Nobunaga T, Toyota T. Inhibition of type 1 diabetes in BB rats with recombinant human tumor necrosis factor-alpha. *J Immunol* 1990; **145**: 1395–9.

44 Takahashi K, Satoh J, Seino H, Shu XP, Sagara M, Masuda T, Toyota T. Prevention of type 1 diabetes with lymphotoxin in BB rats. *Clin Immun Immunopathol* 1993; **69**: 318–23.

45 Oschilewski U, Kiesel U, Kolb H. Administration of silica prevents diabetes in BB rats. *Diabetes* 1985; **34**: 197–9.

46 Kiesel U, Oschilewski M, Kantwerk G, Marutra M, Hanenberg H, Treichel U, Kolb-Bachofen V, Hartung HP, Kolb H. Essential role of macrophages in the development of type I diabetes in BB rats. *Transpl Proc* 1986; **18**: 1525–7.

47 Lee KU, Pak CY, Amano K, Yoon JW. Prevention of lymphocytic thyroiditis and insulitis in diabetes-prone BB rats by the depletion of macrophages. *Diabetologia* 1988; **31**: 400–2.

48 Like AA, Kislauskis E, Williams RM, Rossini AA. Neonatal thymectomy prevents spontaneous diabetes mellitus in the BB/W rat. *Science* 1982; **216**: 644–6.

49 Misra M, Marliss EB. Prevention of diabetes in the spontaneously diabetic BB rat by the glutamine antimetabolite acivicin. *Can J Physiol Pharmacol* 1996; **74**, in press.

50 Thliveris JA, Begleiter A, Kobrinsky NL, Verburg L, Dean HJ, Johnston JB. Prevention of insulin-dependent diabetes mellitus by 2'-deoxycoformycin in the BB Wistar rat. *Biochem Pharmacol* 1993; **46**: 1071–5.

51 Naji A, Silvers WK, Bellgrau D, Barker CF. Spontaneous diabetes in rats: destruction of islets is prevented by immunological tolerance. *Science* 1986; **213**: 1390–2.

52 Naji A, Silvers WK, Bellgrau D, Anderson AO, Plotkin S, Barker CF. Prevention of diabetes in rats by bone marrow transplantation. *Ann Surg* 1981; **194**: 328–38.

53 Naji A, Silvers WK, Kimura H, Anderson AO, Barker CF. Influence of islets and bone marrow transplantation on the diabetes and immunodefiency of BB rats. *Metab Clin Exp* 1983; **32** (Suppl 1): 62–9.

54 Naji A, Silvers WK, Barker CF. Bone marrow transplantation in adult diabetes-prone rats. *Surgical Forum* 1983; **34**: 374–6.

55 Nakano K, Mordes JP, Handler ES, Greiner DL, Rossini AA. Role of host immune system in BB/Wor rat. Predisposition to diabetes resides in bone marrow. *Diabetes* 1988; **37**: 520–5.

56 Rossini AA, Mordes JP, Pelletier AM, Like AA. Transfusion of whole blood prevents spontaneous diabetes mellitus in the BB/W rat. *Science* 1983; **219**: 975–7.

57 Rossini AA, Faustman D, Woda BA, Like AA, Szymanski I, Mordes JP. Lymphocyte transfusions prevent diabetes in the Bio Breeding/Worcester rat. *J Clin Invest* 1984; **74**: 39–46.

58 Burstein D, Mordes JP, Greiner DL, Stein D, Nakaruma N, Handler ES, Rossini AA. Prevention of diabetes in BB/Wor rat by single transfusion of spleen cells parameters that affect degree of protection. *Diabetes* 1989; **38**: 24–30.

59 Mordes JP, Gallina DL, Handler ES, Greiner DL, Nakamura N, Pelletier A, Rossini AA. Transfusions enriched for W3/25+ helper/inducer T lymphocytes prevent spontaneous diabetes in the BB/W rat. *Diabetologia* 1987; **30**: 22–6.

60 Logothetopoulos J, Shumak K, Bailey D. Prevention of spontaneous but not of

adoptively transferred diabetes by injection of neonatal BB/Hooded Hybrid rats with splenocytes or concanavalin A blasts from diabetes-free strains. *Diabetes* 1988; **37**: 1009–14.

61 Kuttler B, Dunger A, Volk HD, Diamanstein T, Hahn HJ. Prevention and suppression of autoimmune pancreatic beta-cell destruction in BB rats by syngeneic lymphocytes obtained from long-term normoglycaemic donors. *Diabetologia* 1991; **34**: 74–7.

62 Georgiou HM, Bellgrau D. Thymus transplantation and disease prevention in the diabetes-prone biobreeding rat. *J Immunol* 1989; **142**: 3400–5.

63 Posselt AM, Barker CF, Friedman AL, Naji A. Prevention of autoimmune diabetes in the BB rat by intrathymic islet transplantation at birth. *Science* 1992; **256**: 1321–4.

64 Posselt AM, Barker CF, Friedman AL, Koeberlein B, Tomaszewski JE, Naji A. Intrathymic inoculation of islets at birth prevents autoimmune diabetes and pancreatic insulitis in the BB rat. *Transpl Proc* 1993; **25**: 301–2.

65 Koevary SB, Blomberg M. Prevention of diabetes in BB/Wor rats by intrathymic islet injection. *J Clin Invest* 1992; **89**: 512–16.

66 Brayman KL, Nakai I, Field MJ, Lloveras JJ, Jessurun J, Najarian JS, Sutherland DE. Evaluation of intrathymic islet transplantation in the prediabetic period. *Surgery* 1992; **112**: 319–26.

67 Battan R, Mordes JP, Abreau S, Greiner DL, Handler ES, Rossini AA. Evidence that intrathymic islet transplantation does not prevent diabetes or subsequent islet graft destruction in RT6-depleted, diabetes-resistant BioBreeding/Worcester rats. *Transplantation* 1994; **57**: 731–6.

68 Suzuki M, Negishi K, Itabashi A, Katayama S, Ishii J, Komeda K, Kawazu S. Effects of PGE1 on the development of diabetes and surface markers of lymphocytes in BB/W/Tky rats. *Diabetes Res Clin Exp* 1991; **18**: 95–9.

69 Lieberman I, Lentz DP, Trucco GA, Seow WK, Thong YH. Prevention of tetrandrine of spontaneous development of diabetes mellitus in BB rats. *Diabetes* 1992; **41**: 616–19.

70 Kida KI, Inoue T, Kaino Y, Goto Y, Ikeuchi M, Ito T, Matsuda H, Elliott RB. An immunopotentiator of beta-1,6;1,3 D-glucan prevents diabetes and insulitis in BB rats. *Diabetes Res Clin Prac* 1992; **17**: 75–9.

71 Rabinovitch A, Suarez WL, Qin HY, Power RF, Badger AM. Prevention of diabetes and induction of non-specific suppressor cell activity in the BB rat by an immunomodulatory azaspirane, SK&F 106610. *J Autoimmun* 1993; **6**: 39–49.

72 Gotfredsen CF, Buschard K, Frandsen EK. Reduction of diabetes incidence of BB Wistar rats by early prophylactic insulin treatment of diabetes-prone animals. *Diabetologia* 1985; **28**: 933–5.

73 Appel MC, O'Neil JJ. Prevention of spontaneous diabetes in the BB/W rat by insulin treatment. *Pancreas* 1986; **1**: 356–68.

74 Vlahos WD, Seemayer TA, Yale J-F. Diabetes prevention in BB rats by inhibition of endogenous insulin secretion. *Metabolism* 1991; **40**: 825–9.

75 Gottlieb PA, Handler ES, Appel MC, Greiner DL, Mordes JP, Rossini AA. Insulin treatment prevents diabetes mellitus but not thyroiditis in RT6-depleted diabetes resistant BB/W rats. *Diabetologia* 1991; **34**: 296–300.

76 Bertrand S, De Paepe M, Vigeant C, Yale J-F. Prevention of adoptive transfer in BB rats by prophylactic insulin treatment. *Diabetes* 1992; **41**: 1273–7.

77 Buschard K, Jorgensen M, Aaen K, Bock T, Josefsen N. Prevention of diabetes mellitus in BB rats by neonatal stimulation of B cells. *Lancet* 1990; **335**: 134–5.

78 Yale JF. Relationship between cytotoxicity against β-cells and insulin secretory activity of the target β-cells. In Shafrir E (ed), *Lessons from Animal Diabetes III*,

Lessons from Animal Diseases III. London: Smith-Gordon, 1990, pp 11–13.

79 Corbett JA, McDaniel ML. Does nitric oxide mediate autoimmune destruction of β-cells? *Diabetes* 1992; **41**: 897–903.

80 Behrens WA, Scott FW, Madere R, Trick K, Hanna K. Effects of dietary vitamin E on the vitamin E status in the BB rat during development and after the onset of diabetes. *Ann Nutr Metab* 1986; **30**: 157–65.

81 Drash AL, Rudert WA, Borquaye S, Wang R, Leiberman I. Effect of probucol on development of diabetes mellitus in BB rats. *Am J Cardiol* 1988; **62**: 27b–30b.

82 Lefkowith J, Schreiner G, Cormier J, Handler ES, Driscoll HK, Greiner D, Mordes JP, Rossini AA. Prevention of diabetes in the BB rat by essential fatty acid deficiency. Relationship between physiological and biochemical changes. *J Exp Med* 1990; **1**: 729–43.

83 Rossini AA, Mordes JP, Gallina DL, Like AA. Hormonal and environmental factors in the pathogenesis of BB rat diabetes. *Metabolism* 1983; **32** (Suppl 1): 33–6.

84 Flechner I, Maruta K, Burkart V, Kawai K, Kolb H, Kiesel U. Effects of radical scavengers on the development of experimental diabetes. *Diabetes Res Clin Exp* 1990; **13**: 67–73.

85 Murthy VK, Shipp JC, Hanson C, Shipp DM. Delayed onset and decreased incidence of diabetes in BB rats fed free radical scavengers. *Diabetes Res Clin Prac* 1992; **18**: 11–16.

86 Roza AM, Slakey DP, Pieper GM, Van Ye TM, Moore-Hilton G, Komorowski RA, Johnson CP, Hedlund BE, Adams MB. Hydroxyethyl starch deferoxamine, a novel iron chelator, delays diabetes in BB rats. *J Lab Clin Med* 1994; **123**: 556–60.

87 Wu G. Nitric oxide synthesis and the effect of aminoguanidine and N^G-monomethyl-L-arginine on the onset of diabetes in the spontaneously diabetic BB rat. *Diabetes* 1995; **44**: 360–4.

88 Lindsay RM, Smith W, Rossiter SP, McIntyre MA, Williams BC, Baird J. N^W-nitro-L-arginine methyl ester reduces the incidence of IDDM in BB/E rats. *Diabetes* 1995; **44**: 365–8.

89 Scott FW and Trick KD. Dietary modification of spontaneous diabetes in the BB Wistar rat. *Proc Can Fed Biol Soc* 1983; **26**: 222.

90 Issa-Chergui D, Guttmann RD, Seemayer TA, Kelley VE, Colle EC. The effect of diet on the spontaneous insulin-dependent diabetic syndrome in the rat. *Diabetes Res* 1988; **9**: 81–6.

91 Hoorfar J, Buschard K, Brogren C-H. Impact of dietary protein and fat source on the development of insulin-dependent diabetes in the BB rat. *Diabetes Res* 1992; **20**: 33–41.

92 Elliott RB, Martin JM. Dietary protein: a trigger of insulin-dependent diabetes in the BB rat? *Diabetologia* 1984; **26**: 297–9.

93 Scott FW. Food, diabetes and immunology. In Forse RA, Bell SJ, Blackburn GL, Kabbash LG (eds), *Diet, Nutrition and Immunity*. Boca Raton, FL: CRC Press, 1994, pp 71–92.

94 Daneman D, Fishman L, Clarson C, Martin JM. Dietary triggers of insulin-dependent diabetes in the BB rat. *Diabetes Res* 1987; **5**: 93–7.

95 Scott FW. Dietary initiators and modifiers of BBrat diabetes: a summary and working hypothesis. In: Shafrir E, Renold AE (eds), *Lessons From Animal Diabetes II.* 2nd International Workshop. London: John Libbey, 1988, pp 34–9.

96 Scott FW. Alterations in single diet constituents and diabetes expression in the BB rat. In Jaworski *et al.* (eds), *Immunology of Diabetes.* Amsterdam: Elsevier, 1986, pp 307–12.

97 Hoorfar J, Scott FW, Cloutier HE. Dietary plant materials and development of

diabetes in the BB rat. *J Nutr* 1991; **121**: 908–16.
98 Scott FW, Sarwar G, Cloutier HE. Diabetogenicity of various protein sources in the diet of the BB rat. In Camerini-Davalos RA, Cole HS (eds), *Prediabetes*. New York: Plenum, 1988, pp 277–85.
99 Dyrberg T, Schwimmbeck PL, Oldstone MBA. Inhibition of diabetes in BB rats by virus infection. *J Clin Invest* 1988; **81**: 928–31.
100 Sadelain MJW, Qin HY, Sumoski W, Parfrey N, Singh B, Rabinovitch A. Prevention of diabetes in the BB rat by early immunotherapy using Freund's adjuvant. *J Autoimmunity* 1990; **3**: 671–80.
101 Satoh J, Shintani S, Oya K, Tanaka S-I, Nobunaga T, Toyota T, Goto Y. Treatment with streptococcal preparation (OK432) suppresses anti-islet autoimmunity and prevents diabetes in BB rats. *Diabetes* 1988; **37**: 1188–94.
102 Kolb H, Kolb-Bachofen V, Roep BO. Autoimmune versus inflammatory type 1 diabetes: a controversy? *Immunol Today* 1995; **16**: 170–2.

20

Lessons from Animal Models: NOD Mouse

AKIRA SHIMADA, BRETT CHARLTON and C. GARRISON FATHMAN

Department of Medicine, Division of Immunology and Rheumatology, Stanford University School of Medicine, Stanford, California, USA

INTRODUCTION

The non-obese diabetic (NOD) mouse is an excellent model of insulin-dependent diabetes mellitus (IDDM) and shows many of the characteristics of human IDDM[1]. In NOD murine diabetes, lymphocytic infiltration into the pancreatic islets, termed insulitis, can be detected by 4–5 weeks of age, and is pronounced by 8 weeks of age. Overt diabetes, however, does not usually occur until after 12–15 weeks of age. Unlike human IDDM the incidence of diabetes differs between females and males—females have a higher incidence than males[1]. The incidence of diabetes is also colony dependent. T lymphocytes[2–7] and macrophages[8–13] are considered to be involved in the disease process. Although many autoantibodies, such as anti-islet cell antibodies (ICAs)[14], insulin autoantibodies (IAAs)[15], anti-heat shock protein antibodies[16] and others, can be detected in NOD serum, it appears that autoantibodies themselves are neither necessary nor sufficient for β-cell destruction[17].

In comparison to human IDDM, animal models of diabetes afford the opportunity to study a wide variety of preventive agents and strategies. These range from highly specific synthesized molecules to simple changes in diet. In this chapter, we will assign preventive therapies into the following categories:

Prediction, Prevention and Genetic Counseling in IDDM. Edited by Jerry P. Palmer.
© 1996 John Wiley & Sons Ltd.

1. Antibodies
2. Cytokines
3. Islet antigen specific
4. Antigen non-specific
5. Cell transfer
6. Genomic alteration—transgenes, gene knockout
7. Drug treatment
8. Environmental agents—virus diet.

ANTIBODIES

Immunohistochemical analysis of the pancreatic islets in NOD mice showed large numbers of T lymphocytes, and in particular those of the Lyt-1+ or L3T4 (CD4)+ subsets, in the islets. Based upon these findings, several groups used anti-CD4 antibodies to prevent diabetes in NOD mice. Continuous administration of a depleting anti-CD4 antibody from the age of 4 weeks to 6 months prevented the occurrence of insulitis and subsequent diabetes[18]. However, in another study, after stopping anti-CD4 treatment insulitis recurred in the treated mice, suggesting that anti-CD4 monoclonal antibody treatment does not induce an islet antigen tolerant state[19]. Although insulitis did recur after cessation of anti-CD4 antibody treatment, the subsequent development of diabetes was shown to be prevented suggesting a tolerance at the post-insulitis stage[2]. Short-term anti-CD4 antibody treatment has subsequently been shown to have a similar effect[20]. The mechanism by which anti-CD4 prevents the progression from insulitis to diabetes remains unknown but it is perhaps related to the generation of a disease suppressing cell population(s). Anti-L3T4 (anti-CD4) monoclonal antibody treatment for the first 6 months after birth reduced diabetes but did not prevent the accumulation of autoreactive cells since cyclophosphamide (CY) injection precipitated diabetes[21]. Also, transfer of splenocytes from short-term anti-L3T4 monoclonal-antibody-treated mice prevented CY-induced diabetes in diabetic cell co-transferred mice, suggesting that the "tolerance" induced by the treatment might not be due to clonal deletion but rather to suppressor cells[20].

CD8+ cells are also present in the insulitis lesion and the transfer of the diabetes requires transfer of both CD4+ and CD8+T cells suggesting that antibodies against CD8 might also prevent diabetes[22]. Anti-CD8 antibodies were able to prevent the development of diabetes after CY administration suggesting that CD8+ cells are necessary for the progression from insulitis to diabetes[9,23]. However, anti-CD8 antibodies did not prevent the recurrence of disease in islets transplanted to diabetic NOD mice which indicates disease might be CD8+ cell independent once diabetes is established[24].

Because of the obvious requirement for T cells in disease, there are several other T-cell-specific antibodies which could also prevent diabetes. The administration of anti-lymphocyte serum to recently diabetic NOD mice reversed diabetes and the effect was long term [25]. Treatment of NOD neonates with anti-CD3 monoclonal antibodies reduced the incidence of diabetes in NOD mice[26]. This protection seemed to be dependent on the age at antibody treatment because the protective effect was observed with treatment at 1 week but not 3 weeks of age. It has now been established that anti-CD3 treatment in older mice can prevent diabetes indefinitely after short-term treatment and further treatment of recently diabetic mice can reverse the disease indefinitely[27]. The current clinical use of anti-CD3 antibodies suggests an immediate opportunity for the treatment of recent-onset IDDM patients.

Administration of monoclonal antibody to the α/β dimer of the T-cell receptor for antigen also suggested potential clinical application. An efficient and durable reversal of recent-onset diabetes in treated NOD mice was observed when the anti-α/β TCR antibodies were injected within 1 week of the development of IDDM[28].

Monoclonal antibody treatment to the $V\beta$ region of the T-cell receptor was also attempted in NOD mice. Anti-$V\beta8$ monoclonal antibody treatment reduced the incidence of diabetes after CY treatment in NOD mice[29]. T-cell vaccination with $V\beta8+$ CD4+T cells isolated from diabetic splenocytes and activated by surface-immobilized anti-$V\beta8$ monoclonal antibodies suppressed adoptive transfer of diabetes to young NOD mice[30]. Because of practical concerns about inducing long-term pan-T-lymphocyte inactivation for prevention of IDDM in humans, selective suppression of specific diabetogenic T-cell populations is ideal. However, it is still not clear if such a specific population can be identified on the basis of TCR $V\beta$ usage.

T lymphocytes do not act to cause diabetes in isolation from other cells in particular antigen-presenting cells and so these might also be targets for antibody-mediated disease prevention. Treatment with anti-class II antibodies specific for the NOD I-A antigen prevented the spontaneous development of IDDM in NOD mice and the protection was transferable using CD4+T cells[31,32]. The fact that protection from diabetes was transferable suggests that treatment not only prevented activation of autoreactive cells but facilitated the generation of a suppressive population.

Anti-MHC class I (K^d) monoclonal antibody treatment in CY-treated male or untreated female NOD mice also reduced the incidence of diabetes[23]. This effect was not simply due to significant reduction of T cells in the treated mice since the T-lymphocyte subset numbers and response to concanavalin A (Con A) was normal. Anti-D^b antibody treatment had no effect which localized the class restricting element to K^d only.

The monoclonal antibody 5C6 is specific for the myelomonocytic adhesion-promoting type 3 complement receptor (CR3) found on macrophages and granulocytes. Blockade of macrophage CR3 *in vivo* prevented intra-islet infiltration by both macrophages and T cells, and inhibited the development of IDDM in NOD mice[13]. This confirmed earlier studies which showed that interference with macrophage function by silica treatment could prevent diabetes[9,10].

Administration of anti-asialo GM1 antibody, which mainly reacts with natural killer cells, prevented the onset of diabetes in CY-injected NOD mice[33]. The role of NK cells, however, is unclear as NK cell function in mice is reported to be very poor.

CYTOKINES

Immune responses involve the interactions of numerous cells and the generation of a multitude of cytokines. These cytokines may be both requisite for disease and useful in the regulation of disease and so are obvious therapeutic targets in the prevention of diabetes. Monoclonal antibody treatment against several cytokines has been assessed in the NOD mouse. Anti-interferon-γ (IFN-γ) monoclonal antibodies prevented the induction of IDDM by CY as well as the adoptive transfer of diabetes by splenocytes from diabetic NOD mice[34,35]. Similarly, the use of anti-IL-6 antibodies prevented CY-induced diabetes[35]. Thus, monoclonal antibody treatment against certain cytokines is effective in preventing IDDM in NOD mice.

Other preventive strategies have employed administration of cytokines themselves. This approach is based upon the speculation that IDDM in NOD mice may involve immune dysregulation resulting from cytokine deficiencies. Long-term treatment with recombinant TNF-α caused a significant reduction in the lymphocytic infiltration and blocked spontaneous diabetes mellitus in NOD mice[36]. Moreover, TNF-α was able to suppress the induction of diabetes in adoptive transfer of lymphocytes from diabetic mice to young non-diabetic mice[36]. Lymphotoxin (TNF-β), which is structurally and functionally related to TNF-α, also prevented IDDM in NOD mice[37].

Treatment with low levels of exogenous interleukin 1 α(IL-1α) for 22 weeks prevented occurrence of insulitis and diabetes in NOD mice during and at least 33 weeks after cessation of the treatment[38]. Even after islet-cell destruction, IL-1α injections in diabetic NOD mice normalized plasma glucose levels when administered in combination with insulin.

Based on speculation that suppressive mechanisms in NOD mice were dysfunctional, Serreze et al. tried to prevent IDDM in NOD mice by injecting IL-2. They injected human recombinant IL-2 (twice weekly) beginning at 6 weeks of age until 20 weeks of age and the treatment suppressed the onset of diabetes[39]. Moreover, treatment of mice with poly I:C, an inducer of IFN-α/β, in conjunction with IL-2 was even more effective in preventing IDDM[39]. However, cessation of the treatment resulted in increased severity of insulitis. They observed increased transcription of IL-1 mRNA in peritoneal macrophages and increased lipopolysaccharide-stimulated IL-1 secretion in IL-2 treated mice. IL-4 secretion by thymocytes from NOD mice was found to be subnormal after treatment with either anti-T-cell receptor α/β, anti-CD3, or Con A compared with thymocytes from control mice. This observation prompted a study of *in vivo* administration of IL-4 into pre-diabetic NOD mice; the treatment also protected the onset of diabetes[40]. Most recently, one group showed that daily subcutaneous administration of IL-10, a known potent inhibitor of IFN-γ production by TH1 T cells, also delayed the onset of diabetes and significantly reduced the incidence of diabetes in this model[41]. However, localized production of IL-10 by islet β cells accelerated the onset and increased the prevalence of diabetes in NOD mice[42], so this issue remains controversial. Thus, administration of certain cytokines such as TNF-α, IL-1, IL-2, and IL-4 can also prevent IDDM in NOD mice. The effect is presumed to result from the activation of disease regulating pathways which are otherwise ineffective in NOD mice.

ISLET ANTIGEN SPECIFIC

The ideal immunotherapy for IDDM would be a precise antigen or even antigenic epitope specific form of immune unresponsiveness—a therapy which might leave the rest of the immune system intact. There are several antigens which are considered to be candidates for islet antigen specific therapy in IDDM. For instance, the two isoforms of glutamic acid decarboxylase (GAD; GAD-65 and GAD-67)[43],[44], insulin[45,46], heat shock protein[16,47,48], gangliosides[49], peripherin[50], carboxypeptidase H[51] are all involved. Which antigens are most relevant to prevention of diabetes is still not clear and so approaches using some or all of these antigens are currently under investigation.

By utilizing whole islets or islet cells as an antigen source, the majority of potential islet antigens are included in the preventive procedure. Several groups have placed this antigenic material directly into the thymus since this is the site for the selection of T cells and hence of the autoreactive repertoire. Intrathymic injection of syngeneic islet cells into 4-week-old female NOD mice produced a significant reduction in the severity of insulitis and development of diabetes[52]. However, the severity of sialitis, which is also usually present in NOD mice, was not reduced, indicating that the protective effect was tissue-specific. Moreover, splenocytes from the treated mice did not transfer diabetes to susceptible recipients.

Another group transplanted islet cells from newborn NOD mice into 10–11-day-old female NOD mice and also observed protective effect for IDDM development[53,54]. In this study, however, after injection of CY into the islet-transplanted mice at 30 weeks, half of the mice developed diabetes, suggesting that peripheral tolerance, rather than removal of reactive T cells, might play a role in preventing the onset of diabetes. Since the disease in NOD mice might begin even earlier than 10 days of age, another group injected islets into the thymus of NOD mice within 24 hours of birth. This treatment prevented insulitis and diabetes and the protection was resistant to CY administration, suggesting that autoreactive cells may have been eliminated[55]. However, antibodies to islet cell antigens were still present in treated mice.

Recently, the intrathymic injection of GAD-65 protein was also assessed. NOD mice receiving intrathymic injection of GAD-65 at 3 weeks of age exhibited markedly reduced T-cell proliferative responses to GAD in addition to remaining free of diabetes[44]. However, intrathymic injection of GAD in NOD mice is controversial for the prevention of IDDM, because it has been reported that intrathymic injection of a GAD peptide accelerates the onset of diabetes (unpublished data). Intravenous GAD-65 administration in 3-week-old NOD mice was also effective in preventing the development of diabetes and in greatly reducing the severity of insulitis[43].

Intensive insulin therapy in patients with recent diagnosed IDDM has been reported to result in a prolonged "honeymoon" period during which endogenous insulin-secreting capacity is sufficient to negate insulin therapy. Because of this, some investigators tested whether prophylactic insulin therapy might prevent IDDM in NOD mice. NOD mice were injected with protamine zinc pork insulin from weaning until 6 months and the treatment significantly reduced the frequency of diabetes and pancreatic insulitis[45]. In an even more unusual but practical approach, the oral administration of porcine insulin was tested in NOD mice. Porcine insulin was given orally twice a week for 5 weeks and then weekly until 1 year of age. Despite having no demonstrable metabolic effect, the treatment reduced the severity of lymphocytic infiltration of pancreatic islets and the incidence of diabetes[46]. Furthermore, splenocytes from oral insulin-treated mice protected against adoptively transferred IDDM. The authors concluded that oral insulin administration generates active cellular mechanisms which suppress disease.

Heat shock proteins are also involved in the immune response to islet antigens. It was reported that a pancreatic β-cell target antigen in NOD mice is a molecule cross-reactive with the 65 kilodalton(kDa) heat shock protein (hsp 65) of *Mycobacterium tuberculosis* and that the hsp 65 antigen can be used to vaccinate against diabetes. The efficacy of this treatment is apparently dependent on the form of hsp 65 administration[16]. Moreover, a functionally important peptide within the sequence of the human variant of the 65 kDa heat shock protein molecule was found and administration of this peptide to NOD mice can also down-regulate immunity to the 65 kDa heat shock protein and prevent the development of diabetes[47]. Most recently, these same investigators reported that a peptide of the 60 kDa heat shock protein, designated p277, administered once, could arrest the autoimmune process even after it was far advanced, and successful therapy was associated with down-regulation of the autoimmune process and regulation of islet inflammation[48].

Some investigators tried to prevent IDDM by administration of gangliosides (Cronassial). Cronassial was administered to NOD mice daily from 5 to 11 weeks of age and the mice were followed until 21 weeks of age. The treatment slowed the rate of rise in glycemia, but the final diabetes incidence was not reduced[49].

Thus, whole islets, GAD-65, insulin, or heat shock protein seem capable of preventing IDDM in NOD mice. The mechanism by which so many different antigens can influence the course of the pathogenic process remains to be determined.

ANTIGEN NON-SPECIFIC

Because of the evidence that either immunostimulation or immunosuppression might be able to affect the disease in NOD mice, there have been a number of "non-specific" agents assessed. The best characterized example of this is the use of complete Freund's adjuvant (CFA). When CFA was injected into the footpads and peritoneum at 5 weeks of age in NOD mice, it prevented the onset of diabetes for the life span of the mice[56]. The regulatory cells in this system seemed to be natural suppressor cells. Another group also reported that CFA treatment in 8–10-week-old pre-diabetic NOD mice prevented IDDM in both females and males[57]. However in this report, splenocytes or Mac1-enriched splenocytes from CFA-treated NOD mice appeared to be regulatory and prevented adoptive transfer of IDDM. Yet other reports suggested that CD4+T cells were responsible for protection by CFA and IDDM could be induced in the CFA-treated (diabetes protected) mice by CY treatment[58].

By using this CFA treatment, some investigators tried to prevent autoimmune destruction and rejection of transplanted islets in diabetic NOD mice[59-61]. CFA treatment extended syngeneic, but not allogeneic, islet graft survival[60]. Since CFA contains mycobacterial cell products with adjuvant properties, 4-week-old NOD mice were injected with *Mycobacterium tuberculosis* or *Mycobacterium bovis* (BCG vaccine)[58]. In this system also, protection from diabetes was found. Similarly, the injection of live BCG organisms intravenously at 5–10 weeks of age in NOD mice also suppressed the occurrence of insulitis and diabetes[62]. The mechanism of the preventive effect appeared to be the generation of suppressor macrophages[63,64]. Based upon these observations, a trial of BCG vaccine in recent-onset IDDM patients has already started[65].

A streptococcal derived immunomodulator, OK-432, also prevented insulitis and diabetes in NOD mice[66]. Splenocytes from OK-432 treated mice were unable to suppress transfer of diabetes by diabetic splenocytes, and CY could not induce diabetes in OK-432 treated mice[67]. These results suggested that OK-432 treatment prevented the development of diabetes by suppressing the generation of the effector cells for pancreatic β-cell destruction. Further, serum from OK-432 treated mice, if injected into NOD mice, could also suppress diabetes in the treated mice[68]. This finding prompted the speculation that the effect might be due to endogenous TNF production.

CELL TRANSFER

Cell populations can be transferred into NOD mice with a resultant effect on diabetes development. In general, the effect seems to be due to either the introduction of non-NOD MHC molecules or the transfer of antigen- or idiotype-specific regulatory cells. Since regulatory cells seem to be an integral part of the disease process in NOD mice, it is not surprising that these cells have been isolated, and in many instances perpetuated *in vitro*, in several laboratories. As has been noted, there exist sex differences in NOD mice, which cause a higher diabetes incidence in females than in males[1]. This phenomenon suggests that there may be more effective regulatory circuits in male NOD mice. Based upon this speculation, splenocytes from young males were tested for their ability to protect from IDDM in NOD mice[69]. Investigators reconstituted irradiated male recipients 6 days before the transfer of diabetic splenocytes and succeeded in preventing the transfer of disease. Moreover, they found that the protective population was present in the CD4+T-cell population. On the other hand, an IL-2-dependent non-cytolytic $V\beta11+$ CD8+T-cell clone from NOD mice can protect from the transfer of IDDM[70].

T lymphocytes from the islets of newly diabetic NOD mice have been isolated and used to generate autoreactive CD4+T-lymphocyte lines. When the lines were injected into NOD mice, they prevented IDDM from occurring[71]. The recipients of protective cell lines had a marked decrease in the incidence of both diabetes and insulitis; no insulitis was present at 1 year of age.

Neonatal tolerance induction to semi-allogenic F1 splenocytes protected from both insulitis and diabetes significantly[72]. This protection was independent of the major histocompatibility complex (MHC) haplotypes of the F1 splenocytes injected at birth, for instance, (C57Bl/6 × NOD)F1, (CBA/Ca × NOD)F1, or (BALB/c × NOD)F1 cells. Further, the injection of MHC-compatible but minor histoincompatible splenocytes at birth also protected from diabetes development. These observations led to the conclusion that the expression of spontaneous T-cell-mediated autoimmunity can be modulated by immune manipulations at birth. Thymus from (CBA × NOD)F1 donor was transplanted to NOD mice by another group and the treatment also reduced the incidence of IDDM in NOD mice[73]. Many groups have succeeded in preventing diabetes in the NOD mouse by transplanting bone marrow from diabetes-resistant mice, both semi and fully allogeneic[74-79]. Irradiated NOD mice were reconstituted with bone marrow cells from young BALB/c nu/nu mice, and both occurrence of insulitis and IDDM were prevented[75]. Lethally irradiated NOD mice reconstituted with B10.BR/cd hematopoietic cell also remained totally free of insulitis, and failed to develop IDDM[76]. Bone marrow transplantation from NOD-E transgenic mice (see transgenic treatment), which express the I-E molecule (absent in NOD mice) and are free from both insulitis and IDDM, into NOD mice also protected from diabetes[78].

Recently it was shown that dendritic cells from the draining lymph nodes of the pancreas (PLN) significantly lowered the level of insulitis and limited the expression of diabetes in NOD mice[80]. Clare-Salzler *et al.* speculated that PLN dendritic cells prevented IDDM by the induction of regulatory cells. Thus many forms of cell transfer can protect from IDDM in NOD mice, suggesting the existence of multiple protective mechanisms.

GENOMIC ALTERATION—TRANSGENES, GENE KNOCKOUT

In the NOD mouse, the MHC class II region has been implicated in disease susceptibility, since the NOD strain expresses a unique I-Aβ chain[81] and no surface I-E molecules due to a lack of I-Eα chain production[82]. Originally, it was found that the selective expression of I-E molecules in NOD mice, by backcrossing on to I-E expressing C57Bl/6 transgenic mice, could prevent the development of autoimmune insulitis[83]. It was indirectly shown that this protection was not simply due to the deletion of self-reactive T cells[84]. To avoid the complications of backcrossing techniques another group directly microinjected the Eα^d gene into fertilized NOD eggs and established I-Eα^d transgenic mice[85]. They showed that transgene expression of the MHC class II I-E molecules prevented insulitis. Moreover, they treated the transgenic NOD mice with CY, which effectively induces diabetes in normal NOD mice, and showed that the I-Eα^d transgenic NOD mice were resistant to CY treatment and did not develop diabetes up to 40 weeks of age[86].

Other groups also showed the protective effect of an I-E transgene in NOD mice with similar CY resistance[87]. However, I-E+ congenic NOD mice have been established and these mice showed insulitis[88]. Moreover, in some mice, CY-induced and spontaneous diabetes developed. Thus, the degree and mechanism of protection afforded by transgenic I-E expression seems to be controversial.

Some investigators made NOD mouse transgenic for I-A^k by microinjecting I-A^k α- and β-genes into fertilized NOD eggs and in this mouse also, insulitis was markedly reduced and the onset of IDDM was prevented[89]. Similarly, Aβ^k expressing transgenic NOD mice were produced by another group and a protective effect was observed[85].

The sequence of I-Aβ chain in the first external domain is unique with His 56 and Ser 57 replacing Pro and Asp, respectively, at these positions. Mutations of the NOD IA molecule have also been transgenically introduced into NOD mice. A transgene encoding a modified Aβ NOD with Pro 56, since Pro 56 might give rise to a different conformation of I-Aβ chain than does His

56, protected NOD mice from IDDM[87]. In this mouse also, protection was not associated with a complete deletion of any T cells expressing commonly used T-cell receptor $V\beta$ genes.

NOD mice were shown to express MHC class I K^d and D^b antigens. Some attempted to express a different type of class I molecule in NOD mice by crossing C57Bl/6 mice transgenic for the class I L^d gene with NOD mice[90]. The expression of the class I L^d antigen significantly reduced the incidence of insulitis.

Recently, NOD-β2m null mice, which lack expression of β2 microglobulin, were developed by backcrossing with a β2 microglobulin gene knockout line[91]. The mice, which lack both class I expression and CD8+T cells in the periphery, not only failed to develop diabetes but were completely devoid of insulitis. These NOD-β2m null mice were also established by other groups and similarly these lines of NOD mice showed neither diabetes nor insulitis[92].

Thus, genetic modification of both MHC class II and class I by transgene insertion or gene knockout can afford protection from IDDM in NOD mice, although there exists some controversy as to how these manipulations are effective.

DRUG TREATMENT

There are many reports of drug trials for prevention of IDDM in NOD mice. Nicotinamide is a precursor for new NAD (nicotinamide adenine dinucleotide) synthesis and an inhibitor of poly (ADP-ribose) synthetase and other ADP-ribosyl transferases. It was shown to have preventive and therapeutic effects on diabetes in NOD mice, and the results suggested it might reverse β-cell damage[93,94]. Nicotinamide therapy in man has already been shown to have a beneficial effect on the remission phase of IDDM, and its use is safe[95,96]. Nicotinamide may also repair β-cell function in high risk subjects although the effect seems not to be mediated by an immune mechanism[97].

Some trials of immunosuppressive drugs for prevention of IDDM are also reported. When cyclosporin was administered to NOD mice, the treatment suppressed the development of insulitis and diabetes as long as the drug was continually administered[98]. However, cyclosporin appeared to have little therapeutic effect when the treatment was started after development of glucose intolerance[98]. This drug has already been used for immunosuppression in IDDM of recent onset in humans[99,100], but has several side-effects[101,102]. One group tried to establish an *in vitro* regimen for cyclosporin A immunosuppression in order to avoid its *in vivo* side-effects[103]. They cultured autologous splenic lymphoid cells from young NOD mice with cyclosporin A plus IL-2 before re-infusing the splenocytes into the animal from which they were isolated. This procedure was reported to prevent IDDM from developing. Long-term treatment with azathioprine was studied in NOD mice to compare the effect with cyclosporin A[104]. Early and prolonged treatment with azathioprine seemed to prevent the onset of IDDM in NOD mice as effectively as cyclosporin A, and it was concluded that azathioprine, which is significantly safer than cyclosporin A, could replace the latter as a potential drug for the immunotherapy of IDDM.

The oral administration of rapamycin in NOD mice has also been studied[105]. This treatment also prevented the onset of disease although intervention therapy with this drug was ineffective at reversing the course of disease after IDDM onset.

FK506, which is a novel immunosuppressive compound isolated from *Streptomyces*, also prevented the progression of insulitis and diabetes in NOD mice[106]. Moreover, both syngeneic and allogeneic islet transplants were accepted in 2–6-week-old NOD mice after FK506 treatment[107]. However, treatment of NOD mice with FK506 was less effective in preventing insulitis and the onset of diabetes when the treatment was started at 4 weeks of age instead of 2 weeks of age[107].

Another newly described immunosuppressive drug, deoxyspergualin[108,109], was also reported to be an effective drug to prevent IDDM in NOD mice. A new class of immunoconjugate, in which a molecular toxin is conjugated to a targeting molecule, has been used to prevent diabetes in NOD mice with some success. The drug combines diphtheria toxin with IL-2 such that activated IL-2 receptor expressing cells are selectively destroyed thereby preventing T cells from destroying the β cells[110]. Results of clinical trials will shed further light on the utility of this form of therapy.

Previous studies in which IDDM was experimentally induced by administration of the oxidant alloxan suggested that specific β-cell damage results from alloxan-induced production of reactive oxygen free radicals in the β cells[111]. Moreover, macrophages in pancreatic islets would produce reactive oxygen and nitrogen free radicals on activation and these reactive intermediates could be directly toxic to β cells[12,112,113]. Based upon these observations, many kinds of antioxidant compounds have been used to prevent IDDM in NOD mice. *In vivo* treatment of NOD mice with the enzymes superoxide dismutase and catalase protected islet tissue from disease recurrence following transplantation into spontaneously diabetic mice[114]. Probucol partially prevented the development of IDDM in NOD mice[115], but the combination of probucol with the anti-inflammatory corticosteroid, deflazacort, could prevent both insulitis and diabetes[116]. Other antioxidants such as lazaroid[117], lipid acid[118], or MDL29311 (4,4'-[methylene bis (thio)]bis [2,6-bis(1,1-dimethylethyl)]-phenol; an analogue of probucol)[119] have also apparently prevented IDDM in NOD mice.

Thus, nicotinamide, immunosuppressive agents, and antioxidant compounds have been successfully employed as drugs for the prevention of IDDM in NOD mice. Other agents such as 1,25-dihydroxy vitamin D_3[120], tolbutamide[121], or monosodium glutamate[122] might also have the potential to protect from diabetes in this model.

ENVIRONMENTAL AGENTS—VIRUS, DIET

Other approaches to the prevention of IDDM in NOD mice include virus infection and dietary treatment. Viruses may act as primary injurious agents to pancreatic β cells or as triggering agents for autoimmunity. However, some viruses are reported to prevent IDDM in NOD mice. Lymphocytic choriomeningitis virus (LCMV)[123–125], lactate dehydrogenase virus (LDV)[11] and encephalomyocarditis virus (EMCV-D)[126] are known to suppress the onset of diabetes in NOD mice.

With respect to dietary treatment, casein hydrolysate could prevent overt diabetes in NOD mice if introduced early into the diety[127,128]. THI (2-acetyl-4-tetrahydroxybutylimidazole), a compound present in ammonia caramel food coloring and a widely used food additive, reduced the incidence of IDDM in NOD mice[129]. THI is a small imidazole-containing compound with structural similarity to histamine and urocanic acid, both known to have immunosuppressive properties.

Epidemiological studies have revealed that children of diabetic mothers have a lower diabetes incidence than children of diabetic fathers[130,131]. One explanation for these observations was that the hyperglycemic environment in diabetic mothers could protect the fetus from developing diabetes. Investigators therefore tried glucose administration to NOD neonates subcutaneously for the first six days of life and found that the treatment did reduce the incidence of diabetes in NOD mice[132]. Since both female and male NOD mice develop insulitis but clinical diabetes occurs mainly in females, some investigators treated NOD females with androgen and this prevented IDDM[133]. Other environmental factors, such as exogenous superantigens, can also protect from IDDM in the NOD mouse[134]. Thus, manipulation of environmental factors including viruses and diet can also prevent IDDM in NOD mice.

CONCLUSIONS

The NOD mouse is a useful model of IDDM in which it is possible to readily investigate the disease etiology and potential therapies. It has been shown in the NOD mouse that there is a requirement for CD4+ and CD8+T cells and macrophages in the disease process; therapies directed at any of these cells are effective in preventing disease progression. Short-term treatment with monoclonal antibodies directed at the CD3 or CD4 molecules has been shown to prevent diabetes developing in the NOD mouse. Since similar monoclonal antibodies are available for clinical use, it seems that this means of disease therapy could soon be applied in human IDDM. More generalized immunosuppression is less attractive in human IDDM due to the associated risks. "Non-specific" therapies such as BCG immunization which are very effective at preventing disease progression in NOD mice, may afford some short-term benefit in IDDM and the risks of treatment are minimal. It is hoped that further understanding of the mechanisms involved in this form of therapy will enable more potent agents to be developed for clinical use in IDDM.

Antigen-specific therapies have been proven to be very effective in the prevention of disease in the NOD mouse and the clinical application of antigen-specific therapies seems requisite. Antigens which are both safe and effective in the NOD mouse, e.g. insulin and GAD, need to be assessed in clinical trials and should provide the most optimism for the future.

REFERENCES

1 Makino S, Kunimoto K, Muraoka Y, Mizushima Y, Katagiri K, Tochino Y. Breeding of a non-obese, diabetic strain of mice. *Jikken Dobutsu* 1980; 29(1): 1–13.
2 Shizuru JA, Taylor-Edwards C, Banks BA, Gregory AK, Fathman CG. Immunotherapy of the nonobese diabetic mouse: treatment with an antibody to T-helper lymphocytes. *Science* 1988; 240(4852): 659–62.
3 Hayward AR, Schreiber M. Neonatal injection of CD3 antibody into nonobese diabetic mice reduces the incidence of insulitis and diabetes. *J Immunol* 1989; 143(5): 1555–9.
4 Bendelac A, Boitard C, Bedossa P, Bazin H, Bach JF, Carnaud C. Adoptive T cell transfer of autoimmune nonobese diabetic mouse diabetes does not require recruitment of host B lymphocytes. *J Immunol* 1988; 141(8): 2625–8.
5 Lehuen A, Bendelac A, Bach JF, Carnaud C. The nonobese diabetic mouse model. Independent expression of humoral and cell-mediated autoimmune features. *J Immunol* 1990; 144(6): 2147–51.
6 Harada M, Makino S. Suppression of overt diabetes in NOD mice by anti-thymocyte serum or anti-Thy 1, 2 antibody. *Jikken Dobutsu* 1986; 35(4): 501–4.
7 Makino S, Harada M, Kishimoto Y, Hayashi Y. Absence of insulitis and overt diabetes in athymic nude mice with NOD genetic background. *Jikken Dobutsu* 1986; 35(4): 495–8.
8 Ihm SH, Yoon JW. Studies on autoimmunity for initiation of beta-cell destruction. VI. Macrophages essential for development of beta-cell-specific cytotoxic effectors and insulitis in NOD mice. *Diabetes* 1990; 39(10): 1273–8.
9 Charlton B, Bacelj A, Mandel TE. Administration of silica particles or anti-Lyt2 antibody prevents beta-cell destruction in NOD mice given cyclophosphamide. *Diabetes* 1988; 37(7): 930–5.
10 Lee KU, Amano K, Yoon JW. Evidence for initial involvement of macrophage in development of insulitis in NOD mice. *Diabetes* 1988; 37(7): 989–91.
11 Takei I, Asaba Y, Kasatani T et al. Suppression of development of diabetes in NOD mice by lactate dehydrogenase virus infection. *J Autoimmun* 1992; 5(6): 665–73.
12 Kasuga A, Maruyama T, Takei I et al. The role of cytotoxic macrophages in non-obese diabetic mice: cytotoxicity against murine mastocytoma and beta-cell

lines. *Diabetologia* 1993; **36**(12): 1252–7.

13 Hutchings P, Rosen H, O'Reilly L, Simpson E, Gordon S, Cooke A. Transfer of diabetes in mice prevented by blockade of adhesion-promoting receptor on macrophages. *Nature* 1990; **348**(6302): 639–42.

14 Supon P, Stecha P, Haskins K. Anti-islet cell antibodies from NOD mice. *Diabetes* 1990; **39**(11): 1366–72.

15 Maruyama T, Takei I, Asaba Y *et al*. Insulin autoantibodies in mouse models of insulin-dependent diabetes. *Diabetes Res* 1989; **11**(2): 61–5.

16 Elias D, Markovits D, Reshef T, van der Zee R, Cohen IR. Induction and therapy of autoimmune diabetes in the non-obese diabetic (NOD/Lt) mouse by a 65-kDa heat shock protein. *Proc Natl Acad Sci USA* 1990; **87**(4): 1576–80.

17 Hodgson RJ, Loudovaris T, Charlton B, Mandel TE. Destruction of transplanted beta cells into diabetic NOD mice is not mediated by antibody alone. *Transpl Proc* 1992; **24**(5): 2300.

18 Koike T, Itoh Y, Ishii T *et al*. Preventive effect of monoclonal anti-L3T4 antibody on development of diabetes in NOD mice. *Diabetes* 1987; **36**(4): 539–41.

19 Charlton B, Mandel TE. Recurrence of insulitis in the NOD mouse after early prolonged anti-CD4 monoclonal antibody treatment. *Autoimmunity* 1989; **4**(1–2): 1–7.

20 Kurasawa K, Sakamoto A, Maeda T *et al*. Short-term administration of anti-L3T4 MoAb prevents diabetes in NOD mice. *Clin Exp Immunol* 1993; **91**(3): 376–80.

21 Hayward AR, Shriber M, Cooke A, Waldmann H. Prevention of diabetes but not insulitis in NOD mice injected with antibody to CD4. *J Autoimmun* 1993; **6**(3): 301–10.

22 Miller BJ, Appel MC, O'Neil JJ, Wicker LS. Both the Lyt-2+ and L3T4+ T cell subsets are required for the transfer of diabetes in nonobse diabetic mice. *J Immunol* 1988; **140**(1): 52–8.

23 Taki T, Nagata M, Ogawa W *et al*. Prevention of cyclophosphamide-induced and spontaneous diabetes in NOD/Shi/Kbe mice by anti-MHC class I Kd monoclonal antibody. *Diabetes* 1991; **40**(9): 1203–9.

24 Wang Y, Pontesilli O, Gill RG, La Rosa FG, Lafferty KJ. The role of CD4+ and CD8+ T cells in the destruction of islet grafts by spontaneously diabetic mice. *Proc Natl Acad Sci USA* 1991; **88**(2): 527–31.

25 Maki T, Ichikawa T, Blanco R, Porter J. Long-term abrogation of autoimmune diabetes in nonobese diabetic mice by immunotherapy with anti-lymphocyte serum. *Proc Natl Acad Sci USA* 1992; **89**(8): 3434–8.

26 Hayward AR, Shriber M. Reduced incidence of insulitis in NOD mice following anti-CD3 injection: requirement for neonatal injection. *J Autoimmun* 1992; **5**(1): 59–67.

27 Chatenoud L, Thervet E, Primo J, Bach JF. Anti-CD3 antibody induces long-term remission of overt autoimmunity in nonobese diabetic mice. *Proc Natl Acad Sci USA* 1994; **91**(1): 123–7.

28 Sempe P, Bedossa P, Richard MF, Villa MC, Bach JF, Boitard C. Anti-alpha/beta T cell receptor monoclonal antibody provides an efficient therapy for autoimmune diabetes in nonobese diabetic (NOD) mice. *Eur J Immunol* 1991; **21**(5): 1163–9.

29 Bacelj A, Charlton B, Mandel TE. Prevention of cyclophosphamide-induced diabetes by anti-V beta 8 T-lymphocyte-receptor monoclonal antibody therapy in NOD/Wehi mice. *Diabetes* 1989; **38**(11): 1492–5.

30 Formby B, Shao T. T cell vaccination against autoimmune diabetes in nonobese diabetic mice. *Ann Clin Lab Sci* 1993; **23**(2): 137–47.

31 Boitard C, Bendelac A, Richard MF, Carnaud C, Bach JF. Prevention of diabetes in nonobese diabetic mice by anti-I-A monoclonal antibodies: transfer of protection by splenic T cells. *Proc Natl Acad Sci USA* 1988; **85**(24): 9719–23.

32 Singh B, Dillon T, Fraga E, Lauzon J. Role of the first external domain of I-A beta

chain in immune responses and diabetes in non-obese diabetic (NOD) mice. *J Autoimmun* 1990; 3(5): 507–21.

33 Maruyama T, Watanabe K, Takei I et al. Anti-asialo GM1 antibody suppression of cyclophosphamide-induced diabetes in NOD mice. *Diabetes Res* 1991; 17(1): 37–41.

34 Debray-Sachs M, Carnaud C, Boitard C et al. Prevention of diabetes in NOD mice treated with antibody to murine IFN gamma. *J Autoimmun* 1991; 4(2): 237–48.

35 Campbell IL, Kay TW, Oxbrow L, Harrison LC. Essential role for interferon-gamma and interleukin-6 in autoimmune insulin-dependent diabetes in NOD/Wehi mice. *J Clin Invest* 1991; 87(2): 739–42.

36 Jacob CO, Aiso S, Michie SA, McDevitt HO, Acha-Orbea H. Prevention of diabetes in nonobese diabetic mice by tumor necrosis factor (TNF): similarities between TNF-alpha and interleukin 1. *Proc Natl Acad Sci USA* 1990; 87(3): 968–72.

37 Seino H, Takahashi K, Satoh J et al. Prevention of autoimmune diabetes with lymphotoxin in NOD mice. *Diabetes* 1993; 42(3): 398–404.

38 Formby B, Jacobs C, Dubuc P, Shao T. Exogenous administration of IL-1 alpha inhibits active and adoptive transfer autoimmune diabetes in NOD mice. *Autoimmunity* 1992; 12(1): 21–7.

39 Serreze DV, Hamaguchi K, Leiter EH. Immunostimulation circumvents diabetes in NOD/Lt mice. *J Autoimmun* 1989; 2(6): 759–76.

40 Rapoport MJ, Jaramillo A, Zipris D et al. Interleukin 4 reverses T cell proliferative unresponsiveness and prevents the onset of diabetes in nonobese diabetic mice. *J Exp Med* 1993; 178(1): 87–99.

41 Penniline KJ, Roque-Gaffney E, Monahan M. Recombinant human IL-10 prevents the onset of diabetes in the nonobese diabetic mouse. *Clin Immunol Immunopathol* 1994; 71(2): 169–75.

42 Wogensen L, Lee MS, Sarvetnick N. Production of interleukin 10 by islet cells accelerates immune-mediated destruction of beta cells in nonobese diabetic mice. *J Exp Med* 1994; 179(4): 1379–84.

43 Kaufman DL, Clare-Salzler M, Tian J et al. Spontaneous loss of T-cell tolerance to glutamic acid decarboxylase in murine insulin-dependent diabetes. *Nature* 1993; 366(6450): 69–72.

44 Tisch R, Yang XD, Singer SM, Liblau RS, Fugger L, McDevitt HO. Immune response to glutamic acid decarboxylase correlates with insulitis in non-obese diabetic mice. *Nature* 1993; 366(6450): 72–5.

45 Atkinson MA, Maclaren NK, Luchetta R. Insulitis and diabetes in NOD mice reduced by prophylactic insulin therapy. *Diabetes* 1990; 39(8): 933–7.

46 Zhang ZJ, Davidson L, Eisenbarth G, Weiner HL. Suppression of diabetes in nonobese diabetic mice by oral administration of porcine insulin. *Proc Natl Acad Sci USA* 1991; 88(22): 10252–6.

47 Elias D, Reshef T, Birk OS, van der Zee R, Walker MD, Cohen IR. Vaccination against autoimmune mouse diabetes with a T-cell epitope of the human 65-kDa heat shock protein. *Proc Natl Acad Sci USA* 1991; 88(8): 3088–91.

48 Elias D, Cohen IR. Peptide therapy for diabetes in NOD mice. *Lancet* 1994; 343(8899): 704–6.

49 Papaccio G, Chieffi Baccari G, Mezzogiorno V. In vivo effect of gangliosides on non-bese diabetic mice. *Acta Anat* 1993; 147(3): 168–73.

50 Boitard C, Villa MC, Becourt C et al. Peripherin: an islet antigen that is cross-reactive with nonobese diabetic mouse class II gene products. *Proc Natl Acad Sci USA* 1992; 89(1): 172–6.

51 Castano L, Russo E, Zhou L, Lipes MA, Eisenbarth GS. Identification and cloning of a granule autoantigen (carboxypeptidase-H) associated with type I diabetes. *J*

Clin Endocrinol Metab 1991; 73(6): 1197–201.
52 Gerling IC, Serreze DV, Christianson SW, Leiter EH. Intrathymic islet cell transplantation reduces beta-cell autoimmunity and prevents diabetes in NOD/Lt mice. Diabetes 1992; 41(12): 1672–6.
53 Nomura Y, Stein E, Mullen Y. Prevention of overt diabetes and insulitis by intrathymic injection of syngeneic islets in newborn nonobese diabetic (NOD) mice. Transplantation 1993; 56(3): 638–42.
54 Nomura Y, Mullen Y, Stein E. Syngeneic islets transplanted into the thymus of newborn mice prevent diabetes and reduce insulitis in the NOD mouse. Transplant Proc 1993; 25(1 Pt 2): 963–4.
55 Charlton B, Taylor-Edwards C, Tisch R, Fathman CG. Intrathymic islet administration in NOD neonates prevents insulitis and diabetes. J Autoimmun 1994; 7: 549–60.
56 Sadelain MW, Qin HY, Lauzon J, Singh B. Prevention of type I diabetes in NOD mice by adjuvant immunotherapy. Diabetes 1990; 39(5): 583–9.
57 McIlnerney MF, Pek SB, Thomas DW. Prevention of insulitis and diabetes onset by treatment with complete Freund's adjuvant in NOD mice. Diabetes 1991; 40(6): 715–25.
58 Qin HY, Sadelain MW, Hitchon C, Lauzon J, Singh B. Complete Freund's adjuvant-induced T cells prevent the development and adoptive transfer of diabetes in nonobese diabetic mice. J Immunol 1993; 150(5): 2072–80.
59 Ulaeto D, Lacy PE, Kipnis DM, Kanagawa O, Unanue ER. A T-cell dormant state in the autoimmune process of nonobese diabetic mice treated with complete Freund's adjuvant. Proc Natl Acad Sci USA 1992; 89(9): 3927–31.
60 Wang T, Singh B, Warnock GL, Rajotte RV. Prevention of recurrence of IDDM in islet-transplanted diabetic NOD mice by adjuvant immunotherapy. Diabetes 1992; 41(1): 114–17.
61 Lakey JR, Wang T, Warnock GL, Singh B, Rajotte RV. Prevention of recurrence of insulin-dependent diabetes mellitus in islet cell-transplanted diabetic NOD mice using adjuvant therapy. Transpl Proc 1992; 24(6): 2848.
62 Harada M, Kishimoto Y, Makino S. Prevention of overt diabetes and insulitis in NOD mice by a single BCG vaccination. Diabetes Res Clin Pract 1990; 8(2): 85–9.
63 Yagi H, Matsumoto M, Suzuki S et al. Possible mechanism of the preventive effect of BCG against diabetes mellitus in NOD mouse. I. Generation of suppressor macrophages in spleen cells of BCG-vaccinated mice. Cell Immunol 1991; 138(1): 130–41.
64 Yagi H, Matsumoto M, Kishimoto Y, Makino S, Harada M. Possible mechanism of the preventive effect of BCG against diabetes mellitus in NOD mouse. II. Suppression of pathogenesis by macrophage transfer from BCG-vaccinated mice. Cell Immunol 1991; 138(1): 142–9.
65 Shehadeh N, Calcinaro F, Bradley BJ, Bruchlim I, Vardi P, Lafferty KJ. Effect of adjuvant therapy on development of diabetes in mouse and man. Lancet 1994; 343(8899): 706–7.
66 Satoh J, Shintani S, Oya K et al. Treatment with streptococcal preparation (OK-432) suppresses anti-islet autoimmunity and prevents diabetes in BB rats. Diabetes 1988; 37(9): 1188–94.
67 Shintani S, Satoh J, Seino H, Goto Y, Toyota T. Mechanism of action of a streptococcal preparation (OK-432) in prevention of autoimmune diabetes in NOD mice. Suppression of generation of effector cells for pancreatic B cell destruction. J Immunol 1990; 144(1): 136–41.
68 Seino H, Satoh J, Shintani S et al. Inhibition of autoimmune diabetes in NOD mice with serum from streptococcal preparation (OK-432)-injected mice. Clin Exp Immunol 1991; 86(3): 413–18.

69 Hutchings PR, Cooke A. The transfer of autoimmune diabetes in NOD mice can be inhibited or accelerated by distinct cell populations present in normal splenocytes taken from young males. *J Autoimmun* 1990; 3(2): 175–85.

70 Pankewycz O, Strom TB, Rubin-Kelley VE. Islet-infiltrating T cell clones from non-obese diabetic mice that promote or prevent accelerated onset diabetes. *Eur J Immunol* 1991; 21(4): 873–9.

71 Reich EP, Scaringe D, Yagi J, Sherwin RS, Janeway C Jr. Prevention of diabetes in NOD mice by injection of autoreactive T-lymphocytes. *Diabetes* 1989; 38(12): 1647–51.

72 Bendelac A, Boitard C, Bach JF, Carnaud C. Neonatal induction of allogeneic tolerance prevents T cell-mediated autoimmunity in NOD mice. *Eur J Immunol* 1989; 19(4): 611–16.

73 Georgiou HM, Mandel TE. Reduced incidence of diabetes in nonobese diabetic mice transplanted with thymus from diabetes-resistant donors. *Transpl Proc* 1992; 24(1): 203–4.

74 Georgiou HM, Slattery RM, Charlton B. Bone marrow transplantation prevents autoimmune diabetes in nonobese diabetic mice. *Transpl Proc* 1993; 25(5): 2896–7.

75 Ikehara S, Ohtsuki H, Good RA *et al*. Prevention of type I diabetes in nonobese diabetic mice by allogenic bone marrow transplantation. *Proc Natl Acad Sci USA* 1985; 82(22): 7743–7.

76 LaFace DM, Peck AB. Reciprocal allogeneic bone marrow transplantation between NOD mice and diabetes-nonsusceptible mice associated with transfer and prevention of autoimmune diabetes. *Diabetes* 1989; 38(7): 894–901.

77 Mathieu C, Vandeputte M, Bouillon R, Waer M. Protection against autoimmune diabetes by induction of mixed bone marrow chimerism. *Transpl Proc* 1993; 25(1 Pt 2): 1266–7.

78 Parish NM, Chandler P, Quartey-Papafio R, Simpson E, Cooke A. The effect of bone marrow and thymus chimerism between non-obese diabetic (NOD) and NOD-E transgenic mice, on the expression and prevention of diabetes. *Eur J Immunol* 1993; 23(10): 2667–75.

79 Serreze DV, Leiter EH. Development of diabetogenic T cells from NOD/Lt marrow is blocked when an allo-H-2 haplotype is expressed on cells of hemopoietic origin, but not on thymic epithelium. *J Immunol* 1991; 147(4): 1222–9.

80 Clare-Salzler MJ, Brooks J, Chai A, Van Herle K, Anderson C. Prevention of diabetes in nonobese diabetic mice by dendritic cell transfer. *J Clin Invest* 1992; 90(3): 741–8.

81 Acha-Orbea H, McDevitt HO. The first external domain of the nonobese diabetic mouse class II I-A beta chain is unique. *Proc Natl Acad Sci USA* 1987; 84(8): 2435–9.

82 Hattori M, Buse JB, Jackson RA *et al*. The NOD mouse: recessive diabetogenic gene in the major histocompatibility complex. *Science* 1986; 231(4739): 733–5.

83 Nichimoto H, Kikutani H, Yamamura K, Kishimoto T. Prevention of autoimmune insulitis by expression of I-E molecules in NOD mice. *Nature* 1987; 328(6129): 432–4.

84 Bohme J, Schuhbaur B, Kanagawa O, Benoist C, Mathis D. MHC-linked protection from diabetes dissociated from clonal deletion of T cells. *Science* 1990; 249(4966): 293–5.

85 Uehira M, Uno M, Kurner T *et al*. Development of autoimmune insulitis is prevented in E alpha d but not in A beta k NOD transgenic mice. *Int Immunol* 1989; 1(2): 209–13.

86 Uno M, Miyazaki T, Uehira M *et al*. Complete prevention of diabetes in transgenic NOD mice expressing I-E molecules. *Immunol Let* 1992; 31(1): 47–52.

87 Lund T, O'Reilly L, Hutchings P *et al*. Prevention of insulin-dependent diabetes mellitus in non-obese diabetic mice by transgenes encoding modified I-A beta-chain or normal I-E alpha-chain. *Nature* 1990; 345(6277): 727–9.

88 Podolin PL, Pressey A, DeLarato NH, Fischer PA, Peterson LB, Wicker LS. I-E+ nonobese diabetic mice develop insulitis and diabetes. *J Exp Med* 1993; **178**(3): 793–803.

89 Slattery RM, Kjer-Nielsen L, Allison J, Charlton B, Mandel TE, Miller JF. Prevention of diabetes in non-obese diabetic I-Ak transgenic mice. *Nature* 1990; **345**(6277): 724–6.

90 Miyazaki T, Matsuda Y, Toyonaga T, Miyazaki J, Yazaki Y, Yamamura K. Prevention of autoimmune insulitis in nonobese diabetic mice by expression of major histocompatibility complex class I Ld molecules. *Proc Natl Acad Sci USA* 1992; **89**(20): 9519–23.

91 Wicker LS, Leiter EH, Todd JA *et al*. Beta 2-microglobulin-deficient NOD mice do not develop insulitis or diabetes. *Diabetes* 1994; **43**(3): 500–4.

92 Serreze DV, Leiter EH, Christianson GJ, Greiner D, Roopenian DC. Major histocompatibility complex class I-deficient NOD-B2mnull mice are diabetes and insulitis resistant. *Diabetes* 1994; **43**(3): 505–9.

93 Yamada K, Nonaka K, Hanafusa T, Miyazaki A, Toyoshima H, Tarui S. Preventive and therapeutic effects of large-dose nicotinamide injections on diabetes associated with insulitis. An observation in nonobese diabetic (NOD) mice. *Diabetes* 1982; **31**(9): 749–53.

94 Reddy S, Bibby NJ, Elliott RB. Early nicotinamide treatment in the NOD mouse: effects on diabetes and insulitis suppression and autoantibody levels. *Diabetes Res* 1990; **15**(2): 95–102.

95 Pozzilli P, Visalli N, Ghirlanda G, Manna R, Andreani D. Nicotinamide increased C-peptide secretion in patients with recent onset type 1 diabetes. *Diabetic Med* 1989; **6**(7): 568–72.

96 Elliott RB, Pilcher CC, Stewart A, Fergusson D, McGregor MA. The use of nicotinamide in the prevention of type 1 diabetes. *Ann NY Acad Sci* 1993; **696**: 333–41.

97 Manna R, Migliore A, Martin LS *et al*. Nicotinamide treatment in subjects at high risk of developing IDDM improves insulin secretion. *Br J Clin Pract* 1992; **46**(3): 177–9.

98 Mori Y, Suko M, Okudaira H *et al*. Preventive effects of cyclosporin on diabetes in NOD mice. *Diabetologia* 1986; **29**(4): 244–7.

99 Stiller CR, Dupre J, Gent M *et al*. Effects of cyclosporine immunosuppression in insulin-dependent diabetes mellitus of recent onset. *Science* 1984; **223**(4643): 1362–7.

100 Feutren G, Papoz L, Assan R *et al*. Cyclosporin increases the rate and length of remissions in insulin-dependent diabetes of recent onset. Results of a multicentre double-blind trial. *Lancet* 1986; **2**(8499): 119–24.

101 Kahan BD, Flechner SM, Lorber MI, Jensen C, Golden D, Van Buren CT. Complications of cyclosporin therapy. *World J Surg* 1986; **10**(3): 348–60.

102 Reznik VM, Jones KL, Durham BL, Mendoza SA. Changes in facial appearance during cyclosporin treatment. *Lancet* 1987; **1**(8547): 1405–7.

103 Formby B, Miller N, Peterson CM. Adoptive immunotherapy of diabetes in autologous nonobese dieabetic mice with lymphoid cells ex vivo exposed to cyclosporin plus interleukin 2. *Diabetes* 1988; **37**(9): 1305–9.

104 Calafiore R, Basta G, Falorni A *et al*. Preventive effects of azathioprine (AZA) on the onset of diabetes mellitus in NOD mice. *J Endocrinol Invest* 1993; **16**(11): 869–73.

105 Baeder WL, Sredy J, Sehgal SN, Chang JY, Adams LM. Rapamycin prevents the onset of insulin-dependent diabetes mellitus (IDDM) in NOD mice. *Clin Exp Immunol* 1992; **89**(2): 174–8.

106 Kurasawa K, Koike T, Matsumura R *et al*. The immunosuppressant FK-506 prevents progression of diabetes in nonobese diabetic mice. *Clin Immunol Immunopathol* 1990; **57**(2): 274–9.

107 Kai N, Motojima K, Tsunoda T, Kanematsu T. Prevention of insulitis and diabetes in nonobese diabetic mice by administration of FK506. *Transplantation* 1993; 55(4): 936–40.

108 Nicoletti F, Borghi MO, Meroni PL *et al*. Prevention of cyclophosphamide-induced diabetes in the NOD/WEHI mouse with deoxyspergualin. *Clin Exp Immunol* 1993; 91(2): 232–6.

109 Strandell E, Sandler S. Protection against hyperglycemia in female nonobese diabetic mice treated with 15-deoxyspergualin. *Autoimmunity* 1992; 14(2): 159–65.

110 Pacheco-Silva A, Bastos MG, Muggia RA *et al*. Interleukin 2 receptor targeted fusion toxin (DAB486-IL-2) treatment blocks diabetogenic autoimmunity in non-obese diabetic mice. *Eur J Immunol* 1992; 22(3): 697–702.

111 Malaisse WJ, Malaisse-Lagae F, Sener A, Pipeleers DG. Determinants of the selective toxicity of alloxan to the pancreatic B cell. *Proc Natl Acad Sci USA* 1982; 79(3): 927–30.

112 Mandrup-Poulsen T, Helqvist S, Wogensen LD *et al*. Cytokine and free radicals as effector molecules in the destruction of pancreatic beta cells. *Curr Topics Microbiol Immunol* 1990; 164: 169–93.

113 Kroncke KD, Kolb-Bachofen V, Berschick B, Burkart V, Kolb H. Activated macrophages kill pancreatic syngeneic islet cells via arginine-dependent nitric oxide generation. *Biochem Biophys Res Commun* 1991; 175(3): 752–8.

114 Nomikos IN, Wang Y, Lafferty KJ. Involvement of O_2 radicals in 'autoimmune' diabetes. *Immunol Cell Biol* 1989; 67(Pt 1): 85–7.

115 Uehara Y, Shimizu H, Sato N, Shimomura Y, Mori M, Kobayashi I. Probucol partially prevents development of diabetes in NOD mice. *Diabetes Res* 1991; 17(3): 131–4.

116 Rabinovitch A, Suarez WL, Power RF. Combination therapy with an antioxidant and a corticosteroid prevents autoimmune diabetes in NOD mice. *Life Sci* 1992; 51(25): 1937–43.

117 Rabinovitch A, Suarez WL, Power RF. Lazaroid antioxidant reduces incidence of diabetes and insulitis in nonobese diabetic mice. *J Lab Clin Med* 1993; 121(4): 603–7.

118 Faust A, Burkart V, Ulrich H, Weischer CH, Kolb H. Effect of lipoic acid on cyclophosphamide-induced diabetes and insulitis in non-obese diabetic mice. *Int J Immunopharmacol* 1994; 16(1): 61–6.

119 Heineke EW, Johnson MB, Dillberger JE, Robinson KM. Antioxidant MDL 29,311 prevents diabetes in nonobese diabetic and multiple low-dose STZ-injected mice. *Diabetes* 1993; 42(12): 1721–30.

120 Mathieu C, Laureys J, Sobis H, Vandeputte M, Waer M, Bouillon R. 1,25-Dihydroxyvitamin D3 prevents insulitis in NOD mic. *Diabetes* 1992; 41(11): 1491–5.

121 Williams AJ, Beales PE, Krug J *et al*. Tolbutamide reduces the incidence of diabetes mellitus, but not insulitis, in the non-obese-diabetic mouse. *Diabetologia* 1993; 36(6): 487–92.

122 Nakajima H, Tochino Y, Fujino-Kurihara H *et al*. Decreased incidence of diabetes mellitus by monosodium glutamate in the non-obese diabetic (NOD) mouse. *Res Commun Chem Pathol Pharmacol* 1985; 50(2): 251–7.

123 Oldstone MB. Prevention of type I diabetes in nonobese diabetic mice by virus infection. *Science* 1988; 239(4839): 500–2.

124 Oldstone MB. Viruses as therapeutic agents. I. Treatment of nonobese insulin-dependent diabetes mice with virus prevents insulin-dependent diabetes mellitus while maintaining general immune competence. *J Exp Med* 1990; 171(6): 2077–89.

125 Oldstone MB, Ahmed R, Salvato M. Viruses as therapeutic agents. II. Viral reassortants map prevention of insulin-dependent diabetes mellitus to the small

RNA of lymphocytic choriomeningitis virus. *J Exp Med* 1990; **171**(6): 2091–100.

126 Hermitte L, Vialettes B, Naquet P, Atlan C, Payan MJ, Vague P. Paradoxical lessening of autoimmune processes in non-obese diabetic mice after infection with the diabetogenic variant of encephalomyocarditis virus. *Eur J Immunol* 1990; **20**(6): 1297–303.

127 Elliott RB, Reddy SN, Bibby NJ, Kida K. Dietary prevention of diabetes in the non-obese diabetic mouse. *Diabetologia* 1983; **31**(1): 62–4.

128 Hoorfar J, Buschard K, Dagnaes-Hansen F. Prophylactic nutritional modification of the incidence of diabetes in autoimmune non-obese diabetic (NOD) mice. *Br J Nutr* 1993; **69**(2): 597–607.

129 Mandel TE, Koulmanda M, Mackay IR. Prevention of spontaneous and cyclophosphamide-induced diabetes in non-obese diabetic (NOD) mice with oral 2-acetyl-4-tetrahydroxybutylimidazole (TH1), a component of caramel colouring III. *Clin Exp Immunol* 1992; **88**(3): 414–19.

130 Rjasanowski I, Heinke P, Michaelis D, Kurajewa TL. The higher frequency of type I (insulin-dependent) diabetes in fathers than in mothers of type I-diabetic children. *Exp Clin Endocrinol* 1990; **95**(1): 91–6.

131 Warram JH, Krolewski AS, Gottlieb MS, Kahn CR. Differences in risk of insulin-dependent diabetes in offspring of diabetic mothers and diabetic fathers. *N Engl J Med* 1984; **311**(3): 149–52.

132 Bock T, Kjaer TW, Jorgensen M, Josefsen K, Rygaard J, Buschard K. Reduction of diabetes incidence in NOD mice by neonatal glucose treatment. *Apmis* 1991; **99**(11): 989–92.

133 Fox HS. Androgen treatment prevents diabetes in nonobese diabetic mice. *J Exp Med* 1992; **175**(5): 1409–12.

134 Kawamura T, Nagata M, Utsugi T, Yoon JW. Prevention of autoimmune type I diabetes by CD4+ suppressor T cells in superantigen-treated non-obese diabetic mice. *J Immunol* 1993; **151**(8): 4362–70.

21

Future Approaches to Prevention

JAY S. SKYLER and JENNIFER B. MARKS
Division of Endocrinology, Departments of Medicine, Pediatrics, and Psychology,
University of Miami, Florida, USA

It is generally accepted that Type 1 or insulin-dependent diabetes mellitus (IDDM) arises as a consequence of immunologically mediated pancreatic islet β-cell destruction in genetically susceptible individuals[1,2]. Yet, the pathogenesis of Type 1 diabetes appears to involve a disruption of the balance between forces propelling the progression of disease and forces retarding or preventing that progression (Figure 21.1). This delicate balance appears to be in place for genetic factors, environmental factors, and immune regulation. Thus, there have been identified genes that confer susceptibility or predisposition to the disease, and genes that confer protection against development of the disease. But, additional susceptibility and protective genes are yet undefined. Likewise, there are apparent environmental insults which have the potential of triggering development of disease in genetically susceptible individuals, while other environmental factors appear to be associated with protection from development of disease. However, it remains unclear which environmental elements stimulate the disease process and which inhibit it. In addition, there seem to be complex regulatory interactions among various elements of the immune response, although it is unclear which elements of the immune circuitry are responsible for β-cell destruction and which are responsible for β-cell protection. The prevalent view is that islet cell destruction is enhanced by CD8+ cytotoxic T lymphocytes stimulated by a T-helper-1 (Th1) subset of CD4+ lymphocytes, with inhibition of islet destruction by a T-helper-2 (Th2) subset of CD4+ T lymphocytes and CD8+ suppressor T lymphocytes[3]. Thus, the pathogenetic sequence can be altered either by down-regulation of

Prediction, Prevention and Genetic Counseling in IDDM. Edited by Jerry P. Palmer.
© 1996 John Wiley & Sons Ltd.

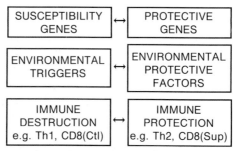

Figure 21.1. Elements in the pathogenesis of Type 1 diabetes. Type 1 diabetes emerges when the elements in the left-hand column outweigh the elements in the right-hand column, i.e. when the balance of forces favors processes which eventuate in immune destruction of islet β cells

destructive forces or by enhancement of protective forces. This explains why both immunosuppressive and immunostimulatory (or immunomodulatory) approaches may be beneficial. In addition, however, it is argued whether Type 1 diabetes is an antigen-specific autoimmune disease or an inflammatory disease which arises because the β cell is inherently less able to withstand local environmental insults than are other cell types[4].

In fact, the development of Type 1 diabetes may involve collaboration among islet-cell specific and non-specific mechanisms, including a complex orchestration of the entire immunologica repertoire[3,4]. Diabetes develops in a highly tissue-specific, cytokine-rich environment of insulitis. Immune activation appears to involve presentation (by antigen presenting cells in the context of MHC class II molecules) to the immune system of a diabetogenic peptide (as yet unknown, although there are several candidates). There is consequent activation of a T-helper-1 (Th1) subset of CD4+T lymphocytes. The cytokines produced by Th1-cell activation, interleukin-2 (IL-2) and interferon-γ (IFN-γ), activate cytotoxic T lymphocytes and cytotoxic macrophages to kill islet β cells by a variety of mechanisms. These killing mechanisms include oxygen free radicals, nitric oxide, destructive cytokines [interleukin-1 (IL-1), tumor necrosis factor-α (TNF-α), tumor necrosis factor-β (TNF-β), and interferon-γ (IFN-γ)], and CD8+ cytotoxic T lymphocytes that interact with a β cell autoantigen–MHC class I complex. Once the initial immune destruction commences, secondary and tertiary immune responses also are activated, with virtually the whole immunologic army attacking β cells. In the process, many β-cell proteins serve as antigens that generate both cellular and humoral immune responses, thus rendering nearly impossible the task of identifying putative "primary" triggering antigens.

The possibility of interrupting this pathogenetic sequence by immune intervention offers us the opportunity to alter the natural history of Type 1 diabetes. Disruption of the sequence at any number of points may interrupt the process by which diabetes ensues. Thus, a vast variety of approaches have been eminently successful in animal models of Type 1 diabetes, such as the NOD (non-obese diabetic) mouse and the BB (Biobreeding) rat. The array of immune interventions used has been both immunosuppressive and immunomodulatory (or immunostimulatory).

In recent years, immune intervention has been attempted in human Type 1 diabetes as well[5-7]. Human experiments have entailed two basic strategies. The first of these is immune intervention begun shortly after diagnosis of Type 1 diabetes, in an effort to: (a) decrease the severity of clinical manifestations; (b) halt destruction of residual β cells; and (c) perhaps allow some recovery of β-cell function. This strategy capitalizes on the fact that it is easy to ascertain a cohort of study subjects at the time of diagnosis, since their identify is known. Yet, at this stage, most β-cell function has already been lost, making the task of finding successful strategies more difficult. Indeed, it is possible that a strategy that could be successful if applied early would be doomed to failure if tested so late in the course of the disease that clinical diabetes was already present. Therefore, much attention has been focused on the second strategy, that which is aimed at prevention or delay of disease onset in susceptible individuals, by altering the pathogenic sequence earlier in its course, prior to clinical manifestations of Type 1 diabetes. Such intervention is contingent on effective case finding. Generally this involves the screening of high risk individuals, e.g. relatives of persons with Type 1 diabetes. Yet, at this stage, individuals are clinically healthy. As a consequence, any intervention to be tested must be reasonably safe.

Type 1 diabetes develops as an insidious process which occurs over years. During the stage of disease evolution, this has led to much effort in prediction of which individuals are destined to develop the disease. Such prediction is crucial for the testing of any intervention strategy. For ease of implementation, many such efforts involve first degree relatives of patients with Type 1 diabetes, since such relatives have a 10- to 20-fold increased empiric risk of Type 1 diabetes (about 3–6% risk of diabetes among first degree relatives) compared to the general population (prevalence about 0.25–0.3%). However, as many as 80–90% of individuals with new-onset Type 1 diabetes do not have a first degree relative with the disease and would be missed by an approach that was only suitable for first degree relatives. Therefore, this has stimulated efforts to identify those in the general population at risk of developing the disease—through combinations of screening for genetic and immune markers. Yet, depending on the nature of a proposed intervention strategy—in terms of risks, costs, convenience, ease of use—prediction may not be essential from a public health standpoint. On a population basis, theoretically it could be easier and less expensive to vaccinate the entire population against Type 1 diabetes, if an extremely safe, inexpensive vaccine were available. On the other hand, applying any therapy to society at large is frought with enormous difficulty in terms of implementation.

With all of this interest, and much ongoing investigation, there now is enormous promise for future prevention of Type 1 diabetes mellitus. Earlier chapters have outlined some of the approaches currently being explored: generalized immunosuppression (e.g. cyclosporine, azathioprine); drugs that protect the β cell from damage (e.g. nicotinamide); antigen-based therapies (e.g. insulin); approaches that alter the balance of elements within the immune repertoire (e.g. oral tolerance); and approaches that would seek to alter neonatal immune development (e.g. exposure to cow's milk proteins). As one examines these approaches currently under investigation, it is evident that they are based on different putative strategies of disease pathogenesis.

In this chapter, we will project future developments for prevention of Type 1 diabetes, recognizing the limitations outlined above, recognizing that we are basing most of our projections on observations in animal models and that we must exert caution in comparing directly animal models and human disease[8], and recognizing the inherent dangers in crystal ball observations. Nevertheless, buoyed by the tremendous advances being made in human studies involving immune modulation of Type 1 diabetes, we will attempt to project the future.

PEPTIDE-MEDIATED IMMUNOTHERAPY

The ultimate goal is to develop vaccine preparations that are capable of generating vigorous memory responses without triggering unwanted side-effects. The development of such vaccines would be greatly facilitated if the IDDM-initiating autoantigen was biochemically defined, such that the relevant antigenic peptides could be isolated and the pathogenetic epitopes identified.

There are several potential mechanisms by which peptides may mediate immunotherapy. Through any of these mechanisms, the use of peptide vaccines may prove to be a singularly important approach in preventing Type 1 diabetes. These are discussed below.

PEPTIDE IMMUNIZATION

Theoretically, one might expect that diabetes could be best prevented by administration, in a protective mode, of the relevant islet β-cell antigen responsible for disease initiation[9,10]. This might involve use of either the antigen itself, some subunit or epitope thereof, or a homologous molecule perhaps synthesized in the laboratory. The identification of relevant initiating or triggering antigens provides the basis for antigen-specific intervention using peptide-mediated immunotherapy. Of the multiple candidate antigens identified to date, most studies have focused on either insulin or glutamic acid decarboxylase (GAD), although the principles might apply to other candidate antigens as well.

Peptides may act via active immune sensitization to the peptide autoantigen, inducing an immunoregulatory network with protective properties. This may involve stimulation of suppressor cells or selective activation of Th2 versus Th1 responses. In the latter circumstance, the peptide-based therapeutic immunization does not require that the peptide be involved in initiation or triggering of the immune response. The peptide may also be effective by "bystander immunosuppression", i.e. an antigen-specific immunoregulatory cell release of cytokines by active T cells (Th2 cells) upon re-encounter with inciting antigen, thus down-regulating other autoreactive immune cells in the islet inflammatory lesion, irrespective of their cognate antigens[11].

Physical form may determine whether the response to a given antigen or peptide is positive or negative, whether it is immunogenic or tolerogenic. This may be because of different epitopes being presented or different affinities of a given peptide for distinct MHC molecules. The dose and route of administration may also influence the nature of the response.

Among the peptides that have been used for vaccination to prevent Type 1 diabetes in animal models are insulin[12], insulin β-chain[13], glutamic acid decarboxylase[14], a peptide (the p227 fragment) of the 60 kDa human heat shock protein (hsp 60)[15], and mycobacterium heat shock protein 65 (hsp 65)[16]. Synthetic peptides also have been used as blocking agents in preventing the transfer of diabetes in NOD mice[10,17,18].

PEPTIDES AS SPECIFIC T-CELL RECEPTOR (TCR) ANTAGONISTS

Synthetic peptides similar in structure to autoantigens may be useful as peptide antagonists[19,20]. These antigen analogs bind to class II MHC molecules but differ from native peptides by a few amino acids[20]. As a consequence, there is peptide competition for binding to class II MHC molecules. This has been demonstrated both in vitro and in vivo. These subtle differences in structure between the peptide competitors and the native molecule result in binding of the analog to class II MHC molecules, thus blocking recognition of self-antigen and consequent T-lymphocyte activation. To accomplish this, an analog should be altered such that the synthetic molecule is incapable of activating T cells specific for the antigenic peptide despite still being capable of effectively competing for T-cell engagement with native antigenic peptide. Such synthetic analogs have been used successfully in the treatment of experimental autoimmune diseases in animals, including Type 1 diabetes[9].

INDUCTION OF ANERGY

Peptides may also be used to induce anergy[21]. For example, if Type 1 diabetes arises, in part, due to failure of self-antigen-induced T-lymphocyte ablation in neonatal life, then early "booster" vaccination with a synthetic peptide may prevent disease by inducing anergy or facilitating T-cell ablation. Caution must be exerted in developing such strategies, however, because the same or similar peptides may also have the potential of inducing disease by triggering proliferative expansion of T cells. Moreover, the effects of peptides in thymocyte selection—positive versus negative—may be related to dose of peptide, the epitope bound and/or the affinity of the peptide presented to class II MHC molecules[22].

HLA-DERIVED PEPTIDES

Synthetic peptides corresponding to linear sequences of HLA class I and class II molecules have been found to be capable of inducing tolerance[23]. Both HLA allele-specific peptides and HLA allele-nonspecific peptides have been identified. Class I peptides that are allele nonspecific have been developed and shown to have potent inhibitory effects, inhibiting generation of cytolytic lymphocytes (CTLs) and inhibiting cytolysis by established CTLs. They have been shown to be capable of inhibiting allograft rejection. More recently, allele nonspecific synthetic class II peptides have also been produced. These, too, have been shown to have the capacity to inhibit T-cell proliferation, generation of CTL precursors, and cytotoxicity by established CTLs. Given the ability of these peptides to inhibit established cytotoxicity, their role in modulating the course of autoimmunity should be explored.

SUPERANTIGEN-BASED VACCINES

If there is restricted T-cell receptor (TCR) usage in Type 1 diabetes, another possible strategy is to inhibit the anti-islet immune response by vaccination with TCR peptides or superantigens[19,24]. In some animal models of autoimmune disease, the use of such TCR peptides can prevent disease occurrence. To date, however, it remains unclear whether there is restricted TCR usage even in animal models of Type 1 diabetes. The available data in human diabetes are confined to two individuals who succumbed from the disease early in its course[25]. However, it is possible that these two individuals may have had an explosive viral etiology for their diabetes and may not have had typical Type 1 diabetes. As a consequence, our interpretation is that superantigens-based vaccines are unlikely to prove fruitful.

INSULIN AND INSULIN PEPTIDES FOR PEPTIDE-MEDIATED IMMUNOTHERAPY

Although a variety of potential candidate antigens have been identified, it should be appreciated that insulin is the best characterized and most β-cell specific molecule. Therefore, a variety of strategies have been proposed based on the use of insulin and insulin peptides to prevent diabetes. Although similar approaches could be used for other candidate antigens in programs of peptide-mediated immunotherapy, it is our bias that insulin is the most suitable and most logical peptide to use for this purpose. Therefore, we extensively discuss its potential use. Nevertheless, similar strategies could be applied to other appropriate peptides.

ANIMAL STUDIES

Insulin-specific T lymphocytes are a predominant part of the islet infiltrate in NOD mice. Indeed, insulin-specific T lymphocytes have been found to be present in high frequency among nominally islet-cell-specific T lymphocytes in the islet infiltrates that accumulate in NOD mice[26]. Insulin-specific T-lymphocyte clones have been propagated from cells obtained from islet infiltrates. All clones tested could mediate β-cell destruction upon adoptive transfer[27]. Most were found to produce IFN-γ, but none produced IL-4. A 15-residue peptide of the insulin β chain (B9-23) is the dominent epitope for this response.

PARENTERAL INSULIN

Insulin injections (subcutaneously or intraperitoneally) have been shown to delay the development of diabetes and to inhibit the appearance and progression of insulitis in animal models of Type 1 diabetes. Injection of young, pre-diabetic BB rats or NOD mice with insulin inhibits the development of both insulitis and diabetes[28-35]. Insulin therapy also prevents adoptive transfer of diabetes in NOD mice[36]. Insulin may be acting immunologically—by immunization, tolerization, or immune modulation[12,13,37-39]. Alternatively, insulin may be acting metabolically—by resting β-cell function, thereby making β cells less susceptible to immune attack. The hypothesis is that by giving insulin before the development of overt disease, it is possible to reduce antigen expression associated with endogenous insulin secretion[40-42]. In vitro, actively secreting β cells are more susceptible to immune attack, including cytotoxic actions of cytokines, than are resting β cells.

INSULIN VACCINATION

Insulin or insulin β-chain immunization, by periodic vaccination in incomplete Freund's adjuvant, has been shown to prevent the development of insulitis and diabetes in NOD mice[12,13]. This appears to be an active immune sensitization to the autoantigen—not anergy induction. The immunization appears to work by induction of a complex lymphocyte immunoregulatory network that has protective properties. It requires both CD4+ and CD8+T lymphocytes to successfully transfer the antidiabetic effect. The near complete protection from diabetes after therapeutic immunization with β-chain insulin is consistent with "bystander immunosuppression".

ORAL INSULIN

Oral administration of insulin to young NOD mice results in less insulitis and delays onset of Type 1 diabetes[12,43–45]. Moreover, spleen cells from animals treated with oral insulin have been shown to prevent the adoptive transfer of diabetes when used in co-transfer experiments. In a variety of experimental models of autoimmune diseases in animals, oral ingestion of soluble antigens has been shown to establish immunological tolerance. This is presumed to result because presentation of antigens to the immune system via the intestinal mucosa stimulates a Th2 subset of helper T lymphocytes, which migrate to the pancreas and secrete inhibitory cytokines which down-regulate ongoing destructive immune cells in the islet inflammatory lesion, irrespective of their cognate antigens, thus working by "bystander immunosuppression"[46].

NASAL INSULIN

Likewise, administration of a 15-residue peptide of the insulin β chain (B9-23) by nose drops to young NOD mice has been shown to prevent the development of insulitis and diabetes[47].

HUMAN STUDIES

In contrast to other candidate antigens, insulin has the advantages of being β-cell specific, of not otherwise affecting the immune system, of being an agent whose effects on people are well understood, and of having side-effects that are well known and can be controlled. As a consequence, it has become the focus of attention in human studies.

In patients with type 1 diabetes, when there is preservation of β-cell function, there is greater metabolic stability and overall management is easier[48–56]. Several clinical studies have suggested that early and more aggressive insulin treatment may result in preservation of β-cell function, better metabolic control, and/or a prolonged honeymoon period[57–59]. However, the results have been inconsistent. In a study from Tampa, intensive insulin therapy in newly diagnosed patients, involving two weeks' treatment with intravenous insulin delivered via an artificial pancreas, preserved β-cell function for at least one year[60]. The response was similar to that seen in studies with conventional immunosuppression using cyclosporin or azathioprine.

Three pilot studies have investigated the use of insulin in relatives of Type 1 diabetic probands at high risk of diabetes. One such pilot study, from Boston, involved 12 subjects, 5 of whom accepted treatment, and 7 of whom declined and were followed as a comparison group[61]. This study suggested that prophylactic parenteral insulin therapy combining 5 days of insulin by intravenous infusion every 9 months and daily subcutaneous insulin injections could preserve β-cell function and may delay the appearance of diabetes. Subsequently, these investigators joined with colleagues in Denver, and continued this approach while enrolling subjects in a randomized fashion, with similar results. Another pilot study, from Munich, has randomized 10 similar subjects to a protocol of intravenous insulin for 7 days every 12 months, combined with daily subcutaneous insulin injections for the first 6 months[62]. It, too, suggests that diabetes may be delayed by such intervention. A third pilot study, from Gainesville, has treated a larger group of relatives, some already with onset of glucose intolerance, with daily subcutaneous insulin injections, and report the approach safe and the preliminary results encouraging[12].

These preliminary results have served as an impetus to the initiation of the *Diabetes Prevention Trial of Type 1 Diabetes* (DPT-1)[63,64]. DPT-1 is a randomized, controlled, nationwide, multicenter clinical trial, designed to test whether intervention with insulin during the prodromal period of the disease can delay the appearance of overt clinical diabetes in high risk relatives. In the "High Risk" group (i.e. $\geq 50\%$ risk over 5 years), the protocol is designed to determine whether parenteral insulin therapy, consisting of periodic courses of continuous intravenous insulin, with accompanying chronic subcutaneous insulin, will delay their expected development of clinical Type 1 diabetes. In those relatives with "Intermediate Risk" (i.e. 25–50% risk over 5 years), the protocol being planned is a randomized, placebo-controlled, double-masked, multicenter clinical trial designed to determine whether oral insulin could induce disease-relevant immunological tolerance, thereby delaying the development of Type 1 diabetes[65].

The idea of testing insulin to prevent diabetes is not new. As early as 1940, in the *New England Journal of Medicine*, Haist et al. suggested:

The prophylactic administration of insulin to potential diabetic patients may become an accepted clinical procedure in the future. We suggest that the incidence of diabetes should be investigated in two large and comparable groups of children with a family history of this disease ... [one] group might receive insulin in the limited amounts which may be safely given under these conditions. We appreciate the difficulties inherent in this type of clinical investigation, but believe that the goal justifies the endeavor[66].

It is likely that insulin or insulin peptides will be prime candidates for peptide-mediated immunotherapy, and may be the mainstay of diabetes prevention. Our prediction is that insulin, insulin β chain, or a peptide fragment of insulin

β chain, will be used in widescale programs of vaccination to prevent Type 1 diabetes mellitus. Whether this will be best accomplished by parenteral administration in a vaccine, oral administration, or nasal administration, will be established by future studies.

MILK-PROTEIN-BASED IMMUNOTHERAPY

One potential environmental influence in human Type 1 diabetes is neonatal and early infancy nutrition. In epidemiological studies, there is a reciprocal relationship between history of breast feeding and the frequency of Type 1 diabetes[67,68]. A small prospective Finnish study has suggested that exclusive breast feeding may reduce the likelihood of disease development[69]. Although consumption of breast milk may lead to disease protection, it has been proposed that consumption of cow's milk proteins, particularly early in life, may lead to the initiation of the immunologic attack against pancreatic islet β cells and increase susceptibility to Type 1 diabetes[70]. This may be operating through molecular mimicry. There is homology between a 69 kDa pancreatic β-cell surface protein known as p69 or ICA 69 and a 17 amino acid sequence (ABBOS) of bovine serum albumin, a major cow's milk protein[71]. In Type 1 diabetes both T-cell activation and anergy to ICA69 have been demonstrated[72]. High affinity recombinant ICA69 as a self-peptide (or an epitope thereof, including a synthetic T-cell epitope Tep69) triggers anergy. In contrast, the low affinity mimicry protein (bovine serum albumin) triggers proliferative expansion of T cells in vitro. Therefore, disease pathogenesis may involve mimicry in which bovine serum albumin prevents self-peptide (ICA69)-induced T-cell ablation in neonatal life.

To test this hypothesis, a multinational experiment is being planned to test whether the frequency of Type 1 diabetes can be reduced by preventing exposure to cow's milk proteins during early life[70]. This randomized prospective trial will involve over 5000 infants, who will be newborns with first degree relatives with Type 1 diabetes. Those genetically determined to be at high risk will be randomized to receive either a formula free of cow's milk or a conventional cows milk based formula. The intervention will be for a 6 month period, with follow-up for 10 years. This would be a "true" primary prevention strategy.

On the other hand, it should be noted that one recent report has found that ICA69 and bovine serum albumin are not antigenically cross-reactive[73]. Nevertheless, if ICA69 is indeed important in disease pathogenesis, it might be possible to use a synthetic T-cell epitope peptide (e.g. Tep69) to induce anergy and thereby prevent disease. Such a strategy might involve early inoculation with this peptide as an infant vaccine. This strategy does not have to be confined to ICA69. It could be used with any islet cell protein found to be important in disease pathogenesis, in which an epitope peptide is shown to be capable of inducing anergy.

IMMUNE SYSTEM STIMULATION

The autoimmune response leading to islet β-cell destruction and consequent diabetes may be amenable to prevention or suppression by therapeutic interventions aimed at stimulating the host's own immunoregulatory mechanisms[4]. The goal is to convert the immune response from a destructive to a non-destructive process. This may be accomplished by the administration of a variety of substances, including microbial agents, adjuvants, and putative β-cell autoantigens, which have diabetes-protective effects. These effects may result from activation of a Th2 subset of T cells that produce the cytokines IL-4 and IL-10 and consequently down-regulate the Th1-cell-mediated autoimmune response.

IMMUNOSTIMULANT VACCINES

Early vaccination with complete Freund's adjuvant (CFA) prevents diabetes in NOD mice[74,75] and BB rats[76]. The protection can be adoptively transferred to other NOD mice[74]. CFA also prevents recurrent diabetes in NOD mice following islet transplantation[77]. Protection also has been reported in NOD mice by vaccination with BCG (bacillus Calmette–Guérin strain of *Mycobacterium bovis*)[78,79]. It may be that stimulation with CFA or BCG induces a generalized activation of protective components of the immune system, thus decreasing the immune attack on β cells. A pilot study with BCG in new-onset diabetes suggested better preservation of β-cell function[80]. This has led to the initiation of several full-scale clinical trials of BCG in new-onset diabetes, now underway in Edmonton, Denver, Ann Arbor, Rome, Australia, and Israel. It is theoretically possible that a program of repetitive vaccination might influence the development of human Type 1 diabetes.

Exposure to a variety of viruses may influence the development of Type 1 diabetes. This is thought to occur because of molecular mimicry involving homology between the structure of a β-cell protein and a viral protein. Such homology has been suggested between glutamic acid decarboxylase (GAD) and coxsackie protein P2-C, between insulin and a retrovirus sequence, and between a 52 kDa islet protein and a rubella protein. The potential role of these viruses in disease pathogenesis is unclear, but a possibility is that they may initiate pathogenetic immune mechanisms. Theoretically, it is possible to develop protective vaccines based on the structure of viral proteins, perhaps using subunits or analogs selected for eliciting protective responses.

LINOMIDE

Linomide, quinoline-3-carboxamide, is a synthetic immunomodulator that up-regulates several T-lymphocyte-dependent functions, including lymphocyte proliferation in response to mitogens, enhancement of cellular immune responses such as delayed type hypersensitivity (DTH) reactions, and increases in the number and function of NK cells[81]. Linomide administration to young NOD mice has been shown to result in complete protection from insulitis and maintenance of normal glucose tolerance for over 40 weeks[82,83]. Linomide suppresses autoreactivity, even in NODs with established insulitis, without causing systemic immunosuppression. Therefore, linomide is now being tested in new-onset Type 1 diabetes[82].

MONOCLONAL ANTIBODY IMMUNOMODULATION

Prevention and reversal of autoimmune disease with a variety of monoclonal antibodies has been demonstrated in animal models[7]. These strategies using MoAbs include: blocking helper T lymphocytes with anti-CD4 MoAb; blocking activated T-lymphocytes with anti-IL-2 receptor MoAb; blocking cytotoxic T-lymphocytes with anti-CD8 MoAb; blocking general T-lymphocyte response with anti-CD2 or anti-CD3 or anti-CD5 MoAbs; blocking antigen presentation or recognition with anti-MHC class II (anti-DQ) MoAb (presumably directed against polymorphic determinants associated with class II gene products) or with anti-Ia MoAb; blocking T-cell receptor (TCR) recognition of antigen either with anti-idiotype MoAb or with anti-TCR MoAb (presumably directed against a specific V_β chain); blocking stimulation of MHC presentation with anti-γ-interferon MoAb; blocking effects of other cytokines with anti-cytokine MoAbs. All of these strategies have been successfully applied in animal models of either Type 1 diabetes or other autoimmune diseases.

Several monoclonal antibodies already have been evaluated for potential effectiveness in pilot studies in new-onset Type 1 diabetes[5]. These have included: an antiblast antibody (CBL1), an anti-CD3 antibody (OKT3), an anti-CD4 antibody, an anti-CD5 immunoconjugate coupled to the α chain of ricin toxin (CD5+), a humanized chimeric anti-CD4 antibody, an anti-interleukin 2 receptor (IL-2R) antibody, and an interleukin 2 receptor (IL-2R) targeted fusion protein, consisting of a diphtheria-toxin-related protein linked to interleukin 2 (IL-2) $(DAB_{486}\text{-}IL2)$[84-90]. (The latter approach, although not using a monoclonal antibody, also specifically targets activated T cells.) Preliminary experience with these agents has generally been suggestive that there is preservation of β-cell function. Unfortunately, full-scale, controlled trials of these or similar therapies have not yet been reported. Other monoclonal antibody strategies are being contemplated. In each of these cases, the strategy of creating conjugate molecules as immunotoxins could be used with any of the MoAbs, as could the strategy of making chimeric "humanized" MoAbs to obviate the immune response against murine immunoglobulin.

A disease-specific approach would be to block antigen recognition by using an anti-β-cell-antigen MoAb, once relevant antigens have been identified. When that is the case, it also may be possible to use purified β-cell antigen itself, linked in a toxin conjugate, to specifically target those cells recognizing that antigen, in a manner analogous to the way the fusion protein DAB_{486}-IL-2 is targeted against the IL-2 receptor of activated T lymphocytes[89,90].

CYTOKINE MANIPULATION

Cytokines and monoclonal antibodies against cytokines have been used in experimental animals to induce diabetes and to inhibit the development of diabetes. Understanding of factors favoring induction of favorable cytokines may offer potential for influencing the course of the disease. For example, the administration of the combination of IL-4 and IL-10 inhibits recurrence of diabetes in NOD mice receiving syngeneic islet transplants[91]. Inhibitors of unfavorable cytokines may also be used. For example, whereas IL-12 administration, by inducing Th1 cells, accelerates the development of massive insulitis and autoimmune diabetes in NOD mice[92], administration of the IL-12 subunit p40 specifically inhibits effects of IL-12[93].

T-CELL VACCINATION

T-cell vaccination involves the use of attenuated autoimmune T cells as vaccines to prevent autoimmune disease[94,95]. Antigen-specific T cells are used for vaccination. Reactive T cells must first be identified, then modified to render them immunogenic yet attenuated, either by the use of chemical cross-linkers (e.g. glutaraldehyde or paraformaldehyde), mitomycin-C, or by gamma irradiation. Immunization with the T-cell clones then stimulates an anti-T-cell response which suppresses the recipient's own autoreactive T cells. Antigen specificity (anti-idiotypic T cells) is of critical importance, since it is possible to generate T-cell clones that are directed against cellular activation markers (so-called anti-ergotypic T cells) which would be non-specific in their immunosuppressive effects. Lymphocyte vaccination has been shown to prevent diabetes in NOD mice[96,97]. In one study, it was demonstrated that vaccination with T cells specific for the p227 fragment of heat shock protein-60 (hsp 60) results in suppression of disease in NOD mice[96].

Theoretically, it is also possible to generate autologous immunoregulatory

T-cell clones with suppressor activity, that could be reinfused in an individual to down-regulate the immune response.

It remains unclear whether cellular vaccination therapy with T lymphocytes will have any real role in the clinical prevention of Type 1 diabetes. Although theoretically exciting, we remain skeptical about the practicalities of this approach.

TOLERANCE INDUCTION

In animal models of Type 1 diabetes, there has been tolerance induction with elimination of disease rendering T cells by islet transplantation into the thymus[98–101]. In addition, the intrathymic injection of the putative islet autoantigen glutamic acid decarboxylase (GAD) has also been shown to induce tolerance in NOD mice[102]. However, the induction of tolerance by injection of islets or antigens into the thymus is a procedure highly unlikely to emerge as a clinical approach. It is thus deemed not very feasible for human beings.

PROSPECTS FOR GENE THERAPY

Genes conferring risk of Type 1 diabetes have been identified at multiple loci[103]. The strongest genetic predisposition is associated with genes in the major histocompatibility complex (MHC), particularly HLA-DR and HLA-DQ region alleles[104,105]. The strongest predisposition to Type 1 diabetes in Europoids is associated with HLA-DR3,DQB1*0201 and with HLA-DR4, DQA1*0501-DQB1*0302. Yet, other DQ alleles, e.g. DQA1*0201-DQB1*0602, confer protection from Type 1 diabetes. That protection is dominant over susceptibility. Thus, DQA1*0201-DQB1*0602 provides protection even in the presence of DQ susceptibility alleles. This offers the potential for gene therapy, which might be envisioned as insertion of protective immune response genes into homologous bone marrow stem cells that are then reinfused into a given individual.

CONCLUSIONS

There are many positive developments which herald the future for the prevention of Type 1 diabetes mellitus. Progress is continuing towards a more complete understanding of the pathophysiology of the disease. This will permit more targeted approaches designed to interdict the disease process by appropriate immune intervention—immunosuppressive or immunomodulatory. Immunosuppressive agents are cytotoxic, by definition; whereas immunomodulating agents act by enhancing or diminishing immune responses, including interrupting or modifying the pathways that mediate β-cell destruction.

Simultaneously, a better understanding of the genetic factors which control predisposition—both susceptibility and protection—to the disease will allow early identification of individuals at risk of developing the disease. Identification and characterization of potential candidate autoantigens will permit the development of assays capable of accurate detection and marking of the onset of immunologic processes. More importantly, molecularly characterized autoantigens will permit the development of specific peptide therapies based on putative pathogenetically important molecules. In development of such approaches, it should be appreciated that diabetes may eventually arise only after β cells suffer progressive damage from a cascade of autoimmune responses against multiple autoantigens. Yet, a therapy based on any of the specific antigens involved in the process, e.g. peptide immunization therapy, may inhibit progression of an important determinant cascade.

In pursuing prevention of Type 1 diabetes, it is important that investigations be confined to carefully designed, randomized, controlled clinical trials. Moreover, it is desirable to test treatments which are relatively innocuous. If successful, prevention of diabetes could spare future generations (and the individuals participating in trials) from a lifelong disease associated with morbid complications. Therefore, the conduct of studies is justifiable.

The ultimate goal of prevention of Type 1 diabetes mellitus is an achievable one.

REFERENCES

1 Atkinson MA, Maclaren NK. The pathogenesis of insulin dependent diabetes mellitus. *New Engl J Med* 1994; **331**: 1428–36.
2 Bach JF. Insulin-dependent diabetes mellitus as an autoimmune disease. *Endocr Revs* 1994; **15**: 516–42.
3 Rabinovitch A. Immunoregulatory and cytokine imbalances in the pathogenesis of IDDM: therapeutic intervention by immunostimulation? *Diabetes* 1994; **43**: 613–21.
4 Kolb H, Kolb-Bachofen V, Roep BO. Autoimmune versus inflammatory Type I diabetes: a controversy? *Immunology Today* 1995; **16**: 170–2.
5 Skyler JS, Marks JB. Immune intervention in Type I mellitus. *Diabetes Revs* 1993; **1**: 15–42.
6 Pozzilli P, Kolb H, Ilkova HM (eds). New trends for prevention and immunotherapy of insulin dependent diabetes mellitus. *Diabetes Metab Revs* 1993; **9**: 237–348.
7 Bach JF. Immunosuppression in insulin-dependent diabetes mellitus: from cellular selectivity towards autoantigen specificity. *Chem Immunol* 1995; **60**: 32–47.
8 Rossini AA, Handler ES, Mordes JP, Greiner DL. Animal models of human disease. Human autoimmune diabetes mellitus: lessons from BB rats and NOD mice—*caveat*

emptor. *Clin Immunol Immunopath* 1995; **74**: 2–9.

9 Fathman CG. Peptides as therapy of autoimmune disease. *Diabetes Metab Revs* 1993; **9**: 239–44.

10 Smilek DE, Lock CB, McDevitt HO. Antigen recognition and peptide-mediated immunotherapy in autoimmune disease. *Immunol Revs* 1990; **118**: 37–71.

11 Hafler DA, Weiner HL. Antigen-specific immunosuppression: oral tolerance for the treatment of autoimmune disease. *Chem Immunol* 1995; **60**: 126–49.

12 Muir A, Schatz D, Maclaren M. Antigen-specific immunotherapy: oral tolerance and subcutaneous immunization in the treatment of insulin-dependent diabetes. *Diabetes Metab Revs* 1993; **9**: 279–87.

13 Muir A, Peck A, Clare-Salzler M, Song YH, Cornelius J, Luchetta R, Krischer J, Maclaren N. Insulin immunization of nonobese diabetic mice induces a protective insulitis characterized by diminished intraislet interferon-γ transcription. *J Clin Invest* 1995; **95**: 628–34.

14 Kaufman D, Clare-Salzler M, Tian J, Forsthuber T, Ting GSP, Robinson P, Atkinson MA, Sercarz EE, Tobin AJ, Lehmann PV. Spontaneous loss of T-cell tolerance to glutamate decarboxylase in murine insulin-dependent diabetes. *Nature* 1993; **366**: 69–72.

15 Elias D, Cohen IR. Peptide therapy for diabetes in NOD mice. *Lancet* 1994; **343**: 704–6.

16 Shehadeh N, Calcinaro F, Bradley BJ, Bruchlim I, Vardi P, Lafferty K. Effects of adjuvant therapy on development of diabetes in mouse and man. *Lancet* 1994; **343**: 706–7.

17 Lock CB, Vaysburd M, McDevitt HO. Characterization of the NOD immune response and prevention of acute transfer of IDDM with a peptide binding to I-A NOD. *Diabetes Res Clin Pract* 1991; **14** Suppl 1): S39.

18 Hurtenbach U, Lier E, Adorini L, Nagy ZA. Prevention of autoimmune diabetes in the non-obese diabetes mice by treatment with a class II major histocompatibility complex blocking peptide. *J Exp Med* 1993; **177**: 1499–504.

19 Brostoff SW, Howell MD. Immunoregulation of autoimmune disease by vaccination with T cell receptor peptides. *Ann NY Acad Sci* 1991; **636**: 71–8.

20 Sette A, Alexander J, Ruppert J, Snoke K, Franco A, Ishioka G, Grey HM. Antigen analogs/MHC complexes as specific T cell receptor antagonists. *Ann Rev Immunol* 1994; **12**: 413–31.

21 Charlton B, Auchincloss H, Fathman CG. Mechanisms of transplantation tolerance. *Ann Rev Immunol* 1994; **12**: 707–34.

22 Sebzda E, Wallace VA, Mayer J, Yeung RSM, Mak TW, Ohashi PS. Positive and negative thymocyte selection induced by different concentrations of a single peptide. *Science* 1994; **263**: 1615–18.

23 Kresnky AM, Clayberger C. Human leukocyte antigen-derived peptides as novel immunosuppressives. *Proc Assn Am Phys* 1995; **107**: 81–5.

24 Conrad B, Trucco M. Superantigens as etiopathogentic factors in the development of insulin-dependent diabetes mellitus. *Diabetes Metab Revs* 1994; **10**: 309–38.

25 Conrad B, Weidmann E, Trucco G, Rudert WA, Ricordi C, Rodriquez-Rilo H, Behboo R, Finegold D, Trucco M. Evidence for superantigens involvement in insulin-dependent diabetes mellitus etiology. *Nature* 1994; **371**: 351–5.

26 Wegmann DR, Norbury-Glaser M, Daniel D. Insulin-specific T cells are a predominant component of islet infiltrates in pre-diabetic NOD mice. *Eur J Immunol* 1994; **24**: 1853–7.

27 Daniel D, Gill RG, Schloot N, Wegmann DR. Epitope specificity, cytokine production profile and diabetogenic activity of insulin-specific T cell clones isolated from NOD mice. *Eur J Immunol* 1995; **25**: 1056–62.

28 Gotfredsen GF, Buschard K, Frandsen EK. Reduction of diabetes incidence of BB Wistar rats by early prophylactic insulin treatment of diabetes-prone animals. *Diabetologia* 1985; **28**: 933–5.

29 Like AA. Morphology and mechanisms of autoimmune diabetes as revealed by studies of the BB/Wor rat. In Hanahan D, McDevitt HO, Cahill GJ (eds), *Perspectives on the Molecular Biology and Immunology of the Pancreatic Beta Cell.* Cold Spring Harbor: Current Communications in Molecular Biology, 1989, pp 81–91.

30 Like AA. Insulin injections prevent diabetes in Bio-Breeding/Worcester (BB/Wor) rats. *Diabetes* 1986; **35**(Suppl 1): 74A.

31 Vlahos WD, Seemayer TA, Yale JF. Diabetes prevention in BB rats by inhibition of endogenous insulin secretion. *Metabolism* 1991; **40**: 825–9.

32 Bertrand S, de Paepe M, Vigant C, Yale JF. Prevention of adoptive transfer in BB rats by prophylactic insulin treatment. *Diabetes* 1992; **41**: 1273–7.

33 Gottlieb PA, Handler ES, Appel MC, Greiner DL, Mordes JP, Rossini AA. Insulin treatment prevents diabetes mellitus but not thyroiditis in RT6-depleted diabetes resistant BB/Wor rats. *Diabetologia* 1991; **34**: 296–300.

34 Atkinson MA, Maclaren NK, Luchetta R. Insulitis and insulin dependent diabetes in NOD mice reduced by prophylactic insulin therapy. *Diabetes* 1990; **39**: 933–7.

35 Stubbs M, Like A. Insulin-releasing implants protect against KRV-induced diabetes in BB/Wor rats. *Diabetes* 1995; **44**(Suppl 1): 164A.

36 Thiovet CH, Goillot E, Bedossa P, Durand A, Bonnard M, Orgiazzi J. Insulin prevents adoptive cell transfer of diabetes in the autoimmune non-obese diabetic mouse. *Diabetologia* 1991; **34**: 314–19.

37 Bowman MA, Campbell L, Ellis TM, Darrow BL, Suresh A, Clare-Salzler M, Atkinson MA. Immunologic and metabolic effects of prophylactic insulin therapy in IDD. *Diabetes* 1995; **44**(Suppl 1): 137A.

38 Helderman JH, Pietri AO, Raskin P. In vitro control of T-lymphocyte insulin receptors by in vivo modulation of insulin. *Diabetes* 1983; **32**: 712–17.

39 Peakman M, Hussain MJ, Millward BA, Leslie RDG, Vergani D. Effect of initiation of insulin therapy on T-lymphocyte activation in Type 1 diabetes. *Diabetic Med* 1990; **7**: 327–30.

40 Aaen K, Rygard J, Josefson K, Petersen H, Brogren C-H, Horn T, Buschard K. Dependence of antigen expression on functional state of cells. *Diabetes* 1990; **39**: 697–701.

41 Bjork E, Kampe O, Andersson A, Karlsson FA. Expression of the 64K/glutamic acid decarboxylase rat islet autoantigen is influenced by the rate of insulin secretion. *Diabetologia* 1992; **35**: 490–3.

42 Bjork E, Kampe O, Karlsson FA, Pipeleers DG, Andersson A, Hellerstrom C, Eizirik DL. Glucose regulation of the autoantigen GAD65 in human pancreatic islets. *J Clin Endocrinol Metab* 1992; **75**: 1574–6.

43 Zhong ZJ, Davidson L, Eisenbarth GS, Weiner HL. Suppression of diabetes in non obese diabetic mice by oral administration of porcine insulin. *Proc Natl Acad Sci* 1991; **88**: 10252–6.

44 Dong J, Muir A, Schatz D, Luchetta R, Hao W, Atkinson M, Maclaren N. Oral administration of insulin prevents diabetes in NOD mice. *Diabetes Res Clin Pract* 1991; **14**(Suppl 1): S55.

45 Bergerot I, Fabien N, Maguer V, Thivolet C. Oral administration of human insulin to NOD mice generates CD4+ T cells that suppress adoptive transfer of diabetes. *J Autoimmunity* 1994; **7**: 655–63.

46 Weiner HL, Friedman A, Miller A, Khoury SJ, Al-Sabbagh A, Santos L, Sayegh M, Nussenblatt RB, Trentham DE, Hafler DA. Oral tolerance: immunologic mechanisms

and treatment of animal human organ-specific autoimmune diseases by oral administration of autoantigens. *Ann Rev Immunol* 1994; **12**: 808–37.
47 Daniel D, Wegmann DR. Intranasal administration of insulin peptide B:9-23 protects NOD mice from diabetes (submitted for publication).
48 Ludvigsson J, Heding LG, Larsen Y. C-Peptide in juvenile diabetics beyond the post-initial remission period: relation to clinical manifestations at onset of diabetes remission and diabetes control. *Acta Paed Scand* 1977; **66**: 177–82.
49 Grajwer LA, Pildes RS, Horwitz DL, Rubinstein AH. Control of juvenile diabetes mellitus and its relationship to endogenous insulin secretion as measured by C-peptide immunoreactivity. *J Ped* 1977; **90**: 42–8.
50 Eff C, Faber O, Deckert T. Persistent insulin secretion assessed by plasma C-peptide estimation in long term diabetics with low insulin requirements. *Diabetologia* 1978; **15**: 169–72.
51 Binder C, Faber OK. Residual beta cell function and its metabolic consequences. *Diabetes* 1978; **27**(Suppl 1): 226–9.
52 Gonen B, Goldman J, Baldwin D, Goldberg RB, Ryan WG, Blix PM, Schanzlin D, Fritz KJ, Rubinstein AH. Metabolic control in diabetic patients: effect of insulin secretory reserve (measured by plasma C-peptide levels) and circulating insulin antibodies. *Diabetes* 1979; **28**: 749–53.
53 Dahlquist G, Blom L, Bolme P, Hagenfeldt L, Lindgren F, Persson B, Thalme B, Theorell M, Westin S. Metabolic control in 131 juvenile-onset diabetic patients as measured by HbA1c: relation to age, duration, C-peptide, insulin dose, and one or two insulin injections. *Diabetes Care* 1982; **5**: 399–403.
54 Madsbad S. Prevalence of residual B cell function and its metabolic consequences in Type I (insulin dependent) diabetes. *Diabetologia* 1983; **24**: 141–6.
55 DCCT Research Group. Effects of age, duration, and treatment of insulin dependent diabetes mellitus on residual B cell function: observations during eligibility testing for the diabetes control and complications trial (DCCT). *J Clin Endocrinol Metab* 1987; **65**: 30–6.
56 Fukuda M, Tanaka Y, Ikegami H, Yamamoto Y, Kumahara Y, Shima K. Correlation between minimal secretory capacity of pancreatic B cells and stability of diabetic control. *Diabetes* 1988; **37**: 81–8.
57 Mirouze J, Selam JL, Pham TC, Mendoza E, Orsetti A. Sustained insulin induced remissions of juvenile diabetes by means of an external artificial pancreas. *Diabetologia* 1978; **14**: 223–7.
58 Madsbad S, Krarup T, Faber OK, Binder C, Regeur L. The transient effect of strict glycemic control on B cell function in newly diagnosed Type I (insulin-dependent) diabetic patients. *Diabetologia* 1982; **22**: 16–20.
59 Perlman K, Ehrlich RM, Filler RM, Albisser AM. Sustained normoglycemia in newly diagnosed Type I diabetic subjects: short term effects and one year follow-up. *Diabetes* 1984; **33**: 995–1001.
60 Shah SC, Malone JI, Simpson NE. A randomized trial of intensive insulin therapy in newly diagnosed Type I insulin-dependent diabetes mellitus. *New Engl J Med* 1989; **320**: 550–4.
61 Keller RJ, Eisenbarth GS, Jackson RA. Insulin prophylaxis in individuals at high risk of Type I diabetes. *Lancet* 1993; **341**: 927–8.
62 Ziegler A, Bachmann W, Rabl W. Prophylactic insulin treatment in relatives at high risk for Type I diabetes. *Diabetes Metab Revs* 1993; **9**: 289–93.
63 DPT-1 Study Group. The Diabetes Prevention Trial of Type 1 Diabetes (DPT-1). *Diabetes* 1994; **43**(Suppl 1): 160A.
64 DPT-1 Study Group. The Diabetes Prevention Trial of Type 1 Diabetes (DPT-1):

Implementation of screening and staging of relatives. *Diabetes* 1995; 44(Suppl 1): 129A.

65 Schatz D for the DPT-1 Study Group. The Diabetes Prevention Trial of Type 1 Diabetes (DPT-1): Design and implementation of the oral antigen (insulin) protocol. *Diabetes* 1995; 44(Suppl 1): 230A.

66 Haist RE, Campbell J, Best CH. The prevention of diabetes. *New Engl J Med* 1940; 223: 607–15.

67 Borch-Johnsen K, Joner G, Mandrup-Paulsen T, Christy M, Zachan-Christiansen B, Kastrup K, Nerup J. Relationship between breastfeeding and incidence rates of insulin dependent diabetes mellitus. *Lancet* 1984; 2: 1083–6.

68 Gerstein H. Cow's milk exposure and Type I diabetes mellitus. *Diabetes Care* 1994; 17: 13–19.

69 Virtanen SM, Rasanen L, Aro A, Lindstrom J, Sippola H, Lounamaa R, Toivanen L, Tuomilehto J, Akerblom HK, Childhood Diabetes in Finland Study Group. Infant feeding in Finnish children <7 yr of age with newly diagnosed IDDM. *Diabetes Care* 1991; 14: 415–17.

70 Akerblom HK, Savilahti E, Saukkonen TT, Paganus A, Virtanen SM, Teramo K, Knip M, Ilonen J, Reijonen H, Karjalainen J, Vaarala O, Reunanen A. The case for elimination of cow's milk in early infancy in prevention of Type I diabetes: the Finnish experience. *Diabetes Metab Revs* 1993; 9: 269–78.

71 Karjalainen J, Martin JM, Knip M, Ilonen J, Robinson BH, Savilahti E, Akerblom HK, Dosch HM. A bovine albumin peptide as a possible trigger of insulin dependent diabetes mellitus. *New Engl J Med* 1992; 327: 302–7.

72 Miyazaki I, Cheung RK, Gaedigk R, Hui MF, van der Muelen J, Rajotte RV, Dosch HM. T cell activation and anergy to islet cell antigen in Type I diabetes. *J Immunol* 1995; 154: 1461–9.

73 Rønningen KS, Atrazhev A, Smith D, Korbutt G, Rajotte RV, Halstensen T, Elliott JF. The 69kD islet cell autoantigen (ICA69) and bovine serum albumin are not antigenically cross-reactive. *Diabetes* 1995; 44(Suppl 1): 78A.

74 Sadelain MWJ, Qin H-Y, Lauzon J, Singh B. Prevention of Type I diabetes in NOD mice by adjuvant immunotherapy. *Diabetes* 1990; 39: 583–9.

75 McInery MF, Pek SB, Thomas DW. Prevention of insulitis and diabetes onset by treatment with complete Freund's adjuvant in NOD mice. *Diabetes* 1991; 40: 715–25.

76 Sadelain MWJ, Qin H-Y, Sumoski W, Parfrey N, Singh B, Rabinovitch A. Prevention of diabetes in the BB rat by early immunotherapy using Freund's adjuvant. *Journal of Autoimmunity* 1990; 3: 671–80.

77 Wang T, Singh B, Warnock GL, Rajotte RV. Prevention of recurrence of IDDM in islet-transplanted diabetic NOD mice by adjuvant immunotherapy. *Diabetes* 1992; 41: 114–17.

78 Guytingco R, Quddus, J, Richardson B, Pek SB. Single administration of Bacillus Calmette-Guerin (BCG) vaccine in nonobese diabetic (NOD) mice results in suppression of in vitro T-lymphocyte proliferation and regression of insulitis. *Diabetes* 1991; 40: (Suppl 1): 152A.

79 Vardi P. Adjuvant administration modulates the process of beta cell autoimmunity and prevents IDDM: introduction to human trials. *Diabetes Metab Revs* 1993; 9: 317–22.

80 Shehadeh N, Calcinaro F, Bradley BJ, Bruchlim I, Vardi P, Lafferty K. Effects of adjuvant therapy on development of diabetes in mouse and man. *Lancet* 1994; 343: 706–7.

81 Kalland T, Alm G, Stalhandske T. Augmentation of mouse natural killer cell activity by LS 2616. A new immunomodulator. *J Immunol* 1985; 134: 3956–61.

82 Slavin S, Sidi H, Weiss L, Rosenmann E, Kalland T, Gross D. Linomide, a new treatment for autoimmune diseases: the potential in Type I diabetes. *Diabetes Metab*

Revs 1993; **9**: 329–36.

83 Gross D, Sidi H, Weiss L, Kalland T, Rosenmann E, Slavin S. Prevention of diabetes mellitus in non-obese diabetic by Linomide, a novel immunomodulating drug. *Diabetologia* 1994; **37**: 1195–201.

84 Culler FL, O'Connor R, Kaufmann S, Jones KL, Roth JC. Immunospecific therapy for Type I diabetes mellitus. *New England Journal of Medicine* 1985; **313**: 695–6.

85 Skyler JS, Lorenz TJ, Schwartz S, Eisenbarth GS, Einhorn D, Palmer JP, Marks JB, Greenbaum C, Saria EA, Byers V, CD5 Diabetes Project Team. Effects of an anti-CD5 immunoconjugate (CD5-Plus) in recent onset Type I diabetes mellitus: a preliminary investigation. *J Diab Comp* 1993; **7**: 224–32.

86 Vallera DA, Carroll SF, Brief S, Blazar BR. Anti-CD3 immunotoxin prevents low-dose STZ/interferon induced autoimmune diabetes in mouse. *Diabetes* 1992; **41**: 457–64.

87 Vialettes B, Vague P. Treatment of diabetes by monoclonal antibodies. Lessons from a pilot study using anti-IL-2 receptor MoAb in recently diagnosed diabetic patients. *Diabetes Prev Ther* 1991; **5**: 21–2.

88 Pacheco-Silva A, Bastos MG, Muggia RA, Pankewycz O, Nichols J, Murphy JR, Strom TB, Rubin-Kelley VE. Interleukin 2 receptor targeted fusion toxin (DAB$_{486}$-IL-2) treatment blocks diabetogenic autoimmunity in non-obese diabetic mice. *Eur J Immunol* 1992; **22**: 697–702.

89 Boitard C, Timset J, Assan R, Mogenet A, Debussche X, Kaloustian E, Attali JR, Chanson P, Chatenoud L, Woodworth T, Bach JF. Treatment of Type I diabetes mellitus with DAB$_{486}$-IL-2, a toxin conjugate which targets activated T-lymphocytes. *Diabetologia* 1992; **35**(Suppl 1): A218.

90 Sanders ME. Clinical trial of chimeric anti-CD4 monoclonal antibody for insulin dependent diabetes mellitus. *Diebetes Prev Ther* 1991; **5**: 28.

91 Rabinovitch A, Suarez-Pinzon WL, Sorenson O, Bleackley RC, Power RF, Rajotte RV. Combined therapy with interleukin-4 and interleukin-10 inbitis autoimmune diabetes recurrence in syngeneic islet-transplanted nonobese diabetic mice: analysis of cytokine mRNA expression in the graft. *Transplantation* 1995 (in press).

92 Tremblau S, Penna G, Bosi E, Mortara A, Gately MK, Adorini L. Interleukin-12 administration induces T Hepler Type 1 cells and accelerates autoimmune diabetes in NOD mice. *J Exp Med* 1995; **181**: 817–21.

93 Mattner F, Fischer S, Guckes S, Jin S, Kaulen H, Schmitt E, Rude E, Germann T. The Interleukin 12 subunit p40 specifically inhibits effects of the interleukin-12 heterodimer. *Eur J Immunol* 1993; **23**: 2202–8.

94 Cohen IR. Regulation of autoimmune disease: physiological and therapeutic. *Immunol Revs* 1986; **94**: 5–21.

95 Cohen IR. T-cell vaccination in immunological disease. *J Int Med* 1991; **230**: 471–7.

96 Elias D, Reshef T, Birk OS, van der Zee R, Walker MD, Cohen IR. Vaccination against autoimmune mouse diabetes with a T-cell epitope of human 64-kDa heat shock protein. *Proc Natl Acad Sci* 1991; **88**: 3088–91.

97 Smerdon RA, Peakman M, Hussain MJ, Vergani D. Lymphocyte vaccination prevents spontaneous diabetes in the non-obese diabetic mouse. *Immunology* 1993; **80**: 498–501.

98 Posselt AM, Barker CF, Friedman AL, Naji A. Prevention of autoimmune diabetes in the BB rat by intrathymic islet transplantation at birth. *Science* 1992; **256**: 1321–4.

99 Gerlin IC, Serreze DV, Christianson SW, Leiter EH. Intrathymic islet cell transplantation reduces beta cell autoimmunity and prevents diabetes in NOD/Lt mice. *Diabetes* 1992; **41**: 1672–6.

100 Koevary SB, Blomberg M. Prevention of diabetes in BB/Wor rats by intrathymic

islet injection. *J Clin Invest* 1992; **89**: 512–16.

101 Herold K, Montag AG, Buckingham F. Induction of tolerance to autoimmune diabetes with islet antigens. *J Exp Med* 1992; **176**: 1107–14.

102 Tisch R, Yang XD, Singer SM, Liblau RS, Fugger L, McDevitt HO. Immune response to glutamate decarboxylase correlates with insulitis in non-obese diabetic mice. *Nature* 1993; **366**: 72–5.

103 Davies JL, Kawaguchi Y, Bennett ST, Copeman JB, Cordell HJ, Pritchard LE, Reed PW, Gough SCL, Jenkins SC, Palmer SM, Balfour KM, Rowe BR, Farrall M, Barnett AH, Bain SC, Todd JA. A genome-wide search for human Type 1 diabetes susceptibility genes. *Nature* 1994; **371**: 130–6.

104 Nepom GT. A unified hypothesis for the complex genetics of HLA associations with IDDM. *Diabetes* 1990; **39**: 1153–7.

105 Sheehy MJ. HLA and insulin dependent diabetes: a protective perspective. *Diabetes* 1992; **41**: 123–9.

Part 4

GENETIC COUNSELING

22

Current Recommendations

CARRIE GARBER, LESLIE J. RAFFEL and JEROME I. ROTTER
Division of Medical Genetics and Medical Genetics Birth Defects Center, Departments of Pediatrics and Medicine, Cedars-Sinai Medical Center, Los Angeles, California, USA

INTRODUCTION

As discussed in previous chapters, much has been learnt regarding the genetics of insulin-dependent diabetes over the past quarter century[1]. This increase in knowledge means that more reliable genetic counseling can now be provided to individuals who have diabetes and to their families.

GENETIC COUNSELING

Before discussing the specific details of counseling for IDDM, it is important to understand what genetic counseling is and what its goals are. Genetic counseling has been defined as "a communication process which deals with the human problems associated with the occurrence, or the risk of occurrence, of a genetic disorder in a family"[2]. There are a number of specific goals which the counselor attempts to achieve in the genetic counseling process. These goals are to assist the individual and/or family as follows:

1. To comprehend the diagnosis, the prognosis and available management.
2. To appreciate the mode of inheritance and the risk of recurrence.
3. To understand the options for dealing with the risk of recurrence.
4. To choose the course of action they perceive as most appropriate.
5. To adjust to the disorder in an affected family member and/or to the risk of recurrence.

Prediction, Prevention and Genetic Counseling in IDDM. Edited by Jerry P. Palmer.
© 1996 John Wiley & Sons Ltd.

The provision of genetic counseling is often a team effort; physicians, nurses, social workers, and genetic associates (university trained, board certified genetic counselors) all contribute to the counseling process. This is particularly true because the complexity and emotional content of the information discussed often make it necessary for the individual and his or her family to hear the same information several times, as well as in different ways. In this chapter, the term genetic counselor will be used to refer to any health care professional who provides genetic counseling.

A precise diagnosis is essential in order to provide accurate genetic counseling[1-3]. Whenever possible, it is helpful to confirm information regarding the patient and his or her relatives by obtaining medical records and/or by examining family members[2,3]. If the individual counseled is the individual with IDDM, verification of the diagnosis is usually straightforward. However, often the individual requesting counseling is an unaffected family member and verification of the diagnosis is not as simple. Occasionally, obtaining medical records requires Herculean efforts; however, verifying that a relative was or was not affected with a particular disorder can make a large difference in determining recurrence risks. Useful medical records are those pertaining to diagnostic tests, pathology reports, autopsy reports, and death certificates.

It is also important to take time to draw the family structure (pedigree), listing both affected and unaffected family members and including pertinent diagnoses. When dealing with a disorder such as IDDM, for example, the occurrence of other autoimmune disorders (i.e. thyroid disease, Addison's disease, autoimmune gastritis leading to pernicious anemia) may help to identify a portion of the extended family which is at higher risk for IDDM. Additionally, because the diagnosis of IDDM may not always be as clear as might be thought, the pattern of affected individuals in the family may help exclude discrete diagnoses with known patterns of inheritance. Maturity-onset diabetes of the young (MODY), for example, exhibits an autosomal dominant pattern of inheritance[4]. There are also forms of diabetes due to mitochondrial mutations, in which all affected family members are related to each other through maternal female relatives, and in which there may be the occurrence of hearing loss in maternal relatives as well[5-7]. The symbols used in pedigree drawing and an example pedigree are given in Figure 22.1.

Once a diagnosis is made or confirmed, the genetic counselor can assist the patient and/or the family in understanding the implications of the disorder[8,9]. This includes discussion of the inheritance pattern, recurrence risks, prognosis, and the risks of possible complications[3,8]. The discussion about risks involves the concept of probability, which may be a difficult concept for some individuals. Each person perceives risk uniquely; their previous experiences impact upon their interpretation of their risks[9]. The genetic counselor's role is to help in the understanding of the probabilities and to present an accurate

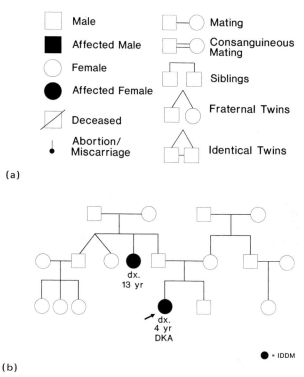

(a)

(b)

Figure 22.1. Pedigree drawing: (a) symbols commonly used in drawing pedigrees; (b) sample pedigree of a family with two members who have insulin-dependent diabetes mellitus. The proband (index case) is denoted by the arrow. DKA = diabetic ketoacidosis

picture of severity[2]. Often it is helpful to express probabilities in different ways; for example using ratios (i.e. 1/20) as well as percentages. Concrete examples, such as tossing a coin and seeing how many times it comes up heads or tails, can also make probabilities more comprehensible.

Perhaps the most overlooked part of genetic counseling is the psychosocial aspect. Every genetic condition creates a burden to the affected individual and his or her family. The burden not only encompasses practical issues, such as financial problems and the need to get the affected individual to frequent medical appointments, but also includes psychological and social problems[3,10]. When a child is diagnosed with a genetic disease, the parents often feel guilty for having contributed the "defective" genes to their son and/or daughter[10-13]. One parent may feel more responsible; occasionally one parent blames the other[10,11]. Parents can also experience feelings of lowered self-esteem following the diagnosis of a genetic condition in their child; many individuals feel that they must be able to produce healthy, "normal" children in order to demonstrate their own worth[13,14]. This can be particularly important in certain cultures. Parents may also grieve the loss of their "normal" child[13–15]. This grief is often poorly understood by others, leaving the parents feeling alone and unsupported in their grief.

The needs of the siblings of a child with a genetic condition must also be addressed; the attention focused on the affected child may cause the unaffected siblings to feel neglected and/or resentful[13,16,17]. They may also feel guilty for being normal or because they imagine that something they did or thought caused the disorder[13,16,17]. With a condition like IDDM, which may not manifest until later in life, the siblings may also be fearful about their own risks for becoming ill. The affected individual may have a low self-esteem due to feelings of being "defective"[13,18]. In the case of a condition such as IDDM, the insulin injections mean the individual is different from most of his peers or her peers; this feeling of difference can be especially pronounced during adolescence when the desire to fit in is very strong.

Directly raising such possibilities in discussion with the family is important[9]; they often will not express their feelings unless asked to do so. A sensitive and empathetic genetic counselor can help the individual and his family to recognize and understand their feelings, thereby facilitating the coping and adaptation processes[8]. It is frequently very helpful to families to have the counselor raise these concerns; learning that such feelings are typical is reassuring to people who may be unaware that others have similar reactions when coping with a genetic diagnosis. When necessary, referrals to outside agencies, such as support groups, can be made[8].

It is widely accepted that genetic counseling should be provided in a non-directive manner, particularly when discussing options related to reproduction[8,13,19,20]. For the health care professional who is used to giving very directed medical instructions to patients, providing non-directive counseling may be difficult and lead to feelings of discomfort and frustration. Most health care professionals have strong feelings about what they would do if faced with a similar situation; it is important to remember that each family must decide what options are best for them, taking into account their cultural, socioeconomic, and religious backgrounds. The individual and/or family should be given all the pertinent information and the various options should be presented to them[8]. The individual/family is then encouraged to make the decisions with which they are most comfortable, rather than being told what to do[8,19]. Individuals who are receiving genetic counseling will frequently ask the counselor what he or she would do; it is best for the counselor to respond by acknowledging that not only is his or her course of action not necessarily relevant for others, but also that no one really knows what they will do until actually faced with the situation. Help can be provided in a number of ways, for example, by comparing and contrasting different situations and discussing potential short- and long-term consequences of each option. Once it becomes clear that a decision has been reached by the individual/family, the role of the genetic counselor is to support that decision, regardless of his or her own personal feelings[8]. If health care professionals give patients and their families the impression that they disagree with the options chosen by the family, it only serves to alienate the family from the medical profession, reduce communication, and, ultimately, compliance with other aspects of patient care.

A good understanding of the nature and etiology of a genetic disorder also frequently results in improved compliance with recommended medical care. When people feel as though they are active participants in their care, they are more likely to follow through with management suggestions. Patients may feel that they are more involved in their care, simply because of the additional time that is taken to be sure they understand the inheritance and recurrence risks of their condition.

COUNSELING IN IDDM

The mode of inheritance in IDDM is not straightforward, since the disorder probably results from the inheritance of different combinations of several susceptibility genes and may require an environmental trigger as well[1]. Alternatively, environment may play a minor role in the development of IDDM and stochastic variation in the immune system may be the explanation for reduced disease expression in genetically at-risk individuals[1]. As a consequence, most genetic counseling for IDDM is based upon empiric risk estimates which have been developed from both population-based and family-based epidemiologic studies. The empiric risk of recurrence for IDDM is dependent upon the relationship of the individual in question to the affected family member. If the father is affected, the risk to his offspring is 4–6%, as compared to 2–3% if the mother is affected[21,22]. In counseling families, it is important to reverse these figures as well, letting them know that 94–96% of the offspring of diabetic fathers and 97–98% of the offspring of diabetic mothers do not develop IDDM. For siblings the empiric risk is approximately 5–10%. Sibling risks can be modified by determining HLA haplotypes (the sequence of HLA, A, B, C and DR alleles inherited on the same chromosome number 6) within the family[23,24]. As discussed in an earlier chapter, the HLA region, especially the class II genes, account for a major portion of the genetic susceptibility to IDDM, even though it is unclear which genes in the region are actually responsible[25–27]. The risks to a sibling of an affected individual are dependent upon whether or not they share 0, 1, or 2 HLA haplotypes in common (formally called 'identical by descent'; that is, inherited from the same parent) (Table 22.1). If two haplotypes are shared, the risk increases to 16–17%, and is 20–25% if the haplotypes contain both DR3

Table 22.1. Impact of HLA haplotype sharing on IDDM risk[a]

Numbers of HLA haplotypes shared with sibling with IDDM	Risk to develop IDDM
0	1%
1	5%
2	16–17%
2 (DR3/DR4)	20–25%

[a] Empiric risk to a sibling of an individual with IDDM is 7%.

and DR4[1]. Siblings who share one haplotype have a risk in the range of 5–7%, while the risk is approximately 1–2% if no haplotypes are shared[1]. It is important to realize that the sibling of an individual with IDDM still has a risk for IDDM that is increased above that of the general population, even when the sib shares no HLA haplotypes in common with the diabetic in the family. The reason for this persistent risk is unclear but there are at least three possible explanations. Since the IDDM gene or genes within the HLA region have not yet been absolutely identified, it is possible for siblings to have inherited the HLA-related IDDM susceptibility genes but, due to recombination, to have inherited different HLA types. Also, because the high risk HLA haplotypes (i.e. those containing DR3 or DR4) occur fairly commonly in the general population, it is possible that one or both parents of a child with IDDM may actually carry two high risk haplotypes. Thus a child may inherit diabetes susceptibility genes, even though he or she shares no HLA haplotypes with the diabetic sibling. Another possibility is that the increased risk is due to non-HLA region susceptibility genes, such as the insulin gene region or chromosome 11[28–30].

There is some concern regarding the benefit of performing HLA typing for the siblings of an individual with IDDM. At this point in time, a proven method of prevention is not available although intervention trials are currently underway[31–34]. There is some thought that immunosuppressive and/or tolerizing therapy may help to prevent or delay the onset of IDDM[34,35]; if this is true, identification of those siblings at highest risk based on HLA typing may enable them to be further evaluated with islet cell autoantibody, anti-insulin autoantibody, and anti-GAD autoantibody assays. If autoantibodies are present, intravenous glucose tolerance testing can be performed to determine if altered first phase insulin secretion, the earliest physiologic abnormality, is present. Prospective studies have shown that high risk relatives who have autoantibodies and altered first phase insulin release have a high probability of developing IDDM in the relatively near future[34]. Such individuals are the most appropriate candidates for intervention. It must be kept in mind, however, that such therapies have not yet been clearly proven to prevent the development of IDDM and have the potential for serious complications. Currently, such therapy is available in research studies only. Therefore, prior to drawing blood for HLA typing and/or autoantibody studies, the advantages and disadvantages of obtaining such information should be thoroughly discussed with the family. Families must discuss how they will adjust if, instead of receiving the reassuring results they are hoping for, they are informed that some family members are at significantly increased risk. Particular attention must be paid to the potential negative effects of stigmatization and the risks of the child being treated as though he is ill; the point must be stressed that HLA testing at best identifies someone to be more susceptible to developing IDDM but in no way guarantees that he or she will become diabetic. The potential for other negative effects, such as possibly being ruled ineligible for health, life, and/or disability insurance due to the presence of a "pre-existing" condition must also be discussed with every family contemplating HLA and autoantibody testing.

SCREENING FOR OTHER AUTOIMMUNE DISORDERS

Diabetes is not the only autoimmune disorder for which relatives of an individual with IDDM are at risk. Family members, as well as the patient, are at increased risk for autoimmune thyroid disease (Hashimoto thyroiditis, Graves' disease), pernicious anemia secondary to autoimmune gastritis, autoimmune adrenal disease (Addison's disease), myasthenia gravis, vitiligo, and coeliac disease[1,36-38]. A study looking at individuals with IDDM and their relatives found that 21% of the diabetics and 22% of their first degree relatives had evidence of autoimmune disease[39]. Of patients with persistent islet cell antibodies (ICAs), 57% had other autoimmune conditions as compared to 15% of those not found to have persistent ICAs[39]. Of the autoimmune disease in relatives, 75% occurred in families in which there was a proband with autoimmune disease[39], indicating that there may be increased genetic susceptibility to other autoimmune disorders in certain IDDM families.

The most common form of autoimmune disease in families with IDDM is thyroid disease[39,40]. Although the proportion of IDDM patients with clinical or subclinical thyroid disease has been reported to be as high as 35%, the actual proportion is thought to be closer to 15–20%[39,41]. In contrast, the prevalence of autoimmune thyroid disease in non-diabetic Caucasians is thought to be 4.5%[42]. The prevalence of clinical or subclinical autoimmune thyroid disease in first degree relatives of individuals with IDDM is estimated to be 15–25%[39,41].

Other autoimmune disorders are also seen with increased frequency in Type 1 diabetic individuals and their relatives. Autoimmune gastritis, as evidenced by the detection of gastric parietal cell autoantibodies or pernicious anemia, is seen in 5–12% of individuals with IDDM and 2.5–6% of their first degree relatives[39,41,42]. The prevalence of Addison's disease or adrenal autoantibodies is 1–3% in individuals with IDDM as compared to a maximum of 0.6% in non-diabetics[39,43].

It is particularly important for the relatives of patients with IDDM to be made aware of this increased risk for autoimmune disease. Although most physicians know of the association of IDDM with other autoimmune diseases, the fact that close relatives are also at risk is not as well appreciated in the medical community. Since many of these autoimmune disorders can have relatively insidious onsets, with fairly non-specific symptoms, making the relatives and their physicians aware of the increased risk may lead to earlier diagnosis.

Given this increased risk for autoimmune diseases, periodic screening of individuals with IDDM and all their first degree relatives is warranted, particularly for thyroid dysfunction (via standard tests such as obtaining T4 and TSH levels) and for vitamin B12 deficiency which if untreated leads to pernicious anemia. In the future, it may also be possible to screen for atrophic gastritis directly by measuring the pepsinogen I/pepsinogen II ratio[44].

PREGNANCY AND IDDM

It is well known that women with IDDM have a higher rate of pregnancy complications than do non-diabetics. The general rule of thumb is the more severe the diabetes, the poorer the pregnancy outcome. This is particularly true of women with vascular complications[45,46]. Also related to pregnancy outcome is the degree of control of the diabetes, i.e. the better the control the better the pregnancy outcome[46–49]. It should be emphasized that although the risks can be lowered by achieving optimal control of the diabetes prior to pregnancy, all diabetic pregnancies must be considered high risk and will benefit from a multispeciality management approach.

As more is learnt about control of IDDM, the frequency of pregnancy complications is diminishing. In diabetic women, the risk for spontaneous abortion (defined as fetal loss prior to 20 weeks' gestation) is greatly increased over the general population rate of approximately 15%[50,51]. This risk has been reported to be as high as 30%[52]; however, it appears that this very high risk applies primarily to women with poor control of their diabetes[46,51]. Better metabolic control has also been associated with lowering the frequency of other complications, such as pre-eclampsia, fetal death, macrosomia, and respiratory distress syndrome in the newborn[53,54].

Women with IDDM are also at increased risk to have a child with congenital anomalies[55,56]. In the general population, the risk to have a child with a birth defect is 2–3%. For women with IDDM, the risk is increased three-fold, to 6–10%[50,53,56]. The malformations seen in infants born to diabetic women tend to be more severe than those seen in infants of non-diabetic women and include abnormalities of the skeletal, renal, cardiac, and central nervous systems[50,55,57-59]. Virtually all anomalies occur with increased frequency in infants of diabetic mothers but those which have the highest relative risk are caudal regression, renal agenesis, transposition of the great vessels, ventricular septal defects, atrial septal defects, situs inversus, and neural tube defects (anencephaly and meningomyelocele). Although these malformations are not specific for diabetes, caudal regression is seen much more often in infants of diabetic mothers than in the general population. The relative risk for caudal regression in the offspring of a diabetic woman has been estimated to be as high as 200 times the risk for offspring of nondiabetic women[58]. The relative risks for the other defects are not as high, due in large part to their higher incidence in the general population[55].

The disruption of embryogenesis leading to the abnormalities occurs prior to the eighth week of pregnancy, i.e. often before a woman realizes that she is pregnant[60]. There is evidence to suggest that elevated glycosylated hemoglobin (HbA1c) levels are associated with a high risk for malformations and vigorous control of blood glucose levels prior to conception has been shown to significantly reduce the incidence of congenital malformations[60-63]. Although it is beneficial to optimize diabetes control even in women who present when they are already pregnant, postconceptional intervention is less likely to reduce the malformation risk. Beginning in early adolescence, diabetic women of childbearing age should be made aware of the risk of congenital malformations and counseled that planning their pregnancies is essential so that optimal metabolic control of their disease can be achieved prior to conception and continued throughout their pregnancy. Unfortunately, this is a topic that is all too often avoided in the management of adolescents and this is the age range in which accidental, unplanned pregnancy is most likely to occur.

Because of the increased risk for major structural malformations, prenatal diagnostic tests should be recommended for all pregnant women who have IDDM. These should be performed during the second trimester (usually between 16 and 20 weeks' gestation), providing women with abnormal results the opportunity to obtain genetic counseling regarding the anomaly (i.e. prognosis, treatment options) and to make informed decisions regarding pregnancy options. For women who have normal results, the information obtained via prenatal diagnosis can be very reassuring and help alleviate anxiety for the remainder of the pregnancy. Ultrasonography can be used to evaluate fetal growth and to rule out major fetal structural anomalies such as renal agenesis, neural tube defects, and caudal regression. Fetal echocardiography, performed at 20-22 weeks following the first day of the last menstrual period, enables prenatal diagnosis of major structural cardiac malformations. Elevations of maternal serum alpha-fetoprotein (MSAFP) have been associated with open neural tube defects such as anencephaly and meningomyelocele[64,65]; thus, MSAFP screening is recommended for all pregnant diabetics. Because MSAFP levels are altered in pregnant diabetics as compared to non-diabetics, tables specific for diabetic women should be used when calculating their MSAFP values and it is therefore important that the laboratory performing the assay be made aware that the patient is diabetic[66-68].

There is evidence that in the general population, folic acid supplementation, begun prior to conception, is helpful in decreasing the risk for neural tube defects[69]. Although studies looking specifically at infants of diabetic mothers have not been reported, folic acid supplementation prior to conception should be strongly considered as the potential benefits (i.e. possibly reducing the risk for neural tube defects), outweigh any known risks.

CONCLUSION

Although our knowledge of the genetic susceptibility to IDDM remains imperfect, there is useful information currently available which should be provided to both those with IDDM and their relatives. Particularly now, with the potential for true prevention of IDDM close to reality, it is imperative that individuals at risk be made aware of their risks so that they can take advantage of new therapies if they would so choose. It is always important to remember that, in order to be effective, the provision of genetic counseling must include counseling and not just risk figures.

ACKNOWLEDGMENT

Supported in part by a grant from the Stuart Foundations and the Cedars-Sinai Board of Governors' Chair in Medical Genetics.

REFERENCES

1 Rotter JI, Vadheim CM, Rimoin DL. Diabetes mellitus. In King RA, Rotter JI, Motulsky AG (eds), *The Genetic Basis of Common Disease*. New York: Oxford University Press, 1992, pp 413–81.
2 Fraser FC. Genetic counseling. *Am J Hum Genet* 1974; **26**: 636–59.
3 Hsia YE, Hirschhorn K. What is genetic counseling? In: Hsia YE, Hirschhorn K, Silverberg RL, Godmilow L (eds), *Counseling in Genetics*. New York: Alan R. Liss, 1979, pp 1–29.
4 Fajans SS. Scope and heterogeneous nature of MODY. *Diabetes Care* 1990; **13**: 49–64.
5 Ballinger SW, Shoffner JM, Hedaya EV, Trounce I, Polak MA, Koontz DA, Wallace DC. Maternally transmitted diabetes and deafness associated with a 10.4 kb

mitochondrial DNA deletion. *Nat Genet* 1992; **1**: 11–15.

6 Reardon W, Ross RJM, Sweeney MG, Luxon LM, Pembrey ME, Harding AE, Trembath RC. Diabetes mellitus associated with a pathogenic point mutation in mitochondrial DNA. *Lancet* 1992; **340**: 1376–9.

7 Kadowaki T, Kadowaki H, Mori Y, Tobe K, Sakuta R, Suzuki Y, Tanabe Y, Sakura H, Awata T, Goto Y-I, Hayakawa T, Matsuoka K, Kawamori R, Kamada T, Horai S, Nonaka I, Hagura R, Akanuma Y, Yazaki Y. A subtype of diabetes mellitus associated with a mutation of mitochondrial DNA. *New Eng J Med* 1994; **330**: 962–8.

8 Kelly TE. *Clinical Genetics and Genetic Counseling*, 2nd edn. Chicago: Year Book Medical Publishers, Inc., 1986.

9 Ekwo EE, Kim J-O, Gosselink CA. Parental perceptions of the burden of genetic disease. *Am J Med Genet* 1987; **28**: 955–63.

10 McCollum AT, Silverberg RL. Psychosocial advocacy. In Hsia YE, Hirschhorn K, Silverberg RL, Godmilow L (eds), *Counseling in Genetics*. New York: Alan R. Liss, 1979, pp. 239–60.

11 Fuhrmann W, Vogel F. *Genetic Counseling*, 3rd edn. New York: Springer-Verlag, 1983.

12 Kessler S, Kessler H, Ward P. Psychological aspects of genetic counseling III. Management of guilt and shame. *Am J Med Genet* 1984; **17**: 673–97.

13 Kessler S. The process of communication, decision making and coping in genetic counseling. In: Kessler S (ed) *Genetic Counseling: Psychological Dimensions*. New York: Academic Press, 1979, pp 35–51.

14 Blacher J. Sequential stages of parental adjustment to the birth of a child with handicaps: fact or artifact. *Ment Retard* 1984; **22**: 55–68.

15 Parks RM. Parental reactions to the birth of a handicapped child. *Health Soc Work* 1977; **3**: 51–66.

16 Kohut SA. The abnormal child: his impact on the family. *J Am Phys Ther Assoc* 1966; **46**: 160–7.

17 Fischman SE. Psychological issues in the genetic counseling of cystic fibrosis. In Kessler S (ed), *Genetic Counseling: Psychological Dimensions*. New York: Academic Press, 1979, pp 153–65.

18 Hayden PW, Davenport SLH, Campbell MM. Adolescents with myelodysplasia: impact of physical disability on emotional maturation. *Pediatrics* 1979; **674**: 53–9.

19 Applebaum EG, Firestein SK (eds). *A Genetic Counseling Casebook*. New York: The Free Press, 1983.

20 Harper PS. *Practical Genetic Counseling*, 4th edn. Oxford: Butterworth-Heinemann, 1993.

21 Warram JH, Krolewski AS, Gottlieb MS, Kahn RC. Differences in risk of insulin-dependent diabetes in offspring of diabetic mothers and fathers. *New Engl J Med* 1984; **311**: 149–52.

22 Warram JH, Krolewski AS, Kahn RC. Determinants of IDDM and perinatal mortality in children of diabetic mothers. *Diabetes* 1988: **37**: 1328–34.

23 Gorsuch AN, Spencer KM, Lister J, Wolf E, Bottazzo GF, Cudworth AG. Can future type I diabetes be predicted? A study in families of affected children. *Diabetes* 1982; **31**: 862–6.

24 Rotter JI, Vadheim CM, Petersen GM, Cantor RM, Riley WJ, Maclaren NK. HLA haplotypes sharing and proband genotype in IDDM. *Genet Epidem* 1986; **3** (suppl 1): 347–52.

25 Rotter JI, Landaw EM. Measuring the genetic contribution of a single locus to a multilocus disease. *Clin Genet* 1984; **26**: 529–42.

26 Erlich H, Rotter JI, Chang J, Shaw S, Raffel LJ, Klitz W, Beshkov Y, Costin R, Pressman S, Bugawan TL. Zeidler A. HLA class II alleles and susceptibility and

resistance to insulin dependent diabetes mellitus in Mexican-American families. *Nat Genet* 1993; 3: 358–64.

27 Erlich HA, Rotter JI, Chang J, Shaw S, Raffel LJ, Klitz W, Bugawan T, Zeidler A. PCR/oligonucleotide probe typing of HLA class II loci in Mexican-American insulin dependent diabetes mellitus (IDDM) families reveals an association of HLA-DPB1*0301 with IDDM. *Am J Hum Genet* 1993; 53: A201.

28 Bell GI, Horita S, Karam JH. A polymorphic locus near the insulin gene is associated with insulin-dependent diabetes mellitus. *Diabetes* 1984; 33: 176–83.

29 Julier C, Hyer RN, Davies J, Merlin F, Soularue P, Briant L, Cathlineau G, Deschamps I, Rotter JI, Froguel P, Boitard C, Bell JF, Lathrop GM. The insulin-IGF 2 region in chromosome 11p encodes a gene implicated in HLA-DR4 dependent diabetes susceptibility. *Nature* 1991; 354: 155–9.

30 Raffel LJ, Hitman GA, Toyoda H, Karam JH, Bell GI, Rotter JI. The aggregation of the 5' insulin gene polymorphism in type I (insulin-dependent) diabetes mellitus families. *J Med Genet* 1992; 29: 447–50.

31 Eisenbarth G. Type 1 diabetes mellitus: a chronic autoimmune disease. *New Engl J Med* 1986; 314: 1360–8.

32 Maclaren NK. How, when and why to predict IDDM. *Diabetes* 1988; 37: 1591–4.

33 Eisenbarth GS. Genes, generator of diversity, glycoconjugates, and autoimmune B-cell insufficiency in Type 1 diabetes. *Diabetes* 1987; 36: 355–64.

34 Skyler JS, Marks JB. Immune intervention in type I diabetes mellitus. *Diabetes Revs* 1993; 1: 15–42.

35 Keller RJ, Eisenbarth GS, Jackson RA. Insulin prophylaxis in individuals at high risk of type I diabetes. *Lancet* 1993; 341: 927–8.

36 Eisenbarth S, Wilson P, Ward F, Lebovitz HE. HLA type and occurrence of disease in familial polyglandular failure. *New Engl J Med* 1978; 298: 92–4.

37 Riley WJ, Maclaren NK, Lezotte DC, Spillar RP, Rosenbloom AL. Thyroid autoimmunity in insulin-dependent diabetes mellitus: the case for routine screening. *J Pediatr* 1981; 98: 350–4.

38 Bottazzo GF, Mann JI, Thorogood M, Baum JD, Doniach D. Autoimmunity in juvenile diabetics and their families. *Br Med J* 1978; ii: 165–8.

39 Betterle C, Zanette F, Pedini B, Presotto F, Rapp LB, Monsciotti CM, Rigon F. Clinical and subclinical organ-specific autoimmune manifestations in type 1 (insulin-dependent) diabetic patients and their first degree relatives. *Diabetologia* 1984; 26: 431–6.

40 Gorsuch AN, Dean BM, Bottazzo GF, Lister J, Cudworth AG. Evidence that type 1 diabetes and thyrogastric autoimmunity have different genetic determinants. *Br Med J* 1980; i: 145–7.

41 Fialkow PJ, Zavala C, Nielson K. Thyroid autoimmunity: increased frequency in relatives of insulin dependent diabetes patients. *Ann Intern Med* 1975; 83: 170–6.

42 Riley WJ, Toskes PP, Maclaren NK, Silverstein JH. Predictive value of gastric parietal cell autoantibodies as a marker for gastric and hematologic abnormalities associated with insulin-dependent diabetes. *Diabetes* 1982; 31: 1051–5.

43 Riley WJ, Maclaren NK, Neufeld M. Adrenal autoantibodies and Addison's disease in insulin-dependent diabetes mellitus. *J Pediatr* 1980; 97: 191–5.

44 Samloff IM, Varis K, Ihamaki T, Siurala M, Rotter JI. Relationships among serum pepsinogen I, serum pepsinogen II, and gastric mucosal histology, a study in relatives of patients with pernicious anemia. *Gastroenterology* 1982; 83: 204–9.

45 Gabbe SG, Mestman JH, Freeman RK, Goebelsmann UT, Lowensohn RI, Nochimson D, Cetrulo C, Quilligan EJ. Management and outcome of pregnancy in diabetes mellitus, classes B to R. *Am J Obstet Gynecol* 1977; 129: 723–9.

46 Jovanovic R, Jovanovic L. Obstetric management when normoglycemia is maintained in diabetic pregnant women with vascular compromise. *Am J Obstet Gynecol* 1984; **149**: 617–23.

47 Nelson RL. Diabetes and pregnancy: control can make a difference. *Mayo Clin Proc* 1986; **61**: 825–9.

48 Karlsson K, Kjellmer I. The outcome of diabetic pregnancies in relation to the mother's blood sugar level. *Am J Obstet Gynecol* 1972; **112**: 213–20.

49 Jovanovic L, Drezin M, Peterson CM. Effect of euglycemia on the outcome of pregnancy in insulin-dependent diabetic woman as compared with normal control subjects. *Am J Med* 1981; **71**: 921–7.

50 Gabbe SG. Congenital malformations in infants of diabetic mothers. *Obstet Gynecol* 1977; **32**: 125–32.

51 Mills JL, Simpson JL, Driscoll SG, Jovanovic-Peterson L, Van Allen M, Aarons JH, Metzger B, Bieber FR, Knopp RH, Holmes LB, Peterson CM, Witham-Wilson M, Brown Z, Ober C, Harley E, Macpherson TA, Duckles A, Mueller-Heubach E, and the National Institute of Child Health and Human Development—Diabetes in Early Pregnancy Study. Incidence of spontaneous abortion among normal women and insulin-dependent diabetic women whose pregnancies were identified within 21 days of conception. *New Engl J Med* 1988; **319**: 1617–23.

52 Miodovnik M, Lavin JP, Knowles HC, Holroyde J, Stys SJ. Spontaneous abortion among insulin-dependent diabetic women. *Am J Obstet Gynecol* 1984; **150**: 372–6.

53 Cousins L. Congenital anomalies among infants of diabetic mothers. Etiology, prevention, prenatal diagnosis. *Am J Obstet Gynecol* 1983; **147**: 333–8.

54 Dandona P, Boag F, Fonseca V, Menan RK. Diabetes mellitus and pregnancy. *New Engl J Med* 1986; **314**: 58.

55 Mills JL. Malformation in infants of diabetic mothers. *Tetratology*: 1982; **25**: 385–94.

56 Kitzmiller JL, Cloherty JP, Younger MD. Diabetic pregnancy and perinatal morbidity. *Am J Obstet Gynecol* 1978; **131**: 560–80.

57 Neave C. Congenital malformations in offspring of diabetics. *Perspct Pediatr Pathol* 1984; **8**: 213–22.

58 Kucera J. Rate and type of congenital anomalies among offspring of diabetic women. *J Reprod Med* 1971; **7**: 73–82.

59 Soler NG, Walsh CH, Malins JM. Congenital malformations in infants of diabetic mothers. *Q J Med* 1976; **45**: 303–13.

60 Mills JL, Baker L, Goldman AS. Malformations in infants of diabetic mothers occur before the seventh gestational week. *Diabetes* 1979; **28**: 292–3.

61 Miller E, Hare JW, Cloherty JP, Dunn PJ, Gleason RE, Soeldner JS, Kitzmiller JL. Elevated maternal hemoglobin A1c in early pregnancy and major congenital anomalies in infants of diabetic mothers. *New Engl J Med* 1981; **304**: 1331–4.

62 Hanson U, Persson B, Thunell S. Relationship between hemoglobin A1c in early type 1 (insulin-dependent) diabetic pregnancy and the occurrence of spontaneous abortion and fetal malformations in Sweden. *Diabetologia* 1990; **33**: 100–4.

63 Kitzmiller JL, Gavin LA, Gin GD, Jovanovic-Peterson L, Main EK, Zigrand WD: Preconception care of diabetes: glycemic control prevents congenital anomalies. *JAMA* 1991; **265**: 731–6.

64 Brock DJH, Sutcliffe RG. Alpha-fetoprotein in the antenatal diagnosis of anencephaly and spina bifida. *Lancet* 1972; **ii**: 197–9.

65 Wald NJ, Cuckle H. Maternal serum alpha fetoprotein measurement in antenatal screening for anencephaly and spina bifida in early pregnancy. United Kingdom Collaborative Study. *Lancet* 1977; **i**: 1323–32.

66 Milunsky A, Alpert E, Kitzmiller JL, Younger MD, Neff RK. Prenatal diagnosis of

neural tube defects VIII. The importance of serum alpha-fetoprotein screening in diabetic pregnant women. *Am J Obstet Gynecol* 1982; **142**: 1030–2.

67 Reece AE, Davis N, Mahoney MJ, Baumgarten A. Maternal serum alpha-fetoprotein in diabetic pregnancy: correlation with blood glucose control. *Lancet* 1987; **ii**: 275.

68 Baumgarten A, Robinson J. Prospective study of an inverse relationship between maternal glycosylated hemoglobin and serum alpha-fetoprotein concentrations in pregnant women with diabetes. *Am J Obstet Gynecol* 1988; **159** 77–81.

69 Czeizel AE, Dudas I. Prevention of the first occurrence of neural tube defects by periconceptional vitamin supplementation. *New Engl J Med* 1992; **327**: 1832–5.

23

Future Prospects

ALICIA SCHIFFRIN and ELEANOR COLLE
The Montreal Children's Hospital, Montreal, Canada

INTRODUCTION

Genetic counseling is a process which attempts to advise individuals (or their relatives) affected with a genetic disorder about: (1) the nature of the disorder; (2) the probability of developing it or transmitting it; and (3) the possibility of preventing the onset of the disease. Type 1 insulin-dependent diabetes (IDDM) is not the best paradigm for the application of genetic counseling because, despite the many publications regarding risks for relatives, the nature of the genetic component is not clear.

What is clear at the present time is that IDMM is a multigenic, multifactorial disease. A combination of genes produce a susceptibility to develop the disease. An interaction of this susceptibility with some agent in the environment is necessary for the development of the full-blown clinical disorder. What is not clear at this time is whether the variation noted in reported studies is due to differences in the prevalence of susceptibility genes, to differences in the presence of environmental factors, or to a combination of the two.

At the moment, we are in a position to describe the nature of the disease process as it is imperfectly understood, to give information on the probability of the occurrence of IDDM in first degree relatives, to refine those probability estimates if certain information on genetic markers is available, and to refine those probability estimates further for those bearing immune markers. At the present time there is little firm data on environmental agents which would allow us to suggest lifestyle changes which could decrease these risks.

Prediction, Prevention and Genetic Counseling in IDDM. Edited by Jerry P. Palmer.
© 1996 John Wiley & Sons Ltd.

NATURE OF THE DISEASE PROCESS

Type 1 (insulin-dependent) diabetes mellitus (IDDM) is a chronic disease with an estimated prevalence of 0.2% in individuals less than 20 years of age[1]. Patients are diagnosed when they present with elevated blood glucose levels and ketonuria following a period of weight loss, poor growth in children, polyuria and polydypsia. In 20% of the cases there is severe dehydration and acidosis leading to diabetic ketoacidosis. Although residual insulin secretion can often be demonstrated, exogenous insulin is required to maintain metabolic homeostasis. However, an asymptomatic prodromal period of varying length precedes the onset of the disease. During this period there is progressive autoimmune destruction of the pancreatic β cells in susceptible individuals[2,3]. This is evidenced by the presence of an inflammatory infiltrate consisting of CD4+ and CD8+T lymphocytes, macrophages and B lymphocytes in the pancreas of newly diagnosed diabetic patients[4], the presence of islet-cell antibodies (ICAs)[5,6], antibodies against glutamic acid decarboxylase (GAD)[7-9], insulin antibodies (IA)[10,11], abnormalities in peripheral T-lymphocyte subsets and their function[12,13], and the association of diabetes with generalized polyendocrine autoimmune syndromes[14,15]. Individuals who have one or more of these immunologic markers have an increased risk of developing insulin dependency.

Epidemiologic surveys have shown the incidence figures for IDDM to range from 3.4 to 35 per 100 000 individuals at risk[16] in various countries. Prevalence figures also vary from one country to another from 0.16 to 0.4%. The crude cumulative-to-age-40 risk for first degree relatives has been calculated in one study to be 5.5%±0.7%[17]. Lifetime risks for first degree relatives have been estimated at 2.9% for parents, 6.6% for siblings and 4.9% for children of IDDM. The risk was higher if the proband was less than 10 years of age[18]. First degree relatives have a greatly increased relative risk, although the absolute risk remains low. Lorenzen *et al.*[19] identified 310 Danish probands older than 50 years of age, with IDDM over 30 years' duration. For those whose age at onset was less than 20 years, the risk of having one first degree relative with IDDM increased from 10.4 to 22.3%. Cumulative recurrence risks from birth were 6.4% for siblings up to 30 years and 9.6% for up to 60 years. The risks of developing IDDM do not rise smoothly, however. Only 25% of the cases occur in children younger than 6 years of age and there is a sharp peak in incidence at the age of puberty. Furthermore, in a study where the offspring of IDDM patients were ascertained through the affected parent, the cumulative risk by age 20 was 6.1±1.8% for the offspring of diabetic fathers but only 1.3±0.9% for diabetic mothers[20]. Thus the risk to first degree relatives depends on the relationship to the index case, on the age of the index case, on the age of the relative, and (in the case of offspring) on the sex of the diabetic parent.

PROBABILITY OF THE OCCURRANCE OF IDDM IN FIRST DEGREE RELATIVES BEARING GENETIC MARKERS OF DISEASE SUSCEPTIBILITY

In animal models of spontaneous IDDM, the diabetic susceptibility is multigenic[21]. In the human, two associations between genetic markers and insulin dependency have been documented.

GENES IN THE HLA REGION

The association of the HLA specificities with IDDM is complex. Of IDDM patients, 95% possess either DR3, DR4, or DR3/DR4 alleles of the HLA-DR region compared to 50% of the non-diabetic population[22]. Heterozygosity for DR3/DR4 which is only found in 1–3% of the general population increases the risk for IDDM even more[23]. HLA-DR1, and DR8 are also positively associated but with decreasing strength of association. Two specificities, DR2 and DR5, are negatively associated and confer resistance[22,23]. Because of the close proximity of the DR genes to the DQ genes, DR specificities are usually associated with a corresponding DQ specificity. There is a well-established synergistic risk associated with the presence of the heterozygote DR3-DQw2/ DR4-DQw8 genotype. It is now generally accepted that the susceptibility associated with DR4 is due to the presence of the DQB1*0302 allele on this haplotype. DR-bearing haplotypes which have instead the DQB1*0301 allele do not confer increased risk of Type 1 diabetes[24]. It has been hypothesized that the differences in the ability of these two different alleles to confer susceptibility is due to the presence of an aspartic acid in position 57. Its presence confers resistance while its absence (Asp57−) is associated with susceptibility. However, this residue alone may be insufficient to determine susceptibility or resistance to IDDM. Indeed, recent studies suggest that the genes coding for the α chain of the DQ peptide may also be important. Khalil *et al.*[25] reported that the susceptibility to IDDM is influenced by the variable expression (dose effect) of the susceptibility HLA-DQ$\alpha\beta$ heterodimers. Extensive DQA1 and DQB1 oligotyping in Caucasian IDDM patients implicated an arginine in position 52 of the α chain (Arg52+) in conferring susceptibility to IDDM. According to this hypothesis susceptibility is increased by the expression on the cell surface of an HLA-DQ $\alpha\beta$ heterodimer in *cis* and/or in *trans*: Arg52+DQα/Asp57−DQβ. The most frequent haplotypes among patients were those consisting of DQB1 and DQA1 susceptibility alleles (S-S; 74% compared with 16% in control subjects, (RR 14, CI 9.31–21.32), mostly including the DQA1*0501-DQB1*0201 and DQA1*0301-DQB*0302 haplotypes associated with DR3-DQw2 and DR4-DQw8, respectively.

The gene frequencies of these DQA1 and DQB1 susceptibility alleles were 80% and 90%, respectively, in IDDM patients and 44% and 45%, respectively, in controls. Only the frequencies of DQA1*0301, 0501 and DQB1*0302 and *0201 alleles were significantly increased in IDDM. Susceptibility was more strongly associated to a DQA1-DQB1 haplotype than to one allele alone. Although 97% of the patients and 46% of controls carried a genotype encoding at least one susceptibility DQ$\alpha\beta$ heterodimer (RR = 34) the highest risks were observed for genotypes exclusively encoding susceptibility heterodimers (RR = 41), followed by those with three susceptibility alleles. Regardless of the immunological mechanisms underlying the HLA associations, the HLA, DR4, DQ*3102 haplotype is found in about 70% of young Type 1 diabetic individuals. A DR3-DQB1*0201 haplotype is found in about 30% of these children. In children with an early onset of disease, it is often found in heterozygosity with the DR4-DQ*3102 haplotype. In addition, siblings who have received the same two parental haplotypes as the index case have the highest risk of disease, those who share only one parental haplotype with the index case have the next highest risk and those who share neither parental haplotype have a risk which is only slightly higher than that of the general population[24]. Despite the observations of a strong association between HLA type and IDDM in families, calculation of the absolute risk for IDDM in populations suggests that other gene(s) either within the HLA region or elsewhere are necessary to provide complete genetic susceptibility. There are presently no markers which are as predictive for IDDM at the population level in contrast with the sensitivity of the haplotypes in family studies.

GENES IN THE INS-IGF-2 REGION

Several groups have now reported an association between IDDM and polymorphic markers on human chrosome 11p[26,27]. These markers span the area from the variable tandem repeat area 5' to the insulin gene to an area 3' of the insulin gene. Recently, it has been shown that the VNTR is the most likely candidate for IDDM2[27]. A "protective" haplotype is present in 45–50% of control subjects but in only 15–20% of diabetic patients. Whether this protection is conferred only when the haplotype is transmitted by the father has been the subject of controversy. Paternal transmission would suggest that the maternal copy is imprinted. This would not only suggest a mechanism by which the epidemiologic data suggesting a higher incidence in offspring of diabetic fathers could be explained, but is also intriguing in view of the known maternal imprinting of the IGF-2 gene which is found only 1.4 kb from the 3' end of the insulin gene.

PROBABILITY OF DEVELOPING IDDM IN THE PRESENCE OF IMMUNE MARKERS

The demonstration that immune intervention can prolong the remission phase of IDDM in approximately 50% of the patients provides evidence for the autoimmune pathogenesis of diabetes[28–31]. Previous studies in animal models and first degree relatives of IDDM patients have led to the consensus that IDDM develops in several stages:

1. A "triggering event" initiates the immune response in a genetically susceptible individual.
2. The presentation of one or more β-cell antigens together with the HLA class II peptide products to a T-cell receptor results in a cellular immune attack against the pancreatic β cells and appearance of antibodies with specificities against various β-cell antigens ICA[32,33], IA[10,11], and anti-GAD[7–9].
3. The duration of the pre-symptomatic stage varies highly depending on individual characteristics, one of them being age, and eventually leads to progressive destruction of the β cells with decreased insulin secretion.
4. When the β-cell mass decreases further, insulin dependency ensues.

At this fourth stage the β-cell mass is so small that immunosuppression is ineffective to reverse the process of insulin dependency. The rate of disappearance of the β-cell mass can be accelerated by a younger age, male sex, younger age of the IDDM sibling and presence in the family of another affected member in addition to the IDDM sibling[34,35]. Following the initiation of insulin therapy, there is a decrease of insulin requirements due to an improvement of the insulin secretory capacity which lasts for a few weeks to several months. However, most patients progress to total or near total insulin dependency within 2 to 5 years after diagnosis. The rate of disappearance of the β-cell function after diagnosis can also be predicted by age, sex, presence of ICA and severity of clinical presentation at diagnosis[35]. The failure of therapeutic intervention during the symptomatic stage of the disease has led to intervention trials in first degree relatives or individuals who have high ICA (with or without decreased insulin response to glucose). Two such ongoing trials are the European nicotinamide trial (ENDID) and the NIH-sponsored Diabetes Prevention Trial (DPT-1) using insulin as treatment. Unfortunately, with the present strategies for early IDDM detection, some of those first degree relatives will be treated relatively late in the course of the diabetic process.[36] Furthermore, by screening first degree relatives only, one could miss the diagnosis of the pre-symptomatic period of IDDM in the general population where 90% of new cases of IDDM arise.

The pre-symptomatic period of IDDM can be identified with the first appearance of antibodies directed against: (a) islet cell antigens (ICAs) not yet completely characterized[5,6]; (b) insulin (IA)[10,11]; and (c) antibodies which precipitate a 64 kDa islet membrane protein, glutamic acid decarboxylase (GAD). GAD proteins share identical amino acid residues with the P2C protein of the coxsackie virus. In genetically susceptible individuals exposed to the virus the viral protein may trigger an immune response which cross-reacts with the GAD antigens, supporting the idea that IDDM may result from molecular mimicry. ICAs are found in about 70–80% of newly diagnosed diabetics, in 2–4% of non-diabetic siblings and in less than 0.5% of the general population[37]. IAs are found in between 45% and 55% of new diabetics. They appear to be more frequent in younger individuals than in those individuals developing diabetes in later life[38]. Antibodies against GAD are present in about 70–95% of newly diagnosed diabetics. It has not yet been established if they are more predictive of IDDM than ICA or IA.

Long-term follow-up of high risk individuals consists of comparisons of the rates of conversion to insulin dependency of those individuals who are ICA+ with those who are ICA− at the time of diagnosis of the index case. Although study designs vary as to the frequency with which antibodies were measured, all studies indicate that individuals who are ICA+ have a higher risk of becoming IDDM than those who are ICA−[39,40] and those individuals with high titer antibodies have higher risks than those with low titers[39]. In addition 80% of individuals whose antibodies stain for both α and β cells rather than β cells alone will progress to IDDM within 5 years[41]. In another study[42], the staining restricted to β cells was completely inhibited by pre-incubation with rat brain homogenate while the diffuse cytoplasmic pattern staining both β and α cells was not affected by pre-incubation with rat brain homogenate. This inhibition was prevented by pre-clearing the brain homogenate with anti-GAD antibody. These data suggest that the specificity of the antibody which gives the β-cell restrictive pattern is most likely directed against GAD.

In other studies, investigators have concentrated on the fate of individuals found to be ICA+ and IA+ in association with the response to intravenous glucose in an effort to predict conversion to IDDM[42,43]. No age difference was found in these studies. The magnitude of the insulin response to intravenous glucose varies with age making this a difficult predictive variable to use in longitudinal studies, especially of very young children. The largest, longest prospective studies assessing the role of ICA in predicting IDDM among first degree relatives (children and adults), are from Windsor (UK)[39], Boston[43] and Gainsville[39]. These data show that ICA are highly specific (95%) and of high negative predictive value (95%) for IDDM but sensitivity and positive predictive value vary according to the degree of ICA positivity: the higher the ICA (JDF) the higher the predictive value. By life-table analysis, approximately 70% of subjects with an ICA level > 40 JDF on first screening were projected to be diabetic within 5 years. In addition, individuals who were older than 10 years of age were less likely to become diabetic, even when antibody positive, than those younger than 10 years and the presence of another IDDM in the family (in addition to the index case) increased the risk. In our study of children younger than 17 years of age[35], siblings of IDDM, we also found that the age of the index case (as opposed to the age of the non-affected relative) influenced the appearance of IDDM in the subject. We observed a 4%

incidence of ICA+ in 562 children in whom analysis was completed. Of those who developed IDDM, 90% were ICA positive before or at diagnosis[35].

ENVIRONMENTAL FACTORS

The low concordance rate of twins, the migrant effect on incidence rates, and the suggestions of increasing incidence rates in Europe but not in North America have suggested a major role for environmental factors interacting with susceptibility genes to produce insulin dependency[42–44]. There is a large body of epidemiological data showing that the disease has an increased incidence during the first decade of life with a peak in incidence at the age of puberty. There is a slight seasonal effect, in that fewer cases occur in the summer months than in the autumn and winter months. Cases occur in clusters but the clusters do not occur at the same time in successive years. There are marked variations in incidence between geographic areas[44].

As regards the pathogenesis of IDDM, two broad hypotheses have been proposed: (a) the initial event is a direct injury to the β cell by a β-cell cytotrophic virus or toxin[45]; (b) the initial event is directed against some other antigen which has a shared specificity with an islet cell component, the so-called "molecular mimicry" model. In both the spontaneously diabetic rat and mouse models, diet has been implicated as increasing or decreasing the prevalence of disease[46,47]. Milk products and gluten have been implicated in increasing incidence of disease and it has been suggested, at least in the rat, that the dietary insult must be introduced early in the life of the animal. There is relatively little relevant literature regarding the effect of diet on human disease. Some of the studies published so far found that the incidence of breast feeding was less in IDDM than in controls, but in all studies[48,49], the effect was weak. Karjalainen *et al.* found that IgG anti-BSA antibodies were present in all 144 IDDM Finnish children studied while they were present in only 2% of controls[50]. So far, these results have not been confirmed in other populations[51]. Kostraba *et al.*[52] in a case-control study concluded that exposure to whole cow's milk and solid foods before 3 months of age increased the risk of IDDM in children who carried at least one HLA-DQB1 non-Asp57 molecular marker. The attributable risk of exposure to whole cow's milk was low in high and low risk individuals (0.09 and 0.11 respectively). The relatively low attributable risk may be related to the low exposure to cow's milk which occurs at that age. In a recent study done in Sardinia[53], an island with the second largest incidence of IDDM in the world, where the incidence of IDDM is also rising, it has been estimated that no more than one-third of actual IDDM incidence could be accounted for by cow's milk consumption. This finding points to other still unidentified environmental factors. The data discussed above underline the importance of the need for additional research into the diabetogenic effects of dietary components before embarking on long-term trials using dietary manipulation.

Other environmental factors such as chemicals agents and/or several viruses may also have a role in initiating the disease process. A viral etiology for Type 1 diabetes has been suggested by the trends observed in age of onset and the closeness of time of onset which are greater than that expected by chance in studies of sib-pairs[54]. In animal models, infectious agents can cause insulin-dependent diabetes by a direct infection of the β cell (EMC and reovirus models), by structural alterations leading to abnormalities of the insulin secretion (VE model), through persistent infection leading to decreased life span of the β cell (LCB model) and through autoimmune mechanisms (rubella model)[5,55]. In the human, studies are controversial. One study suggested a role for cytomegalovirus (CMV) infections by detection of human CMV genes after molecular hybridization with a specific CMV probe[56]. They found infection in 22% of IDDM patients compared to 2.6% of controls. Another study suggested that coxsackie B3 and B4 titers were actually decreased in new-onset IDDM[57]. The best human model for the viral etiology of IDDM is congenital rubella. Affected patients have an increased incidence of IDDM. Those patients have been found to have increased frequency of HLA-DR3 and DR4, decreased frequency of HLA-DR2 T-cell subset abnormalities, and autoimmune antibodies like anti-islet, anti-thyroglobulin, anti-thyroid microsomal suggesting an autoimmune response to a prenatal infection as is found in non-rubella IDDM[58]. Viruses may modify the course of the prodromal period although there is no direct evidence bearing on this.

PRESENT AND FUTURE PROSPECTS

All of the studies hitherto described suffer from the fact that the proband is identified at the time of diagnosis of the index case. Thus, there is no way of knowing how long the subject has been antibody positive. Since antibody positivity appears to mark most individuals with pancreatic β-cell disease, our approach has been to follow the events surrounding the conversion from an antibody negative to an antibody positive state. To this end, we have established a cohort of first degree relatives of IDDM identified at birth and followed prospectively to monitor environmental events (diet, febrile illnesses, and reactions to immunizations) and antibody status. There are currently 130 children in 101 families in the study—26 are siblings of Type 1 diabetics, 36 are offspring of diabetic mothers and 19 are offspring of diabetic fathers. The eldest of the cohort is currently 7 years old. One child has developed IDDM. He was ICA− at 1 year of age, ICA+ at age 2 and IDDM at age 3 when ICA were still positive. His father has IDDM. Three other children have developed ICA. Two are offspring of diabetic mothers and one is a sibling of a diabetic child who developed IDDM at the age of 2 years. This study will permit the description of the natural history of IDDM in IDDM-related and non-IDDM-related children and the correlation of specific genetic, immune and metabolic markers to the progression of the disease.

NEWBORN SCREENING

Newborn genetic screening has been in place in many countries for many years for the diagnosis of PKU, tyrosinemia, and hypothyroidism. Other diseases are being added: screening for hemoglobinopathies, cystic fibrosis, Duchenne's muscular dystrophy, α-antitrypsin deficiency and neuroblastoma are being offered in some centers.

Although the first degree relative studies are intriguing, the major question of whether one can prevent the development of IDDM in the pre-clinical stage in genetically susceptible individuals remains unresolved. In individuals less than 18 years of age, 25% of IDDM cases are diagnosed before the age of 6. Therefore, successful prevention of IDDM may require detection of the pre-clinical phase as early as the neonatal period. Although we feel that for ethical reasons[59–62] there should be a basic presumption against newborn genetic screening, the need for a study looking at the natural history of IDDM is great. Potential benefits of such screening are: (a) the early diagnosis of IDDM before the onset of severe symptomatology; and (b) the feasibility of early detection of individuals at risk of developing IDDM in case the ongoing therapeutic trials are successful in preventing or delaying the onset of IDDM. Because of the irreversibility of the destruction of the pancreatic β cells, the only hope for a cure rests with an intervention that could arrest the diabetic process at its earliest stage when there would be sufficient β cells to preserve. At the present time, the only reasonable strategy for screening is to identify individuals at high risk through HLA-DR and DQ typing and ongoing evaluation of the antibody status.

Potential psychological consequences of neonatal screening were postulated previously[63] but to the best of our knowledge they have not been extensively measured. Depending on the sensitivity of the test some patients with positive tests will subsequently be found not to have the disease and the anxieties may remain for a long time. Results of psychological evaluations through semi-structured telephone interviews have been reported in 102 unselected Swedish families with newborns who had false positive hypothyroidism detected in mass screening[64]. Results showed initial intense psychic stress in the majority of families. The stress was positively solved by most of the families 6 to 12 months later. However 17% of the parents who remained insecure about their babies' health at that time also worried about their child 4 years later. Ten children showed behavioural problems. It was not clear from the studies whether those families and their children were truly affected by the screening or whether they were sensitive to strain because of habitual maladjustment. In contrast, parents of infants retested for false positive tests of metabolic diseases in the Massachusetts Screening Program[65] did not show severe emotional reactions or depression. Furthermore, the authors report that providing information about the process of screening before recruitment reduced parental anxiety. Because we can anticipate that in the future genetic screening will be a large part of our health care system, unmasking psychic long-term distress by positive screening should still be a matter of medical concern. The importance of counseling before screening is often acknowledged but there are few data showing whether adequate information is given before the screening and whether supportive follow-up will minimize adverse emotional effects[66]. To avoid psychological adverse effects it has been proposed that people be adequately informed before participation, in writing, of the possibility of both false positive and false negative results. Results should be given for both negative and positive tests and supportive therapy should be provided to those who test positive[67].

CONCLUSION

Thus, at the present time the family coming for counseling can be given information on the nature of the disease and on the probability of development of the disease in other members of the family. They can be offered the possibility of participating in one of the many prevention/natural history studies being carried on all over the world. If families elect to participate, counseling at each stage of the genetic and immune studies must be available. As well, we would suggest that all intervention studies incorporate validated questionnaires to monitor the effects of the necessarily incomplete information which is being offered.

REFERENCES

1 Bach JF. Mechanisms of autoimmunity in insulin-dependent diabetes mellitus. *Clin Exp Immunol* 1988; **72**: 2–8.
2 Lernmark A, Barmeier H, Dube S, Hagopian W, Karlsen A, Wassmuth R. Autoimmunity of diabetes. *Endocrin Metab Clin North Am* 1991; **20**: 589–617.
3 Rossini A, Greiner D, Friedman H, Mordes J. Immunopathogenesis of diabetes mellitus. *Diabetes Rev* 1992; **1**: 43–75.
4 Gepts, W. Pathology and anatomy of the pancreas in juvenile diabetes mellitus. *Diabetes* 1965; **14**: 619–33.
5 Gleichman H, Bottazzo GF. Progress toward standardization of cytoplasmic islet-cell antibody assay. *Diabetes* 1987; **36**: 578–84.

6 Gleichman, H, Bottazzo, GF, Progress towards standardization of cytoplasmic islet cell antibody assays. *Diabetes* 1987; **36**: 578–84.

7 Baekkeskov S, Neilsen J, Marner B, Bilde T, Ludvigsson J, Lernmark A. Autoantibodies in newly-diagnosed diabetic children immuno-precipitate human pancreatic islet cell proteins. *Nature* 1982; **298**: 167–9.

8 Atkinson M, Maclaren N, Scharp D, Lacy P, Riley W. 64000 Mr autoantibodies as predictors of insulin-dependent diabetes. *Lancet* 1990; **335**: 1357–60.

9 Rowley M, Mackay I, Chen Q, Knowles W, Zimmet P. Antibodies against glutamic acid decarboxylase discriminate major types of diabetes mellitus. *Diabetes* 1992; **41**: 548–52.

10 Palmer J, Asplin C, Clemons P, Lyen K, Tatpati O, Raghu P, Paquette T. Insulin antibodies in insulin-dependent diabetics before insulin treatment. *Science* 1983; **222**: 1337–9.

11 Arslanian SA, Becker DJ, Rabin B, Atchison R, Eberhardt M, Cavender D, Dorman J, Drash AL. Correlates of insulin antibodies in newly diagnosed children with insulin-dependent diabetes before insulin therapy. *Diabetes* 1988; **34**: 926–30.

12 Jackson RA, Morris MA, Haynes BF, Eisenbarth GS. Increased circulating Ia antigen-bearing T cells in type I diabetes mellitus. *New Engl J Med* 1982; **306**: 785–8.

13 Legendre CM, Schiffrin A, Weitzner G, Colle E, Guttmann R. Two-color flow-cytometry analysis of activated T-lymphocyte subsets in type I diabetes mellitus. *Diabetes* 1988; **37**: 792–5.

14 Bottazzo GF, Florin-Christensen AF, Doniach D. Islet cell antibodies in diabetes mellitus with autoimmune polyendocrine deficiencies. *Lancet* 1974; **2**: 1279–82.

15 Tarn A, Dean B, Schwarz G, Thomas J, Ingram D, Bottazo GF. Predicting insulin-dependent diabetes. *Lancet* 1988; **I**: 845–50.

16 Spencer KM, Mann JI, Pyorala K, Teuscher A. Diabetes in epidemiological perspective. In Mann JI, Pyorala K, Tsuscher A (eds), *Diabetes in Epidemiological Perspective*. New York: Churchill Livingstone, 1983, pp 99–121.

17 Chern MM, Anderson VE, Barbosa J. Empirical risk for insulin-dependent diabetes (IDD) in sibs. Further definition of genetic heterogeneity. *Diabetes* 1982; **31**: 1115–18.

18 Tillil H, Kobberling J. Age-corrected empirical genetic risk estimates for first-degree relatives of IDDM patients. *Diabetes* 1987; **36**: 93–9.

19 Lorenzen T, Pociot F, Hougaard P, Nerup J. Long-term risk of IDDM in first-degree relatives of patients with IDDM. *Diabetologia* 1994; **37**: 321–7.

20 Warram JH, Krolewski AS, Gottlieb MS, Kahn CR. Differences in risk of insulin dependent diabetes in offspring of diabetic mothers and fathers. *New Engl J Med* 1984; **311**: 149–51.

21 Colle E, Fuks A, Poussier P, Edouard P, Guttmann R. Polygenic nature of spontaneous diabetes in the rat. Permissive MHC haplotype and presence of the lymphopenic trait of the BBrat are not sufficient to produce susceptibility. *Diabetes* 1992; **41**: 1617–23.

22 Todd JA, Bell JI, McDevitt HO. HLA-DQ beta gene contributes to susceptibility and resistance to insulin-dependent diabetes mellitus. *Nature* 1987; **329**: 599–604.

23 Nepom GT. A unified hypothesis for the complex genetics of HLA associations with IDDM. *Diabetes* 1990; **39**: 1153–7.

24 Trucco M. To be or not to be ASP57, that is the question. *Diabetes Care* 1992; **15**: 705–15.

25 Khalil I, Deschamps I, Lepage V et al. Dose effect of cis- and trans- encoded HLA-DQ$\alpha\beta$ heterodimers in IDDM susceptibility. *Diabetes* 1992; **41**: 378–84.

26 Julier C. Insulin Igf-2 region on chromosome 11 encodes a gene implicated in HLA-DR4-dependent diabetes susceptibility. *Nature* 1991; **354**: 155–9.

27 Undlien D, Bennett Simon, Todd J, Akselsen H et al. Imsulin gene region-encoded

susceptibility to IDDM Maps upstream of the insulin gene. *Diabetes* 1995; **44**: 620–5.
28 Stiller CR, Dupre J, Gent M *et al.* Effects of cyclosporine immunosuppression in insulin-dependent diabetes mellitus. *Science* 1984; **223**: 1362–7.
29 Bougneres PF, Landais P, Boisson C, Carel JC, Frament N, Boitar C, Chaussain JL, Bach JF. Limited duration of remission of insulin dependency in children with recent overt Type 1 diabetes treated with low-dose cyclosporin. *Diabetes* 1990; **39**: 1264–72.
30 Lewis C, Canafax D, Sprafka JM, Barbosa J. Double-blind randomized study of nicotinamide on early-onset diabetes. *Diabetes Care* 1992; **15**: 121–3.
31 Elliott RB, Chase HP. Prevention of Type 1 (insulin-dependent) diabetes mellitus in children using nicotinamide *Diabetologia* 1991; **34**: 362–5.
32 Marrack P, Kappler J. The T cell receptor. *Science* 1987; **238**: 1073–8.
33 Sinha AA, Lopez MT, McDevitt MO. Autoimmune disease: the failure of self tolerance. *Science* 1990; **248**: 1380–8.
34 Poussier P, Colle E, Schiffrin A, Lalla D, Ciampi A, Belmonte MM, Ysm E, du Berger R. The risk for siblings of patients with insulin-dependent diabetes mellitus of developing disease. *Clin Invest Med* 1991; **14**: 1–8.
35 Schiffrin A, Colle E, Ciampi A, Hendricks L, Poussier P. Different rates of conversion to IDDM in siblings of type 1 diabetic children: the Montreal family study. *Diabetes Res Clin Pract* 1993; **21**: 75–84.
36 Schiffrin A, Ciampi A, Hendricks L, Rozen R, Weitzner G. Evidence for different clinical subtypes of Type I diabetes mellitus: a prospective study. *Diabetes Res Clin Pract* 1994; **23**: 95–102.
37 McLaren NK. How, when, and why to predict IDDM. *Diabetes* 1988; **37**: 1591–4.
38 Riley WJ, Maclaren NK, Krishcer J, Spillar RP, Silverstein JH, Schatz DA, Schwartz S, Malone J, Shah S, Vadheim C, Rotter JI. A prospective study of the development of diabetes in relatives or patients with insulin-dependent diabetes. *New Engl J Med* 1990; **323**: 1167–72.
39 Bonifacio E, Bingley PJ, Shattock M, Dean BM, Dunger D, Gale EAM, Bottazzo GF. Quantification of islet-cell antibodies and prediction of insulin-dependent diabetes. *Lancet* 1990; **335**: 147–9.
40 Bleich D, Jackson RA, Soeldner JS, Eisenbarth GS. Analysis of metabolic progression to Type I diabetes in ICA+ relatives of patients with Type I diabetes. *Diabetes Care* 1990; **13**: 111–18.
41 Gianani R, Pugliese A, Bonner-Weir S, Schiffrin A, Soeldner S *et al.* Prognostically significant heterogeneity of cytoplasmic islet cell antibodies in relatives of patients with Type I diabetes. *Diabetes* 1992; **41**: 347–53.
42 Genovese S, Bonifacio E, McNally JM, Wagner R, Bosi E, Gale E, Bottazzo GF. Distinct cytoplasmic antibodies with different risks for Type 1 (insulin-dependent) diabetes mellitus. *Diabetologia* 1992; **35**: 385–8.
43 Siemiatycki J, Colle, Campbell S, Dewar R, Aubert D, Belmonte MM. Incidence of IDDM in Montreal by ethnic group and social class and comparisons with ethnic groups living elsewhere. *Diabetes* 1988; **37**: 1096–102.
44 Epidemiology Research International Group. Geographic patterns of childhood insulin-dependent diabetes mellitus. *Diabetes* 1988; **37**: 1113–19.
45 Muller U, Jongeneel CV, Nedospasov SA, Lindahl KF, Steinmetz M. Tumour necrosis factor and lymphotoxin genes map close to H = 2D in the mouse major histocompatibility complex. *Nature* 1987; **325**: 265–7.
46 Daneman D, Fishman L, Clarson C, Martin JM. Is there a critical period for exposure to dietary triggers for the expression of diabetes in the BB rat? In Jaworski M, Moeller G (eds), *Immunology of Diabetes*. Elsevier, 1988, pp 307–12.

47 Scott FW, Mongeau R, Kardish M, Hatina G *et al*. Diet can present diabetes in the BB rat. *Diabetes* 1985; **34**: 1054–62.
48 Siemiatycki J, Colle E, Campbell S, Dewar RAD, Belmonte M. Case-control study of IDDM. *Diabetes Care* 1989; **12**: 209–16.
49 Mayer EJ, Hamman RF, Gay EC, Lezotte DC, Savitz DA, Klingensmith GJ. Reduced risk of IDDM among breast-fed children: the Colarado IDDM Registry. *Diabetes* 1988; **37**: 1625–32.
50 Karjalainen J, Martin J, Knip M, Ilonen J, Robinson B, Savilahti E, Akerblom H, Dosch H-M. A bovine serum albumin peptide as a possible trigger of insulin-dependent diabetes mellitus. *New Engl J Med* 1992; **327**: 302–7.
51 Atkinson MA, Bowman M, Kuoo-Jang Kao MS, Campbell L, Shah S, Simell O, MacLaren NK. Response of peripheral monuclear cells to BSA and ABBO-S or serum IgG anti-BSA antibodies in insulin-dependent diabetic patients. *New Engl J Med* 1993; **329**: 1853–8.
52 Kostraba J, Cruickshanks K, Lawler-Heavner J, Jobim L, Rewers M, Gay E, Chase P, Klingesmith G, Hamman R. Early exposure to cow's milk and solid foods in infancy, genetic predisposition, and risk of IDDM. *Diabetes* 1993; **42**: 288–95.
53 Muntoni S, Songini M. Sardinian collaborative group for epidemiology of IDDM: high incidence rate of IDDM in Sardinia. *Diabetes care* 1992; **15**: 1317–22.
54 Gamble DR. The epidemiology of IDDM with particular reference to the relationship of viral infections to its etiology. *Epidemiol Revs* 1980 **2**: 49–70.
55 Rayfield EJ, Ishimura K. Environmental factors and insulin-dependent diabetes mellitus. *Diabetes/Metab Revs* 1987; **3(4)**: 925.
56 Pak CY, Eun HM, McArthur RG, Yoon JW. Association of cytomegalovirus infection with autoimmune Type I diabetes. *Lancet* 1988; **ii**: 1–4.
57 Palmer JP, Cooney MK, Ward RH. Reduced Coxsackie antibodies titres in Type I (insulin-dependent) diabetic patients presenting during an outbreak of Coxsackie B3 and B4 infection. *Diabetologia* 1982; **22**: 426–9.
58 Rubinstein P, Walker ME, Fedun B, Witt ME, Cooper LZ, Ginsberg-Feldner F. The HLA system in congenital rubella patients with and without diabetes. *Diabetes* 1982; **31**: 1088.
59 Nyhan W. Neonatal screening for inherited disease. *New Engl J Med* 1985; **313**: 43–4.
60 Townes P. Newborn screening: "A potpourri of policies". *Am J Pub Health* 1986; **76**: 1191–2.
61 United States National Institutes of Health. Consensus development conference on newborn screening for sickle cell disease and other hemoglobinopathies. *JAMA* 1987; **258**: 1205–9.
62 Meerman GJ, Dankert- Roelse J. Pros and cons for neonatal screening for cystic fibrosis. *Adv Exp Med Biol* 1991; **190**: 83–92.
63 Slonit AJ. The risks of neonatal screening. *J Pediatr* 1976; **256**: 646–7.
64 Bodegard G, Fyro K, Larsson A. Psychological reactions in 102 families with a newborn who has a falsely positive screening test for hypothyroidism. *Acta Paed Scand* (suppl) 1983; **304**: 2–21.
65 Sorenson J, Levy H, Mangione T, Sepe S. Parental response to repeat testing of infants with false positive results in a newborn screening program. *Pediatrics* 1984; **73**: 183–7.
66 Marteau T. Psychological costs of screening. *BMJ* 1989; **299**: 527.
67 Marteau T. Screening in practice: reducing the psychological costs. *Br Med J* 1990; **301**: 26–8.

Index

Note: page numbers in *italics* refer to figures and tables

Index compiled by Jill Halliday

Titles of Related Interest ...

WILEY

■ Diabetes in Old Age

Edited by P. FINUCANE and A.J. SINCLAIR

Comprehensively reviewing the major aspects of diabetes in old age, from its epidemiology and pathophysiology to diagnosis and management, this timely compilation brings a fresh approach to the care of the elderly diabetic patient.

0471 95344 X   312pp   April 1995

■ Diabetes Complicated Pregnancy

The Joslin Clinic Method
Second Edition

Edited by F.M. BROWN and J.W. HARE

A concise and convenient volume, this second edition provides practical information and presents a unified team approach for the clinical management of the diabetic pregnancy.

0471 11031 0   220pp June   1995

■ Causes of Diabetes

Genetic and Environmental Factors
Edited by R.D.G. LESLIE

Providing essential reading for clinicians and researchers, this extensive assessment of the causes of NIDDM and IDDM pays particular attention to the environmental factors involved in disease pathogenesis.

0471 94040 2   370pp   September 1993

■ The Foot in Diabetes

Second Edition

Edited by A.J.M. BOULTON, H. CONNOR and P.R. CAVANAGH

The second edition of this textbook on modern diabetic foot care has a multi-disciplinary authorship who provide up-to-date reviews and revision of what is known about diabetic foot disease.

"The Foot in Diabetes' is essentially a practical book and as such is compulsory reading for all those involved in the care and treatment of such patients".

CHIROPODY REVIEW

0471 94259 6   268pp   April 1994

■ Growth Hormone and Insuline-Like Growth Factor 1 in Humanand Experimental Diabetes

Edited by A. FLYVBJERG

This book brings together a group of renowned experts to collect current knowledge of GH and IGF-I, and their role in various aspects of diabetes, into a single volume. At the same time basic aspects of GH and IGFs have been covered in order to provide a clear understanding of the experimental and clinical pathophysiology of the subject area.

0471 93720 7   336pp   January 1993

JOHN WILEY & SONS LTD, BAFFINS LANE, CHICHESTER, WEST SUSSEX, PO19 1UD, UK

Titles of Related Interest ...

WILEY

■ From Obesity to Diabetes

Edited by J-P. FELBER

Introducing a metabolic approach to the study of diabetes and obesity, this text concentrates particularly on the metabolic effects of obesity, the reversibility of the phenomena, as well as prevention and therapy observations.

0471 92765 1   312pp   October 1992

■ Diabetic Medicine

Editor: STEPHANIE AMIEL

Providing a multidisciplinary forum combining original articles, reviews and comment, this journal is of interest to everyone helping diabetic patients, whether through fundamental research or better health care. In this way it helps to increase knowledge about the aetiology and pathogenesis of diabetes and its complications, and promotes new ideas about management and education.

0742 3071   Published Monthly

■ Diabetes/Metabolism Reviews

Editor-in-Chief: DOMENICO ANDREANI

Committed to providing an ongoing debate of clinical and basic advances in the most important areas of diabetes and metabolism, this journal is of essential interest to clinicians and researchers.

0742 4221   Published Quarterly

Due in 1996 ...

■ The International Textbook of Diabetes Mellitus

Second Edition

Edited by K.G.M.M. ALBERTI, R.A. DEFRONZO and P. ZIMMET

Honorary Editor: H. KEEN

From the Reviews of the First Edition...

"Professor K.G.M.M. Alberti and his colleagues have assembled a most distinguished panel of experts to produce a comprehensive volume covering all aspects of modern diabetes. All in all, this is a splendid reference book in two volumes.
The specialist in diabetes will find a chapter on any aspect of diabetes on which he wants to up date himself. There is good uniformity of style despite the number of authors involved. The chapters are extensively reinforced. There are many beautiful and informative illustrations and diagrams. I am confident that every diabetologist will want to have one in his study for reference. This book represents excellent value."

JOURNAL OF THE ROYAL SOCIETY OF MEDICINE

0471 939307   Approx 2000pp
due September 1996

JOHN WILEY & SONS LTD, BAFFINS LANE, CHICHESTER, WEST SUSSEX, PO19 1UD, UK